Series editor
Wilf Yeo
BMedSc, MB ChB, MD,
MRCP,
Section of Clinical
Pharmacology
Department of
Pharmacology &
Therapeutics,
Royal Hallamshire
Hospital,
Sheffield

D0800715

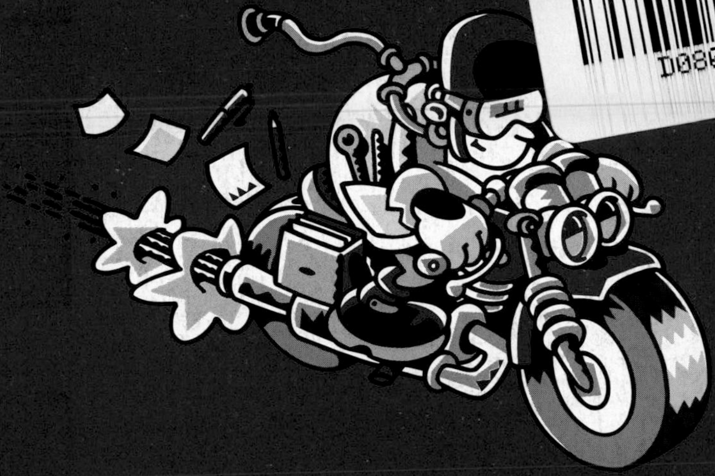

Paediatrics

Christine Budd
MB BS DCH
Royal Free and University
College Medical School
London

Mark Gardiner
MD FRCP FRCPCH
Professor of Paediatrics
Royal Free and University
College Medical School
London

Dr. Peter Cardon

Mosby
London Edinburgh New York
Philadelphia Sydney Toronto

Managing Editor	Louise Crowe
Development Editor	Linda Horrell
Project Manager	Claire Brewer
	Jane Tozer
Designer	Greg Smith
Layout	Robert Curran
Illustration Management	Danny Pyne
Illustrators	Deborah Gyan
	Sandie Hill
	Deborah Maizels
	Mick Ruddy
	Jeremy Theobald
Cover Design	Greg Smith
Production	Andrea Ford
Index	Janine Ross

ISBN 0 7234 3139 6

Copyright © Harcourt Brace and Company Limited, 1999.

Published by Mosby, an imprint of Harcourt Brace and Company Limited, Lynton House, 7–12 Tavistock Square, London WC1H 9LB, UK.

Printed by GraphyCems, Navarra, Spain.
Text set in Crash Course–VAG Light; captions in Crash Course–VAG Thin.

All rights reserved. No part of this publication may be reproduced, stored in a retrieval system or transmitted in any form or by any means electronic, mechanical, photocopying, recording or otherwise, without the prior written permission of the publisher or in accordance with the provisions of the Copyright, Designs and Patents Act 1988, or under the terms of any licence permitting limited copying issued by the Copyright Licensing Agency, 33–34 Alfred Place, London, WC1E 7DP, UK.

Any person who does any unauthorized act in relation to this publication may be liable to criminal prosecution and civil claims for damages.

The rights of Christine Budd and Mark Gardiner to be identified as the authors of this work have been asserted by them in accordance with the Copyright, Designs and Patents Act, 1988.

Every effort has been made to contact holders of copyright to obtain permission to reproduce copyright material. However, if any have been inadvertently overlooked, the publishers will be pleased to make the necessary arrangements at the first opportunity.

Cataloguing in Publication Data
A catalogue record for this book is available from the British Library.

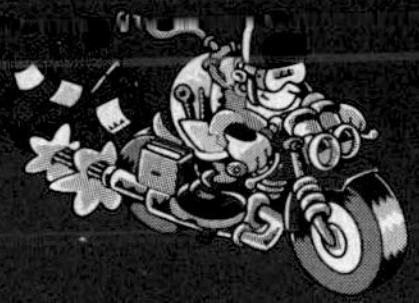

Preface

The beginner in medicine faces a daunting task: how to identify and master in a few short weeks the essentials of subjects each of which would take more than one lifetime to master completely.

This short book is designed to make that task easier for students embarking on the study of paediatrics. We have asked ourselves: what should a newly qualified doctor know about the care of infants and children, both in health and illness? We hope that we have succeeded in focusing on what most teachers of undergraduates would regard as the absolute essentials and in being guided by the ethos of the new curriculum.

The format is in the style of this series, and is therefore rather different from a standard textbook. Part I provides a clinically oriented approach to the symptoms, signs, and problems with which an infant or child may present to their doctor. Part II sets out the basic skillls of history taking and physical examination together with an overview of the special investigations used in paediatric practice. Part III considers the diseases and disorders of childhood in standard fashion, either by organ system or according to the subdivisions—such as the newborn—into which paediatrics divides. Important points are emphasised in Hints & Tips boxes, and key facts are presented in memorable form as tables and algorithms. Lastly, there is a self assessment section, including MCQs, case-based questions, and model short-answer questions designed to test core knowledge.

Of course, no clinical speciality can be learned from books alone. As Osler said 'To study medicine without the aid of books is to set sail without a chart. To study medicine only from books is never to go to see at all'. Venturing on to the wards and into the clinics in total ignorance can be a bewildering and demoralising experience. This book is a chart to help the student on his or her first voyages in the fascinating and rewarding world of children and their illnesses. It is short enough to be read at the beginning of a paediatric attachment, and small enough to carry for easy referral.Good luck!

Christine Budd and Mark Gardiner

So you have an exam in medicine and you don't know where to start? The answer is easy—start with *Crash Course*. Medicine is fun to learn if you can bring it to life with patients who need their problems solving. Conventional medical textbooks are written back-to-front, starting with the diagnosis and then describing the disease. This is because medicine evolved by careful observations and descriptions of individual diseases for which, until this century, there was no treatment. Modern medicine is about problem solving, learning methods to find the right path through the differential diagnosis, and offering treatment promptly.

This series of books has been designed to help you solve common medical problems by starting with the patient and extracting the salient points in the history, examination, and investigations. Part II gives you essential information on the physical examination and investigations as seen through the eyes of practising doctors in their specialty. Once the diagnosis is made, you can refer to Part III to confirm that the diagnosis is correct and get advice regarding treatment.

Throughout the series we have included informative diagrams and hints and tips boxes to simplify your learning. The books are meant as revision tools, but are comprehensive, accurate and well balanced and should enable you to learn each subject well. To check that you did learn something from the book (rather than just flashing it in front of your eyes!), we have added a self-assessment section in the usual format of most medical exams—multiple-choice and short-answer questions (with answers), and case studies for self-directed learning. Good luck!

Wilf Yeo
Series Editor (Clinical)

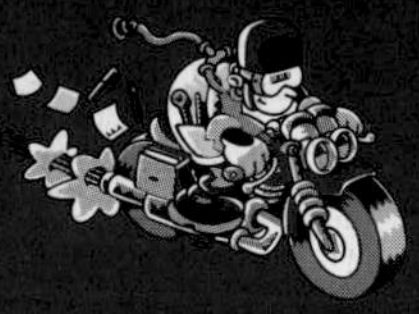

Acknowledgements

We are extremely grateful to Dr Margaret Meeks for assiduously reading the entire manuscript and for providing very helpful and constructive comments. Numerous other colleagues helped with certain sections including in particular Dr Caroline Fertleman, Dr Jane Watkeys, Dr Diana Baralle, Dr Louise Bate, Dr Collette Lewin, Dr Carolyn Coverley, Professor John Wyatt, and Professor Brent Taylor.

Dr Penny Shaw very kindly provided most of the imaging illustrations.

Lucy Milner, Emma Slater, and Louise Harman did an excellent job in producing the manuscript.

Any errors of omission or commission are our own.

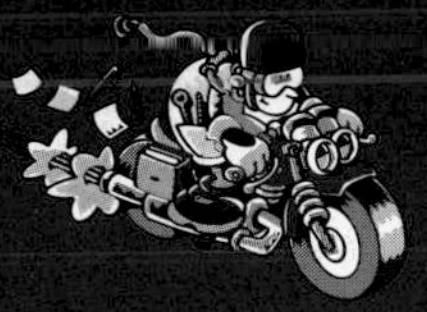

Contents

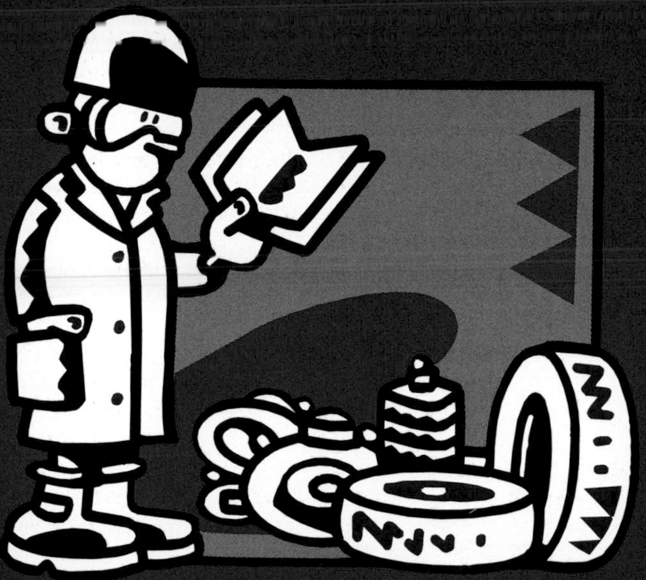

THE PATIENT PRESENTS WITH...

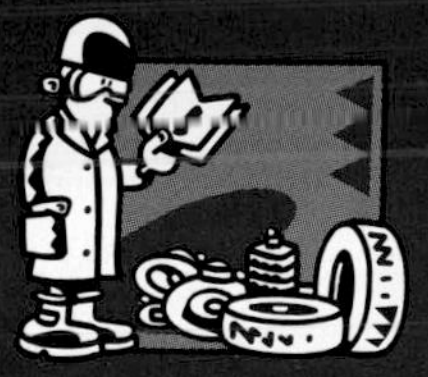

1. Fever or Rash

FEVER

A fever is the most common presenting problem in paediatric practice and nearly all febrile illnesses in children are due to infection (Fig. 1.1). The challenge is to establish the causative agent (in particular, to distinguish between bacterial and viral diseases) and to identify the site of a localized infection (Fig. 1.2).

The diagnosis in a febrile child, or infant, may be apparent at a glance (e.g. if a characteristic rash is present) or may resist the most detailed investigation. In children between 6 months and 6 years, a convulsion may be the first manifestation of a febrile illness.

In a minority of children, especially those with protracted fever, a non-infectious cause may be present, e.g. autoimmune diseases such as juvenile chronic arthritis and systemic lupus erythematosus.

History

How long has the child been febrile?

A duration of more than a week or two suggests diseases such as TB, malaria, typhoid, and auto-immune non-infectious disorders.

Are there any localizing symptoms?

An infection in certain systems will advertise itself:

- Cough—suggests respiratory tract infection.
- Vomiting and diarrhoea—suggests gastrointestinal tract infection.
- A painful limp—suggests infection of the bones or joints.

Common causes of a fever	
Minor illnesses	**Major illnesses**
upper respiratory tract infections (coryza, otitis media, tonsillitis)	bacterial meningitis
viral exanthemata	urinary tract infection
gastroenteritis	pneumonia
	malaria

Fig. 1.1 Common causes of a fever.

In other sites, such as the urinary tract or the meninges (especially in babies), localizing clues may not emerge in the history.

Has there been recent foreign travel?

Malaria or typhoid may be overlooked if recent travel abroad is not declared.

Examination

Is the child systemically unwell?

Severe bacterial infection (especially if there is spread into the bloodstream) causes a 'septic state' characterized in its severe form by circulatory failure.

Is there a rash?

A rash involving the skin or mucous membranes may provide the diagnósis.

Are there local signs of infection?

Tonsillitis, otitis media, pneumonia, meningitis, and septic arthritis may all be revealed on examination (Fig. 1.2).

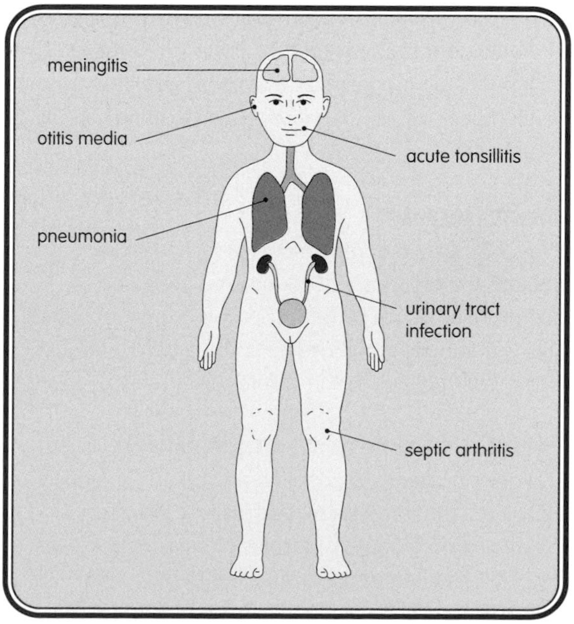

Fig. 1.2 Fever: important sites of local bacterial infection.

- **Look for the purpuric rash of meningococcal septicaemia in all febrile children.**
- **Localization suggests bacterial infection.**

Investigations

In a well child in whom a confident clinical diagnosis has been possible, no investigation is required. However, certain investigations are appropriate in any ill febrile child. These include:

- The full blood count (FBC)—an increase in the total circulating white blood cell count (WBC) indicates infection, and a predominance of neutrophils suggests bacterial infection. In a severe infection (e.g. meningitis, septicaemia) the total WBC may actually fall.
- Samples for microbiological examination (microscopy and culture)—these may include blood cultures, urine for microscopy and culture, throat swab, and cerebrospinal fluid.
- Imaging—a chest X-ray (CXR) should be taken if there is any suspicion of lower respiratory tract infection.
- A 'septic screen'—babies suspected of severe infection without localizing signs on examination are investigated with a standard battery of investigations before starting antibiotic therapy. These include: blood culture, FBC, lumbar puncture, urine sampling, and CXR.

Management

If an attempt is made to return the temperature to normal, the child feels better and the likelihood of complications such as febrile convulsions are reduced. This is done using antipyretics such as paracetamol. Ibuprofen may be used in children over 1 year.

Pyrexia of unknown origin (PUO)

The designation PUO should be reserved for a child with a documented protracted fever (more than 7 days) and no diagnosis despite initial investigation (Fig. 1.3). It is frequently misapplied to any child presenting with a fever of which the cause is not immediately obvious.

Causes of PUO	
Type	**Cause**
infections	malaria TB typhoid Kawasaki disease
non-infectious	juvenile chronic arthritis SLE
malignancy	leukaemia
fictitious	malingering child Munchausen by proxy

Fig. 1.3 Causes of pyrexia of unknown origin (PUO).

RASHES

A rash is a temporary eruption involving the skin. The history and examination often allow a clinical diagnosis without special investigations. Although an exact diagnosis is not always possible, or even necessary, on occasion it may be life-saving, as in the case of meningococcal septicaemia.

History

The history of a rash should ascertain the following:

- Duration, site of onset, evolution, and spread.
- Does it come and go (e.g. urticaria)?
- Does the rash 'itch' (e.g. eczema, scabies)?
- Has there been any recent drug ingestion or exposure to provocative agents (e.g. sunlight, food, allergens, detergents)?
- Are any other family members or contacts affected (e.g. viral exanthems, infestations)?
- Are there any other associated symptoms (e.g. sore throat, upper respiratory tract infection?
- Is there any family history (e.g. atopy, psoriasis)?

Examination

Check for systemic features such as:

- Fever.
- Lymphadenopathy.
- Splenomegaly.

Describe the rash in 'dermatological language' observing the morphology, arrangement, and distribution of the lesions.

Morphology

Describe the shape, size, and colour of the lesions. There may be:

- Macules, papules, or nodules.
- Vesicles, pustules, or bullae.
- Petechiae, purpura, or ecchymoses.

Most lesions are pink or erythematous.

Arrangement

Are they diffusely scattered, well circumscribed, or confluent?

Distribution

The distribution is important (Fig. 1.4). It can be local or generalized (flexor surfaces—eczema, or extensor surfaces—Henoch–Schönlein purpura (HSP) or psoriasis) or may involve mucous membranes (measles, Kawasaki disease, Stevens–Johnson syndrome).

Palpation

Feel the rash for scale, thickness, texture, and temperature.

Investigations

Investigations are rarely required but may include skin scrapings for fungi or scabies.

Causes of a rash

The main causative categories are shown in Fig. 1.5.

Diagnostic features of the more common generalized rashes.

The common generalized rashes are: maculopapular rash, vesicular rash, haemorrhagic rash, and urticarial rash.

Maculopapular rash

This is most likely a viral exanthem, but may be a drug-induced eruption. Common diagnostic features are:

- Measles—prodrome of fever, coryza, and cough. Just before the rash appears, Koplik's spots appear in the mouth. The rash tends to coalesce.
- Rubella—discrete, pink macular rash starting on the scalp and face. Occipital and cervical lymphadenopathy may precede the rash.
- Roseola infantum—occurs in infants under 3 years. After 3 days of sustained fever, a pink morbilliform (measles-like) eruption appears as the temperature subsides. It is due to human herpesvirus 6 (HHV-6).
- Enteroviral infection causes a generalized, pleomorphic rash and produces a mild fever.
- Glandular fever—symptoms include malaise, fever, and exudative tonsillitis. Lymphadenopathy and splenomegaly are commonly found.

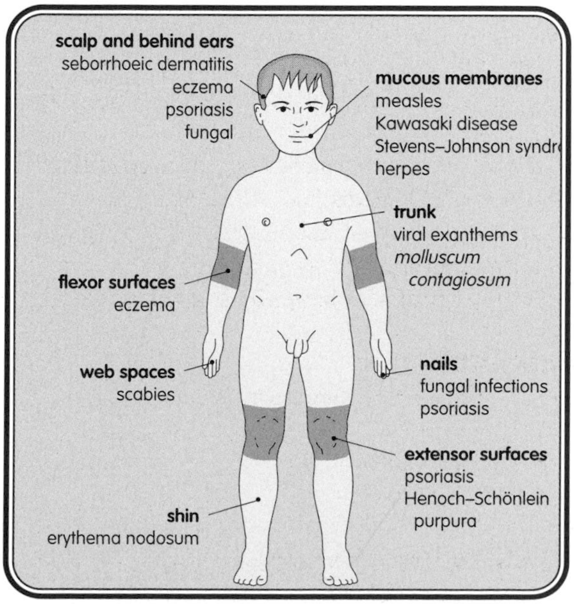

Fig. 1.4 Distribution of rashes.

Causes of a rash	
Type	**Cause**
infections	viral exanthems bacterial toxins
infestations	scabies
dermatitis	atopic dermatitis (eczema) seborrhoeic dermatitis
allergy	urticaria drug eruptions

Fig. 1.5 Causes of a rash.

- Kawasaki disease—causes a protracted fever, generalized rash, red lips, and conjunctival inflammation.
- Scarlet fever—causes fever and sore throat. The rash starts on the face and may include a 'strawberry' tongue.

Vesicular rash

Common causes of vesicular rash are:

- Chickenpox—successive crops of papulovesicles on an erythematous base which become encrusted. Lesions present at different stages. The mucous membranes are involved.
- Eczema herpeticum—exacerbation of eczema with vesicular spots caused by a herpes infection.

Haemorrhagic rash

Due to extravasated blood these lesions do *not* blanch on pressure. Lesions are classified by size:

- Petechiae (smallest).
- Purpura.
- Ecchymoses (largest).

Common diagnostic features are:

- Meningococcal septicaemia—petechial rash (may be preceded by maculopapular rash).
- Acute leukaemia—look for pallor and hepatosplenomegaly.
- Idiopathic thrombocytopenic purpura—the child looks well but may have bruising with, or without, nose bleeds.
- Henoch-Schönlein purpura—distribution is usually on the legs and buttocks. Arthralgia and abdominal pain may be present.

Urticarial rash

Urticaria (hives), a transient, itchy rash characterized by raised weals, appears rapidly and fades. It may recur. Causes include:

- Food allergy—e.g. shellfish, eggs, cow's milk.
- Drug allergy—e.g. aspirin, penicillin.
- Infections—e.g. viral, urinary tract infections (UTIs).
- Contact allergy—e.g. plants, grasses, animal hair.

Two other distinctive rashes that occur in childhood and require special consideration are erythema multiforme and erythema nodosum.

Erythema multiforme

A distinctive, symmetrical rash characterized by annular target (iris) lesions and various other lesions including macules, papules, and bullae. The severe form is Stevens–Johnson syndrome. Causes include infections (most commonly: herpes simplex, *Mycoplasma*, or Epstein–Barr virus) and drugs (especially sulphonamides).

Erythema nodosum

Red, tender, nodular lesions usually occur on the shins. Important causes include streptococcal infections and TB.

2. Heart, Lung, or ENT Problems

HEART

Congenital heart malformations account for most cardiovascular disease in paediatric practice. Rare causes include rheumatic fever, viral myocarditis or pericarditis, arrhythmias, and Kawasaki disease.

Heart disease presents in a limited number of ways:

- An abnormality detected on prenatal ultrasound.
- A murmur noted on routine examination in an asymptomatic infant or child.
- Cyanosis.
- Cardiac failure with or without low cardiac output.

History

Cardiac symptoms may include:

- Poor feeding, cough, and difficulty breathing—cardiac failure in babies.
- Syncope—caused by arrhythmias and on rare occasions by severe aortic stenosis (AS).
- Headache—caused by hypertension due to coarctation of aorta (COA).

Examination

The major physical signs are:

- Cyanosis.
- Murmurs.
- Signs of cardiac failure.

Cyanosis

Several varieties of congenital heart disease may present with central cyanosis (a 'blue' baby) at, or soon after, birth. Central cyanosis is visible if the concentration of deoxygenated haemoglobin (Hb) in the blood exceeds 5 g/dL. Peripheral cyanosis—blueness of the hands and feet (due to a sluggish peripheral circulation) is a normal finding in babies who are cold, or crying, or unwell from some non-cardiac cause.

Central cyanosis due to congenital heart disease is distinguished from that due to respiratory disease by the failure of right radial artery pO_2 to rise above 15 kPa after breathing 100% O_2 for 10 minutes.

Causes

In most patients, there is an abnormality that allows a portion of the systemic venous return to bypass the lungs and enter the systemic circulation directly (i.e. a right to left shunt).

Right to left shunts result from two general types of cardiac malformation:

- Lesions with abnormal mixing—desaturated systemic venous blood is mixed with oxygenated pulmonary venous blood so that the blood discharged into the systemic circulation is not fully saturated. Pulmonary vascularity is increased and pulmonary plethora is apparent on chest X-ray (CXR), e.g. transposition of the great arteries (TGA) (Fig. 2.1).
- Lesions with inadequate pulmonary blood flow—these infants often have right outflow tract obstruction and may depend on blood flowing to the lungs from left to right across a patent ductus arteriosus (PDA). Severe cyanosis develops when the duct closes, pulmonary vascularity is diminished and oligaemic lung fields are apparent on CXR, e.g. Fallot's tetralogy (Fig. 2.2).

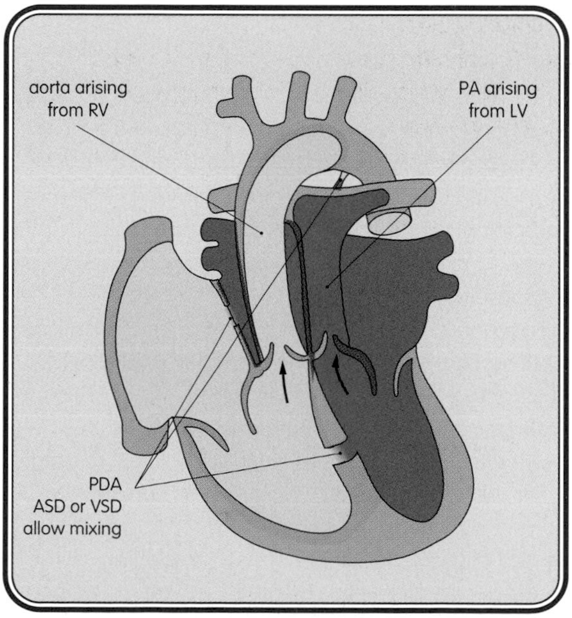

Fig. 2.1 Transposition of the great arteries. There has to be mixing between the two circulations to be compatible with life. As the foramen ovale and the ductus arteriosus begin to close, progressive cyanosis develops.

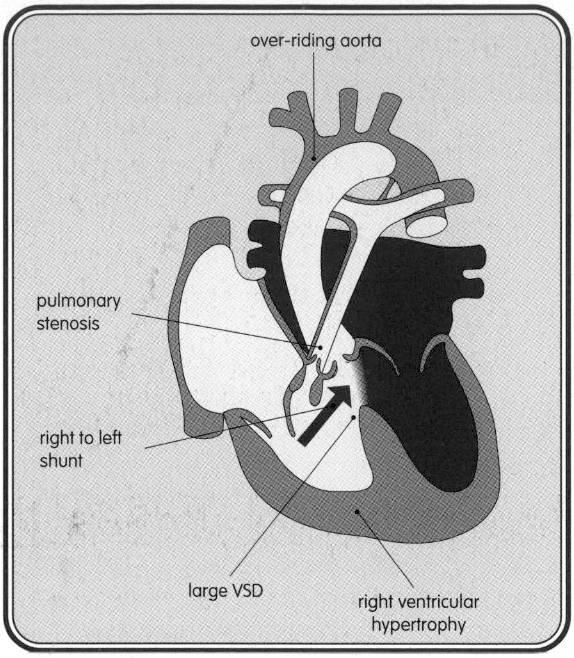

Fig. 2.2 Tetralogy of Fallot: the stenosis of the pulmonary valve causes resistance to flow and shunting of blood through the large ventricular septal defect.

Murmurs

A cardiac murmur discovered during an examination carried out either routinely or during an intercurrent illness represents a common problem. Many of these murmurs are innocent and do not reflect any underlying cardiac disease. Most haemodynamically significant cardiac lesions will present with cyanosis or cardiac failure. However, children with ventricular septal defects (VSDs) or pulmonary stenosis (PS) may be asymptomatic and discovered incidentally.

Evaluation of a murmur

A murmur is merely one component of the information obtained by examination of the cardiovascular system and cannot be interpreted in isolation.

Important features of a murmur include:

- The timing—is it systolic or diastolic? (Most murmurs in children are systolic; diastolic murmurs are rare and always pathological.)
- The character—is it pansystolic or ejection systolic?
- The loudness—grade out of 6. Loud murmurs may be palpable, called a 'thrill'.
- The radiation—a murmur that radiates from its site of maximal loudness is more likely to be significant.

Innocent murmurs

In most children with a murmur, the heart is normal and the murmur is innocent. Innocent murmurs are generated by turbulent flow in a structurally normal cardiovascular system (CVS).

There are two main varieties of innocent murmurs, the ejection murmurs and the venous hums.

The ejection murmurs are:

- Generated in the outflow tract of either side of the heart.
- Soft, blowing, systolic.
- Heard in the second or fourth left intercostal space.

The venous hums are:

- Generated in the head and neck veins.
- Continuous low-pitched rumble.
- Heard beneath the clavicle.
- Disappear on lying flat.

An innocent murmur is more likely to be noted during tachycardia, e.g. with fever, excitement, or exercise.

Significant murmurs

A murmur with any of the following features is significant:

- Symptoms—syncope, episodic cyanosis.
- CVS signs—abnormal pulses, heart sounds, blood pressure (BP), or cardiac impulse.
- Murmur—diastolic, associated with a thrill.

Significant murmurs, which may be difficult to distinguish from an innocent murmur, include those caused by PS and PDA. Refer for echocardiography if in doubt.

Cardiac failure

Cardiac failure is rarely seen in paediatric practice and is usually encountered in babies. The clinical features are different from those in adults, i.e. babies do not climb stairs or need extra pillows at night! Feeding is the only exertion they undertake and not being ambulant bipeds, at this time of life, their ankles do not swell up.

Clinical features

The symptoms and signs of cardiac failure are as follows (Fig. 2.3):

- Symptoms—the parents may notice poor feeding and breathlessness, excessive sweating, and recurrent chest infections. There may be failure to thrive.

- Signs—tachycardia, cool periphery, tachypnoea, and hepatomegaly. CVS signs may include an enlarged heart, murmur, and abnormal pulses.

Causes

In haemodynamic terms, the cause of cardiac failure is either pressure overload (obstructive lesions) or volume overload (left to right shunts):

- Obstructive lesions usually present in the neonate (e.g. severe COA or hypoplastic left heart syndrome).
- Volume overload usually presents in infants. The left to right shunt increases (e.g. VSD, PDA) as the pulmonary vascular resistance falls.

Cardiac failure may be confused with the more common respiratory causes of tachypnoea, e.g. bronchiolitis or wheezing associated with a viral infection. A CXR will clarify the situation. Less common causes include supraventricular tachycardia and viral myocarditis.

Investigations

Useful investigations include:

- CXR.
- ECG.
- Echocardiography.

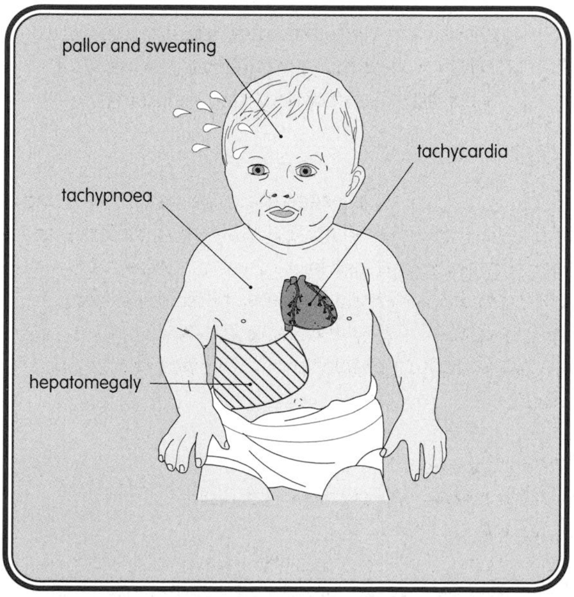

Fig. 2.3 Signs of cardiac failure in an infant.

The hallmarks of an innocent murmur are:

- **Asymptomatic child.**
- **Normal cardiovascular examination including normal heart sounds.**
- **Systolic or continuous (a diastolic murmur by itself is never innocent).**
- **No radiation.**
- **Variation with posture.**

LUNG

Several noises of great diagnostic value emanate from the respiratory tract. A cough is the most obvious. Stridor and wheeze, two other noises associated with breathing and caused by airway narrowing, are also of vital importance.

Cough, stridor, and wheeze

Cough

A cough is a reflex, involuntary explosive expiration that generates a sound familiar to all. A cough in babies or children is rarely productive. The majority are dry and if any sputum is produced, it is usually promptly swallowed.

In most instances, the cough is due to an acute illness, but there are important causes of a persistent cough. The cough itself is rarely diagnostic except in two instances:

- The 'barking' sea lion cough of croup (acute laryngotracheobronchitis).
- The paroxysmal prolonged bouts of coughing sometimes ending in a sharp intake of breath (the 'whoop') which occurs in pertussis.

History

Find out the following information:

- Duration of the cough—this is usually brief, e.g less than a week. A persistent cough raises the possibility of disorders such as asthma, whooping cough, inhaled foreign body, or TB.
- Dry or productive—a productive cough is rare in children and a persistent productive cough raises the suspicion of cystic fibrosis.

- Trigger factors—a nocturnal cough, or cough on exposure to animals, suggests atopy with asthma.

Common causes of a cough are shown in Fig. 2.4.

Stridor and wheeze

Differences between stridor and wheeze

Stridor is a noise associated with breathing due to narrowing of the *extra*thoracic airway. Wheeze is a noise associated with breathing due to narrowing of the *intra*thoracic airway. Either noise can occur at any phase of the respiratory cycle. The differences are:

- Stridor is usually worse on inspiration when extrathoracic airways naturally collapse.
- Wheeze is usually worse on expiration when intrathoracic airways naturally collapse.

It is very important to make a clear distinction between these signs as the likely cause and management of stridor is very different from that of wheeze. Stridor implies an upper airway obstruction which may be life threatening.

Stridor

There are two types of stridor: the acute and the persistent (Fig. 2.5).

Causes of acute stridor are:

- Acute laryngotracheobronchitis (croup).
- Acute epiglottitis.
- Inhaled foreign body.
- Angioneurotic oedema (rare).

Causes of persistent stridor in an infant are:

- Laryngomalacia ('floppy' larynx).
- Anatomical obstructions, e.g. vascular ring (rare).

The different features of epiglottitis and croup shown in the Hints & Tips boxes reflect the differences in pathology. In epiglottitis, there is rapid onset of supraglottic swelling (the swollen epiglottis is painful and makes swallowing difficult) and bacteriaemia. In croup, involvement of the larynx generates the characteristic hoarse voice and barking cough.

Features of epiglottitis

- **Appearance: toxic.**
- **Cough: slight/absent.**
- **Voice: muffled.**
- **Drooling: yes.**
- **Able to drink: no.**

Features of croup

- **Appearance: well.**
- **Cough: barking.**
- **Voice: hoarse.**
- **Drooling: no.**
- **Able to drink: yes.**

Causes of cough	
type of cough	**cause**
acute	viral URTI acute bronchiolitis (babies) pneumonia measles (prodrome) foreign body
chronic	recurrent URTIs (± postnatal drip) asthma (esp. nocturnal, exercise induced) TB cystic fibrosis pertussis foreign body

Fig. 2.4 Causes of cough.

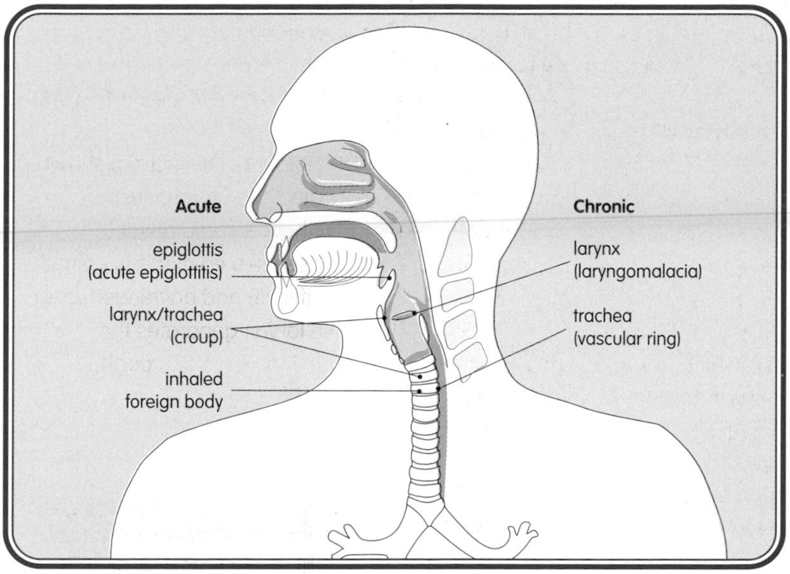

Fig. 2.5 Causes of stridor.

Wheeze

Wheeze is very common. The usual causes are viral lower respiratory tract infections and asthma. In children under 1 year old, the tiny airways are easily narrowed by oedema and secretions, making wheeze a common feature of infections that involve the bronchi and bronchioles. In children over 1 year old, asthma is the most common cause of wheeze. Asthma may have its onset in the first year of life, however, it can be difficult to distinguish from the episodic wheezing induced by recurrent viral lower respiratory tract infections.

Less common causes of recurrent or acute wheezing in childhood include:

- Cystic fibrosis.
- Cardiac failure.
- Inhaled foreign body.

EAR, NOSE, AND THROAT (ENT)

Infections of the ears and the throat are very common in childhood, therefore, ENT examination is essential in any febrile child.

Ear

Pain or discharge

Earache is usually caused by infection of the middle ear (acute otitis media). Less common causes include otitis externa, a foreign body, or referred pain from teeth. A discharge may be of wax or purulent material (from otitis externa, otitis media with perforation, or a foreign body).

Hearing impairment

Hearing impairment is classified into two main types—conductive and sensorineural hearing loss (SNHL). The causes of both are illustrated in Fig. 2.6.

Conductive hearing loss is very common and usually due to otitis media with effusion (OME, also known as 'glue ear'). Over half of all pre-school children have at least one episode of OME. A much smaller percentage

Causes of impaired hearing

Type	Cause
conductive	otitis media with effusion foreign body wax
sensorineural	congenital infection prematurity (<32/40) risk factors: hypoxia jaundice ototoxic drugs meningitis genetic (rare)

Fig. 2.6 Causes of impaired hearing.

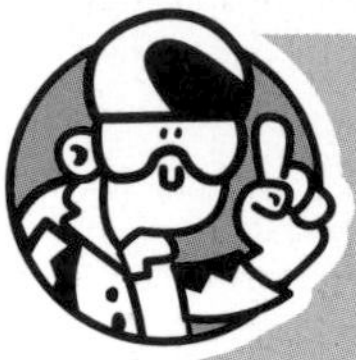

A small child may not localize pain to the ear. The ears must be examined carefully in any febrile child.

Any child with delayed speech must have a hearing test.

have persistent OME with hearing impairment, which may delay language acquisiton. Impedance tests are used to assess middle ear function (Fig. 2.7). They are not a direct measure of hearing.

Sensorineural hearing loss is less common. There is no routine screening in the newborn period but babies with high risk factors are tested (Fig. 2.8) Not all cases will be detected in the neonatal period as, for example, congenital infections and some genetic causes of SNHL are progressive and may not be detectable at this age.

Meningitis is the most important cause of acquired hearing loss. The numbers of cases may be falling since the introduction of the Hib vaccine. All children and babies should have audiological tests after recovery.

Nose

Noses may discharge or bleed. The common cold accounts for most acute watery discharges. A chronic discharge may be due to allergic rhinitis or a unilateral foreign body.

Causes of epistaxis include:

- Trauma.
- Nose picking.
- Bleeding disorders (especially low platelets).

Throat

Sore throat (pharyngitis)

In two-thirds of cases, inflammation of the pharynx, with or without involvement of the tonsils, is viral. Clinically, it is very difficult to distinguish between viral and bacterial pharyngitis and tonsillitis:

- Constitutional upset, tonsillar exudate, and lymphadenopathy suggest a bacterial infection: group A β-haemolytic streptococci is a common pathogen ('Strep. throat').
- Rarely a peritonsillar abscess (quinsy) may develop which requires incision and drainage.
- Epstein–Barr virus (infectious mononucleosis) is an important cause of exudative tonsillitis.

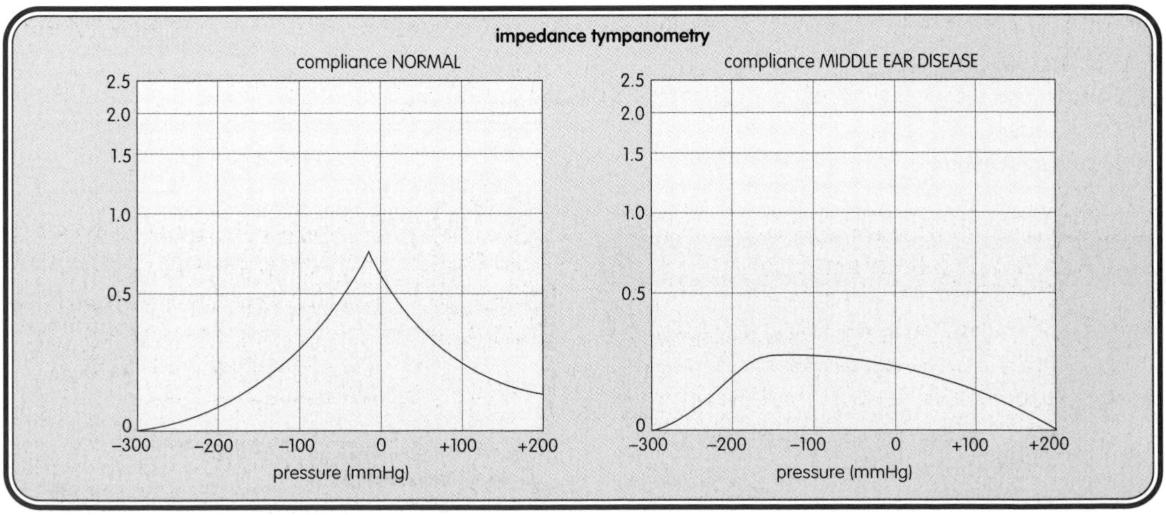

Fig. 2.7 Impedance tympanometry. This tests for middle ear disease. Sound is transmitted across the tympanic membrane if it is compliant (i.e. equal pressure either side). The test measures reflected sound at different pressures. In serous otitis media, compliance is reduced at all pressures because of the fluid present resulting in a flattened curve.

Test of auditory function		
Age	**Test**	Indication
newborn	otoacoustic emission brainstem-evoked potential audiometry response cradle	presence of hig-risk factors, e.g. prematurity
7–9 months	parental questionnaire distraction test	screen all infants
18–24 months	speech discrimination tests threshold audiometry (<3 years) impedance audiometry	children with suspected hearing loss children with repeated middle ear disease
school entry	'sweep test' (modified pure tone audiogram–Fig. 2.9)	screen all children

Fig. 2.8 Tests of auditory function.

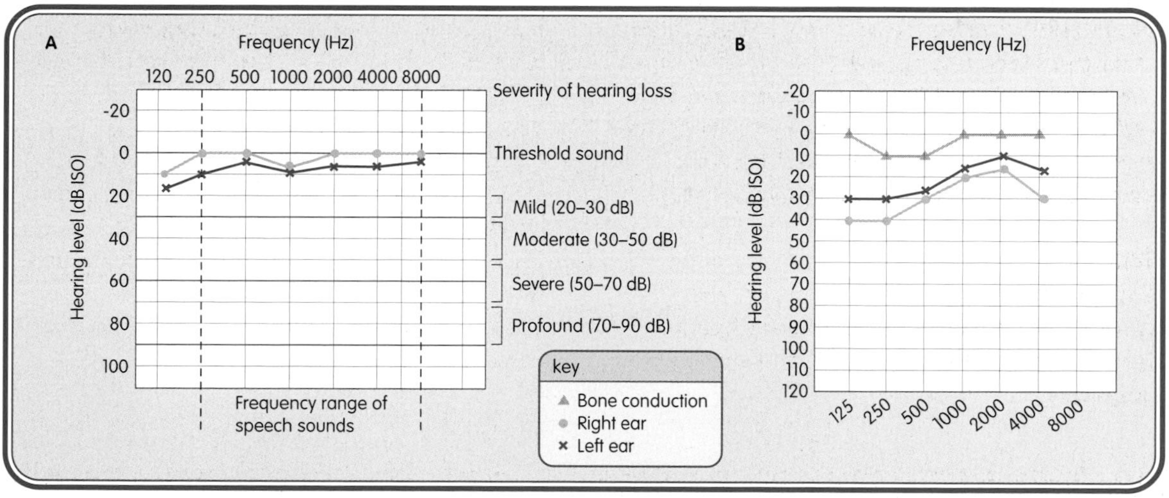

Fig. 2.9 Audiogram demonstrating: (A) normal hearing and (B) bilateral conductive hearing loss. In (B), there is a 20–40 dB hearing loss in both the right and left ears.

- **Speech uses frequencies of 400–4000 Hz.**
- **Hearing thresholds (in decibels = db):**

>70 db = profound hearing loss.
20–70 db = mild–severe hearing loss.
<20 db = normal hearing.

- **Parental suspicions about possible hearing loss should be taken seriously with early referral for audiological testing.**
- **Children with significantly impaired language development, behavioural problems, or those with a history of repeated middle ear disease, should also be referred.**

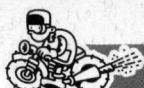

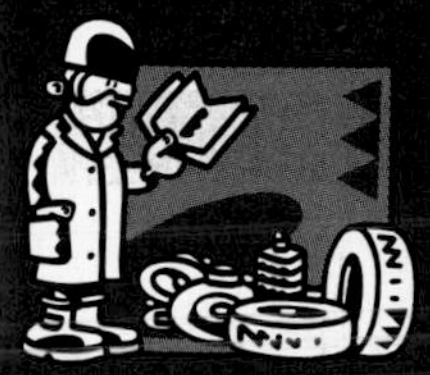

3. Gut or Liver Problems

GUT

Disorders of the gut present with a limited number of symptoms including abdominal pain, vomiting, diarrhoea or constipation, failure to thrive, and bleeding.

Abdominal pain

Acute abdominal pain

The most important issue is whether the pain is being caused by a condition requiring urgent surgical intervention (Figs 3.1 and 3.2).

History

In babies, abdominal pain is inferred from episodic screaming and drawing up of the legs. In older children, important features in the history are:

- Duration: pain lasting more than 4 hours is likely to be significant.
- Location: the further away from the umbilicus the more likely to be significant.
- Nature: constant or intermittent/colicky.
- Associated symptomatology: vomiting (is there obstruction or gastroenteritis?), stools (pain and bloody stools suggest intussusception in an infant, inflammatory bowel disease in older children), dysuria (urinary tract infection), cough (pneumonia), anorexia (a normal appetite is a sign of wellbeing).

Physical examination

Careful systemic examination is important if the many traps for the unwary are to be avoided. Look for:

- Fever—present in appendicitis, but also in mesenteric adenitis and urinary tract infections [UTIs].
- Jaundice—infectious hepatitis causes abdominal pain.
- Rash—the abdominal pain of Henoch–Schönlein purpura (HSP) may precede the characteristic purpuric rash.
- Respiratory tract—is there a right lower lobe pneumonia?
- Hernial orifices—is there a strangulated hernia?
- Genitalia—is there a torsion of the testis?

Surgical causes of acute abdominal pain
acute appendicitis intussusception torsion of testis strangulated hernia

Fig. 3.1 Surgical causes of acute abdominal pain.

Medical causes of acute abdominal pain	
Abdominal causes	**Systemic causes**
colic constipation mesenteric adenitis gastroenteritis hepatitis pancreatitis acute pyelonephritis/UTI	diabetic ketoacidosis sickle-cell disease Henoch–Schönlein purpura lower lobe pneumonia

Fig. 3.2 Medical causes of acute abdominal pain.

Investigations

Consider the following:

- Full blood count (FBC)—a neutrophil leucocytosis may be present in acute appendicitis or bacterial infection of the urine, lung, or throat. A sickling test should be done in children of African or Afro-Caribbean origin.
- Urinalysis—dipstick for glucose and ketones, urine microscopy and culture.
- Imaging—a plain abdominal film may reveal constipation, renal calculi, or signs of intestinal obstruction. Abdominal ultrasound may reveal obstructive uropathy, an appendix mass, or ovarian cysts.
- Urea and electrolytes—in a vomiting child, electrolyte disturbances must be identified in advance of anaesthesia and surgery.
- Blood glucose.

- **Acute appendicitis is uncommon under 2 years.**
- **Consider intussusception in vomiting infants aged 6–12 months.**
- **Not all abdominal pain originates in the abdomen.**
- **Diabetic ketoacidosis is often associated with abdominal pain.**
- **Consider gynaecological causes in a teenage girl.**

Recurrent abdominal pain

In 90% of children, recurrent abdominal pain does *not* have an organic cause. In most cases, a positive diagnosis of 'functional' abdominal pain can be made without investigations (Fig. 3.3). The exact basis of this phenomenon, which also includes so-called 'periodic syndrome' and 'abdominal migraine', is uncertain. It may be triggered by stress and certainly generates anxiety.

There is a long list of *rare* causes of recurrent abdominal pain (Fig. 3.4). Careful history and examination will usually provide a clue. Further investigations to exclude a possible organic cause may include:

- Urine microscopy and culture.
- Plain abdominal film.
- Abdominal ultrasound.
- FBC, erythrocyte sedimentation rate (ESR).

Vomiting

Vomiting is the forceful ejection of gastric contents and is a common symptom in babies and children. In babies, it should be distinguished from posseting (the normal effortless return of small amounts of milk during winding after a feed) and regurgitation (the non-forceful return of larger quantities of milk which accompanies gastro-oesophageal reflux).

Vomiting may be caused by a host of illnesses and often indicates disease outside the gastrointestinal tract.

History

Important points to establish include:

- Does the vomit contain blood or bile?
- Duration—is vomiting an acute or a persistent problem?
- Associated symptoms—is vomiting accompanied by abdominal pain, constipation, or diarrhoea?

Examination

Examine for the following:

- Signs of dehydration.
- Fever.
- Abdomen—distension (visible peristalsis), tenderness, or masses.
- Hernial orifices and genitalia.

Common and important causes, considered by age group and divided into medical and surgical conditions, are discussed below.

Vomiting is a non-specific symptom of infection in children.

Features of 'functional' recurrent abdominal pain
• pain is periumbilical, worse on waking, and short-lived • no associated appetite loss or bowel disturbance • family history of migraine, irritable bowel syndrome, or recurrent abdominal pain • healthy, thriving child with normal physical examination

Fig. 3.3 Features of 'functional' recurrent abdominal pain.

Rare 'organic' causes of recurrent abdominal pain
UTI urinary calculus obstructive uropathy inflammatory bowel disease duodenal ulcer malrotation recurrent pancreatitis

Fig. 3.4 Rare 'organic' causes of recurrent abdominal pain.

The neonate

Vomiting may be a sign of systemic infection (e.g. meningitis, urinary tract infection) or certain inborn errors of metabolism (e.g. congenital adrenal hyperplasia).

Surgical causes include bowel obstruction, which may be either small or large bowel obstruction.

Causes of small bowel obstruction include:

- Duodenal atresia (associated with Down syndrome).
- Malrotation with volvulus.
- Meconium ileus due to cystic fibrosis.

Causes of large bowel obstruction include:

- Hirschsprung's disease (absence of the myenteric plexus in the rectum and colon). Passage of meconium is often delayed beyond 48 hours.

Infants—1 month to 1 year

The most common cause of persistent vomiting in babies up to 1 year is gastro-oesophageal reflux. There is a functional immaturity of the lower oesophageal sphincter that resolves spontaneously. Thickening the feeds and positioning head up after feeds are useful manoeuvres. Severe reflux is uncommon (it occurs in cerebral palsy and babies with chronic lung disease) and may be complicated by failure to thrive, oesophagitis, and recurrent aspiration pneumonia.

Acute medical causes of vomiting include:

- Gastroenteritis.
- Respiratory tract infections such as tonsillitis, otitis media, and whooping cough.
- UTI.
- Meningitis.

Important surgical causes include pyloric stenosis and intussusception:

- Pyloric stenosis causes non-bile-stained projectile vomiting, more commonly in baby boys between the age of a few weeks and 3 months.
- The peak age of intussusception is around 6 months. The vomiting is associated with episodic severe abdominal pain and the eventual passage of bloodstained, 'redcurrent jelly' stools.

Older children

Acute vomiting may occur in infections as described or may be one of the symptoms of acute appendicitis.

In the older child, recurrent vomiting may occur as part of the symptom complex of abdominal migraine.

Any infant with bile-stained vomit requires a surgical opinion.

Rare but important causes include raised intracranial pressure, malrotation of the intestine, inborn errors of metabolism, and eating disorders such as bulimia nervosa.

Diarrhoea

Acute diarrhoea

The most common cause is infective viral gastroenteritis. It commonly occurs in combination with vomiting (the well-known entity D&V).

Some infections cause pathology in the lower GI tract. In this case, there may be no vomiting and diarrhoea often with blood and mucus dominates the clinical presentation (Fig. 3.5). Bloody diarrhoea should raise suspicion of specific pathogens and of non-infective conditions such as intussusception.

On examination, high fever suggests a bacterial gastroenteritis, especially shigella infection. Assessment of dehydration is most important (see Chapter 17).

Chronic diarrhoea

The most common cause of persistent loose stools in a well, thriving, preschool child is so-called 'toddler diarrhoea'. A maturational delay in intestinal mobility

Infective causes of acute diarrhoea
Viral
rotavirus
small round structured virus (SRSV)
adenovirus
Bacterial
E. coli
Campylobacter spp.
Salmonella spp.
Shigella spp.
Vibrio cholerae
Protozoa
Giardia lamblia
Entamoeba histolytica
cryptosporidium parvum

Fig. 3.5 Causes of acute diarrhoea.

causes intermittent explosive loose stools with undigested vegetables often present ('peas and carrots' syndrome).

An acute diarrhoeal episode may become protracted (duration more than 2 weeks) because of 'postgastroenteritis' syndrome due to secondary lactose intolerance. Watery diarrhoea returns when a normal diet, including milk, is reintroduced. Stools give a positive clinitest result for reducing substances.

Some infective agents such as *Giardia* also cause protracted diarrhoea.

Chronic diarrhoea in a child who is failing to thrive raises the possibility of several important diagnoses (Fig. 3.6). A description of the stools may suggest steatorrhoea (pale, bulky, and offensive) and the presence of blood or mucus suggests infective causes or inflammatory bowel disease.

Physical examination

Key points include assessment for evidence of malabsorption—anaemia, poor weight gain, abdominal distension, and buttock wasting. A thriving child with no associated symptomatology is unlikely to have significant disease. Faecal soiling due to constipation with overflow can be mistaken for diarrhoea (confirm by rectal examination).

Investigations

These are directed towards the suspected cause and may include:

- Stool microscopy and culture.
- Tests for reducing substances.
- Tests for nutrient malabsorption—Hb estimation, serum iron, and red cell folate.
- Jejunal biopsy (coeliac disease).
- Sweat test (cystic fibrosis).

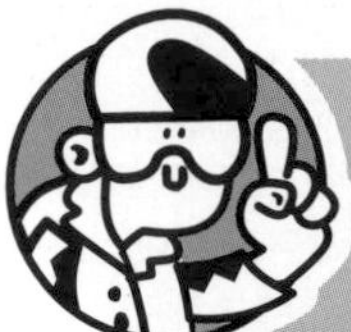

Bloody diarrhoea—consider:

- **Infective causes—*Campylobacter*, *Shigella*, amoeba.**
- **Intussusception—especially 6–9 months.**
- **Haemolytic–uraemic syndrome—check renal function and BP.**
- **Ulcerative colitis (rare).**

Constipation

The term constipation refers to infrequent passage of stools, passage of abnormally hard stools, or pain or discomfort on defecation. It may be accompanied by soiling caused by involuntary passage of faeces (overflow incontinence), or voluntary passage of faeces in an unacceptable place (encopresis).

In infants and children, constipation is often acute and transient and it is important to remember the wide normal variation in stool pattern. Constipation may follow an acute febrile illness and may be prolonged if the hard stools cause a small, superficial anal tear.

Organic causes of constipation are rare (Fig. 3.7). An organic cause is more likely in infants, with onset at birth, or when constipation occurs in the context of additional problems such as failure to thrive.

In childhood, the most common cause of chronic constipation is so-called 'simple' constipation (Fig. 3.8) associated with acquired megacolon. Short-segment Hirschprung's may present late and may be considered in severe or intractable simple constipation (Fig. 3.9).

Causes of chronic diarrhoea	
infective causes	giardiasis amoebiasis
food intolerance	disaccharides—lactose intolerance proteins—cow's milk protein intolerance
malabsorption	coeliac disease (gluten enteropathy) cystic fibrosis
inflammatory bowel disease	Crohn's disease ulcerative colitis

Fig. 3.6 Causes of chronic diarrhoea.

Organic causes of constipation	
local causes	Hirschsprung's disease neuromuscular disorders, e.g. cerebral palsy
systemic causes	hypothyroidism hypercalcaemia renal tubular disorders

Fig. 3.7 Organic causes of constipation.

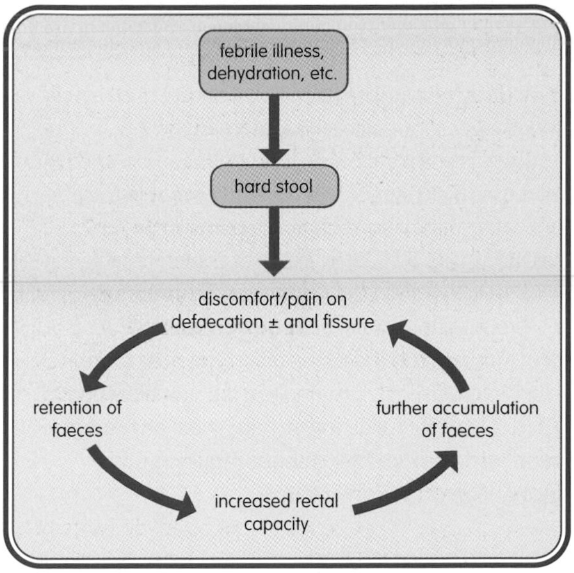

Fig. 3.8 The cycle of simple constipation.

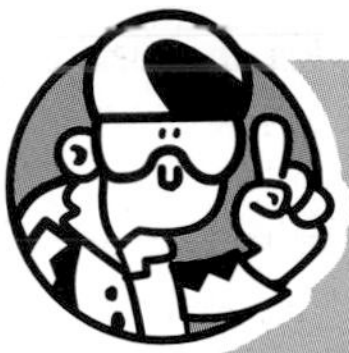

Hard stools in a baby may occur with:
- **Inadequate milk intake.**
- **Overstrength formula feeds.**
- **Changing to cow's milk.**

History
Enquire about:
- Frequency and consistency of stools.
- Presence of pain or blood on defecation.
- Presence or absence of soiling (in children).
- Any history of delay in passage of meconium.

Physical examination
Check for the following:
- Systemic signs of failure to thrive or dehydration.
- Abdominal distension, palpable descending colon.
- Presence of anal fissure.
- Rectal examination: anal tone, rectum empty or loaded?

Failure to thrive
The phrase 'failure to thrive' is used to describe an inadequate weight gain during the first year of life. Although this may be associated with poor linear growth and short stature, it is better to consider this as a separate problem.

It is the rate of weight gain that is important and this can only be judged by plotting serial weights on a centile chart over a period. A single observation is difficult to interpret. Much unnecessary anxiety is expended on normal small infants who are proceeding steadily up the third centile. It is also important to remember that birthweight is determined by the intrauterine environment, and the infant's weight may fall from its birth centile to a lower, genetically determined centile (catch down) in the first year. Normal small infants have small appetites, a feature that may cause inappropriate parental anxiety.

Globally, the most common cause of failure to thrive is inadequate intake of food (i.e. starvation). In the UK, most cases have a non-organic cause and are associated with psychosocial and environmental deprivation. Organic causes include inadequate food

Differences between simple constipation and Hirschsprung's disease

	Simple constipation	Hirschsprung's disease
frequency	common	rare—1:4500 live births
onset	late	85% in first month of life
passage of meconium	normal (<24 h)	delayed
soiling	usual	uncommon
abdomen	faecal mass	distended
rectum	loaded and distended	narrow and empty

Fig. 3.9 Differences between simple constipation and Hirschprung's disease.

intake, defective absorption of food from the GI tract (malabsorption), protein loss from the gut, and increased energy expenditure (Fig. 3.10).

Extensive investigation is not usually required. The constitutionally small normal child should be recognized (see Hint & Tips), and non-organic failure to thrive can be positively diagnosed. A brief hospital admission to document weight gain on a measured dietary intake may be helpful.

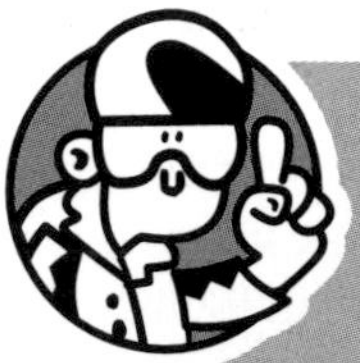

Recognition of the constitutionally small child:

- **Small parents.**
- **Low birthweight for gestational age.**
- **Proportionally small: low centile for height, weight, and head circumference.**
- **Normal height and weight velocities.**
- **Asymptomatic.**
- **Normal physical examination.**

LIVER

Liver disease is uncommon in childhood and usually manifests as jaundice or hepatomegaly.

Jaundice is a yellowish discolouration caused by an increase in circulating bilirubin. The bilirubin may be unconjugated or conjugated depending on the aetiology (Fig. 3.11). Mild jaundice is best detected in the sclerae rather than the skin.

Infectious hepatitis is the most common cause of acute jaundice in the older child. However, jaundice is encountered most commonly in the newborn period, at which time its causes range from trivial physiological changes to severe liver disease requiring early recognition and intervention.

Neonatal jaundice

Please refer to Chapter 9.

Jaundice or hepatomegaly after infancy

Jaundice

Jaundice in childhood usually has an infective cause. Viral hepatitis accounts for most, but other pathogens can involve the liver.

Infective hepatitis can be caused by:

- Hepatitis viruses.
- Epstein–Barr virus (EBV).

Causes of failure to thrive	
organic	non-organic
inadequate food intake: • breast feeding-insufficient milk, poor technique • bottle feeding-milk too dilute • insufficient diet offered • anorexia: due to chronic illness • unable to feed: cleft palate, cerebral palsy • vomiting: gastro-oesophageal reflux malabsorption: • coeliac disease • cystic fibrosis • short gut (post-operative) protein-losing enteropathy: • cow's milk protein intolerance increased energy requirements: • chronic illness-cystic fibrosis, congenital heart disease, chronic renal failure	• psycho-social/enviromental deprivation • inadequate or inappropriate feeding is usually a component

Fig. 3.10 Causes of failure to thrive.

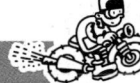

- Malaria or bilharzia.
- Leptospirosis (Weil's disease).

Liver injury may be caused by a variety of drugs (e.g. sodium valproate, halothane), and in overdose, paracetamol and iron are toxic to the liver. Jaundice with pallor suggests a haemolytic episode (e.g. glucose-6-phosphate dehydrogenase deficiency, spherocytosis).

Hepatomegaly

Isolated hepatomegaly is uncommon. In association with jaundice, the causes include biliary atresia and infective hepatitis. In babies, hepatomegaly is an important feature of cardiac failure.

Hepatosplenomegaly may occur in advanced liver disease and in a number of important haematological diseases (e.g. leukaemia, thalassaemia) and rare storage disorders (e.g. mucopolysaccharidosis).

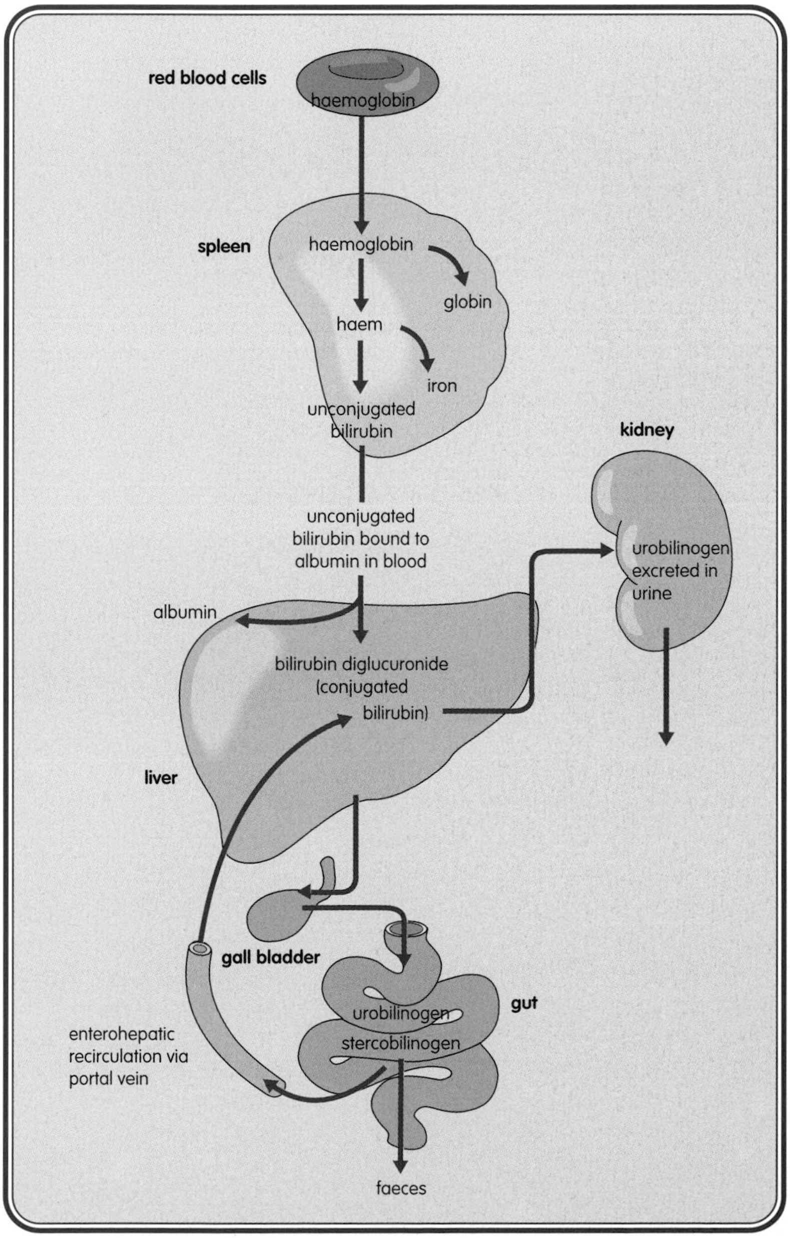

Fig. 3.11 Bilirubin metabolism.

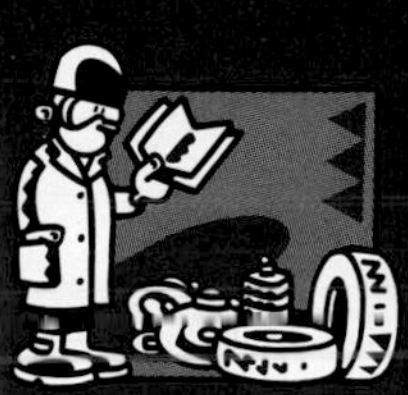

4. Haematuria or Proteinuria

In childhood, disorders of the kidneys or urinary tract are often manifested by changes in the urine. Urine analysis is therefore of prime importance (Fig. 4.1). In the infant or younger child, urinary tract infection (UTI) is the most common disorder encountered and it often presents without specific symptoms or signs.

Important symptoms:

- Polyuria, frequency, enuresis suggesting UTI or diabetes mellitus.
- Dysuria suggesting UTI.
- Oliguria suggesting dehydration or acute renal failure.
- Discoloured urine (Fig. 4.1).
- Fever with or without rigors suggests UTI or pyelonephritis.

Important signs are:

- Hypertension suggesting glomerulonephritis.
- Oedema suggesting nephrotic syndrome.
- Palpable bladder or kidneys which suggest anatomical abnormalities.

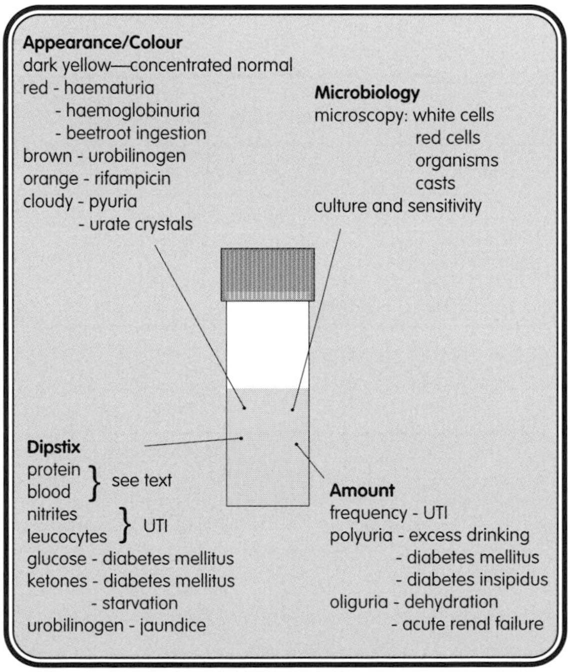

Fig. 4.1 Information available from urine.

HAEMATURIA

Test strips are very sensitive. Haematuria should be confirmed by urine microscopy and it is defined as >10 red blood cells (RBCs) per high power field. The causes are listed in Fig. 4.2.

History

Find out the following:

- Duration and recurrence.
- Dysuria and frequency (UTI).
- Associated loin pain (pyelonephritis).
- Recent foreign travel (schistosomiasis).

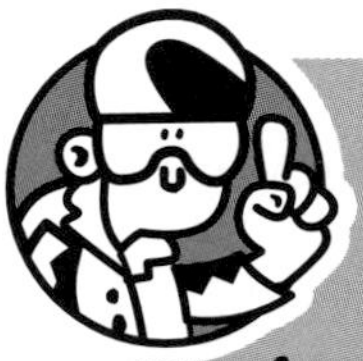

- **Polyuria and polydipsia suggest diabetes mellitus—test the urine for glucose and ketones.**
- **Excessive drinking is a more common cause of polyuria and polydipsia in a toddler than diabetes insipidus.**
- **Polyuria may present as secondary enuresis.**

Causes of haematuria	
Glomerular	**Non-glomerular**
presence of red cell or white cell casts and proteinuria suggests a glomerular source of the blood—glomerulonephritis: • acute, poststreptococcal • Henoch–Schönlein nephritis • IgA nephropathy (Berger's disease) • Alport syndrome (familial deafness and nephritis)	infection: • bacterial UTI • TB • schistosomiasis trauma stones Wilms tumour bleeding disorders, esp: thrombocytopenia

Fig. 4.2 Causes of haematuria.

- Recent sore throat (post-streptococcal glomerulonephritis).
- Family history of stones or deafness (Alport syndrome).

Examination

Examine for:

- Fever (UTI).
- Hypertension (acute nephritis).
- Rash and joint swelling (Henoch–Schönlein purpura).
- Bruises and purpura (idiopathic thrombocytopenic purpura).
- Abdominal mass (Wilms tumour).

Investigations

The investigations are as follows:

- Microscopy and culture of urine.
- Imaging—plain abdominal X-ray and ultrasound scan.
- Haematology—full blood count, coagulation screen, and sickle cell screen.
- Biochemistry—urea and electrolytes (U&E), creatinine (Cr), Ca^{2+}, PO_4^{3-}, and urate.
- Throat swab.
- Anti-streptolysin O titre (ASOT), C3, and Hepatitis B antigen.

Transient, benign haematuria may occur but is a diagnosis of exclusion. A renal biopsy may be indicated when there is:

- Persistent microscopic haematuria or recurrent macroscopic haematuria.
- Abnormal renal function.
- Abnormal complement levels.
- Associated heavy proteinuria.

UTI may present with fever and no clues to its origin, especially in infants and young children. Urine microscopy and culture should be undertaken in any infant with unexplained fever.

PROTEINURIA

Urinalysis dipstix are very sensitive. Transient, mild proteinuria is mostly benign. The nephrotic syndrome causes persistent heavy proteinuria. The causes of proteinuria are listed in Fig. 4.3.

Examination

Physical examination should include evaluation for the presence or absence of signs of renal disease (especially the nephrotic syndrome) which include:

- Oedema—especially periorbital, scrotal, leg, and ankle.
- Ascites.
- Pleural effusions (unusual).
- Blood pressure: low or high.

Investigations

The investigations include:

- Urine dipstix (Fig. 4.4).
- Renal function—U&E, Cr.
- Plasma albumin.
- Midstream urine for microscopy, culture, and sensitivity.
- Throat swab, ASOT.
- Complement C3, C4.

Causes of proteinuria	
Transient	**Persistent**
fever exercise orthostatic—proteinuria during the day (stops when recumbent at night)	nephrotic syndrome (>1 g/m^2/24 h) UTI glomerulonephritis

Fig. 4.3 Causes of proteinuria.

Albustix values	
Stix reading	**Albumin concentration g/L**
+	0.3
+ +	1.0
+ + +	3.0
+ + + +	>20

Fig. 4.4 Albustix values

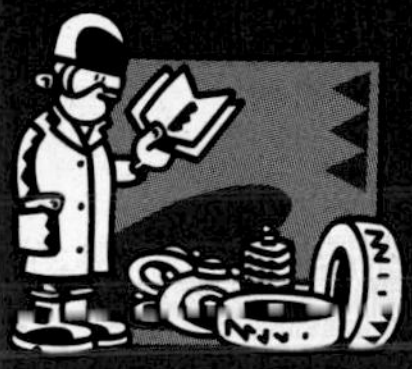

5. Neurological Problems

Important symptoms are:

- Paroxysmal episodes (fits, faints, and funny turns).
- Headache.
- Vomiting and ataxia.

Important signs are:

- Focal neurology.
- Altered consciousness or coma.

Global or specific developmental delay may be a manifestation of neurological disease, as may abnormalities of head size or shape. These are discussed in Chapters 8 and 19.

FITS, FAINTS, AND FUNNY TURNS

Transient episodes of altered consciousness, abnormal movements, or abnormal behaviour are a common presenting problem. The first task is to distinguish true epileptic seizures (fits) from faints and funny turns. An accurate account from a witness is essential.

History

Provoking events

Find out exactly when and where the episode occurred.

Description of the episodes

Get an exact description of:

- Any altered consciousness or awareness.
- Abnormal movements (involving limbs or face?).
- Altered tone (rigidity or sudden fall?).
- Altered colour (pallor or cyanosis?).
- Eye movements (did they 'roll up'?).
- Duration of the episode.
- Any trigger factor, e.g video

Other important features to establish in the history include:

- Previous history—was the birth normal, was there any recent head injury?
- Family history—both epilepsy and febrile convulsions run in families.

The paroxysmal episodes (faints and funny turns) which must be distinguished from epileptic seizures are listed in Fig. 5.1 and described below.

Seizures (fits)

Generalized tonic–clonic seizures

These are characterized by:

- Tonic phase of rigidity with loss of posture followed by clonic movements of all four limbs.
- Loss of consciousness.
- Duration 2–20 minutes.
- Postictal drowsiness.

Febrile seizures are usually of this sort.

Absence seizures

These are characterized by:

- Brief unawareness lasting a few seconds.
- No loss of posture.
- Immediate recovery.
- May be very frequent.
- Associated with automatisms (e.g. blinking and lip-smacking).

Differential diagnosis of seizures by age

Age	Differential diagnosis
infants	jitteriness benign myoclonia apnoeas gastro-oesophageal reflux
toddlers	breath-holding attacks reflex anoxic seizures rigors
children	vaso-vagal syncope (faints) tics day-dreaming migraine panic attacks, tantrums night terrors

Fig. 5.1 Differential diagnosis of seizures by age.

Faints (vasovagal syncope)

Features include the following:

- Usually occurs in teenagers.
- Provoked by emotion, hot environment.
- Preceded by nausea and dizziness.
- Sudden loss of consciousness and posture.
- Rapid recovery.

Funny turns

Breath-holding attacks

Have the following characteristics:

- Provoked by temper or frustration.
- The screaming toddler holds their breath in expiration, goes blue, then limp, and then makes a rapid spontaneous recovery.

Reflex anoxic seizures

Have the following characteristics:

- Provoked by pain or fear.
- The infant or toddler becomes pale and loses consciousness (reflecting syncope, secondary to vagal-induced bradycardia).
- The subsequent hypoxia may induce a tonic–clonic seizure.

Rigors

Rigors are transient exaggerated shivering in association with high fever.

Examination

The well child

Physical examination is often normal in a well child with idiopathic epilepsy (the majority). However, particular attention should be paid to:

- Skin—neurocutaneous syndromes are associated with epilepsy, especially tuberous sclerosis and neurofibromatosis.
- Optic fundi—fundal changes may be apparent in congenital infections and neurodegenerative diseases.

The convulsing child

Physical examination of an infant or child presenting acutely with generalized tonic–clonic seizures (convulsions) has a different emphasis reflecting the likely causes (Fig. 5.2).

- **A 'seizure' is a transient episode of abnormal and excessive neuronal activity in the brain which is apparent either to the subject or an observer.**
- **The term 'fit' is synonymous with 'seizure'.**
- **The term 'convulsion' refers to a subset of 'seizure' in which there is abnormal *motor* activity.**

Important features on examination include:

- Fever—febrile convulsions or intracranial infection.
- Anterior fontanelle—tense or bulging if raised intracranial pressure (ICP).
- Meningism.
- Optic fundi—papilloedema in raised ICP (changes may occur in congenital infections and neurodegenerative diseases).
- Focal neurological signs.
- Altered level of consciousness.

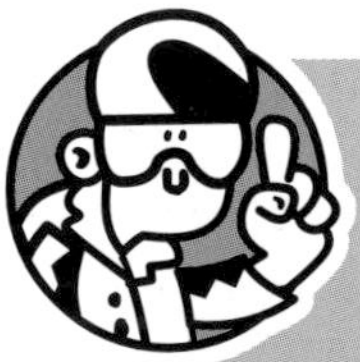

Regarding the convulsing child:

- **Remember ABC—airway, breathing, circulation.**
- **Always measure blood glucose urgently in a convulsing child to identify and treat hypoglycaemia.**

Causes of acute convulsions	
Common	**Less common**
febrile seizures meningitis hypoglycaemia	encephalitis vascular episode: thrombosis/haemorrhage hypocalcaemia hypomagnesaemia head injury hypertension

Fig. 5.2 Causes of acute convulsions.

HEADACHE

An acute headache commonly occurs as a non-specific feature of any febrile illness in a child but is of course a specific feature of meningitis.

Recurrent headaches are very common in children and their causes range from the trivial to the sinister (Fig. 5.3). Serious causes are rare.

History

Important features include:

- Site—frontal, temporal, or unilateral?
- Intensity—severe, throbbing?
- Duration and frequency.
- Provoking factors—stress, food?
- Associated symptoms—weakness, paraesthesia, nausea, or vomiting?

Simple tension headaches are characterised by the following:

- Affect ten per cent of school children.
- Symmetrical and band-like in nature.
- Gradual onset, duration less than 24 hours.
- No associated nausea or vomiting.
- Often recur frequently.

Migraine:

- May be unilateral and throbbing in nature.
- With or without visual aura, area of visual loss, or fortification spectra.
- Associated nausea, vomiting, abdominal pain.
- Duration several hours.
- Trigger factors—stress or relaxation, foods (cheese, chocolate).
- Family history.

Headache from raised intracranial pressure is:

- Worse in recumbent position, i.e. during the night or early morning.
- Associated with nausea and vomiting.
- Pain is severe in nature.
- Personality changes may develop.

Examination

Attention should be paid to the following signs in a child with recurrent headache:

- Blood pressure—hypertension (e.g. aortic coarctation is a rare cause of headache).
- Pulse—radial-femoral delay (coarctation).
- Visual acuity—refractive errors cause headache.
- Papilloedema—a late sign of raised ICP.
- Focal neurological deficit—especially cerebellar signs (posterior fossa tumour).

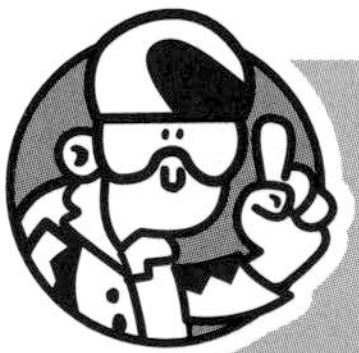

Migraine can be classified as:

- **Common—no aura.**
- **Classical—aura (often visual).**
- **Complex—transient neurological deficit, e.g. hemiplegia, ophthalmoplegia.**

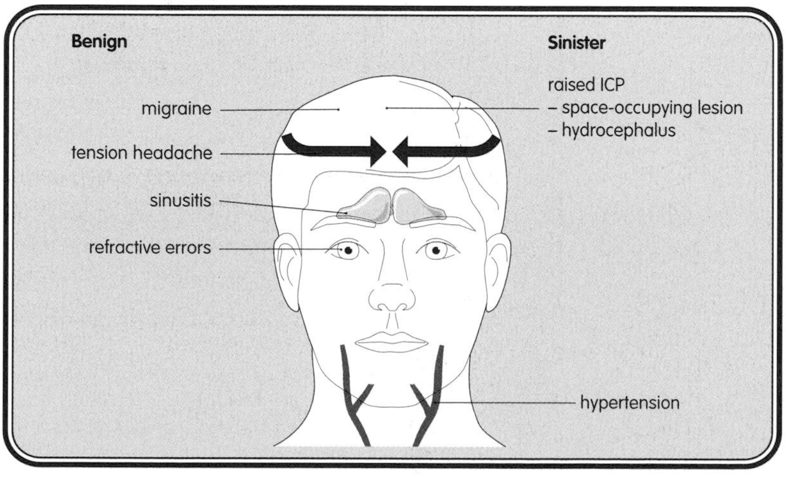

Fig. 5.3 Causes of recurrent headache.

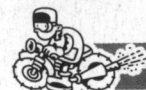

Headache is rarely caused by a brain tumour, but 70% of children with a brain tumour present with headache. The headache is severe and associated with vomiting. Most are in the posterior fossa and cause secondary hydrocephalus with raised ICP.

COMA

The acute development of a diminished level of consciousness that persists (coma) is a medical emergency. In the majority of cases a systemic problem rather than a primary brain disorder is responsible (Fig. 5.4).

The cause may be evident from the history, but if not, clinical evaluation is the key after emergency management. For investigation and management see Chapter 28.

Examination

Systemic examination

Check the following:

- Airway, Breathing, and Circulation (ABC).
- Febrile?
- Ketotic breath?
- Hypertension, bradycardia, irregular respiration (signs of coning).
- Signs of physical abuse.

Neurological examination

For a neurological examination, check the AVPU Score—four categories:

- A = alert.
- V = responds to voice.
- P = responds to pain.
- U = unresponsive.

Check also:

- The Glasgow coma scale (Fig 5.5).
- The pupils—small pupils (may indicate opiate or barbiturate poisoning), large pupils (may indicate a postictal state), and unequal pupils (may indicate severe head injury or intracranial haemorrhage).
- Meningism

Causes of coma

Cause	Differential diagnosis
trauma	head injury
infection	meningitis encephalitis
poisoning	barbiturates opiates alcohol
seizures	post-ictal state
metabolic	hypoglycaemia hyperglycaemia (diabetic ketoacidosis) hepatic encephalopathy
vascular	intracranial haemorrhage (rare)

Fig. 5.4 Causes of coma.

Glasgow coma scale

Score	Eye opening	Best motor response	Best verbal response
1	no response	no response	no response
2	open to pain	extension	non-verbal sounds
3	open to verbal command	inappropriate flexion	inappropriate words
4	open spontaneously	flexion with pain	disorientated and conversing
5		localizes pain	orientated and conversing
6		obeys command	

Fig. 5.5 The Glasgow coma scale: top score = 15.

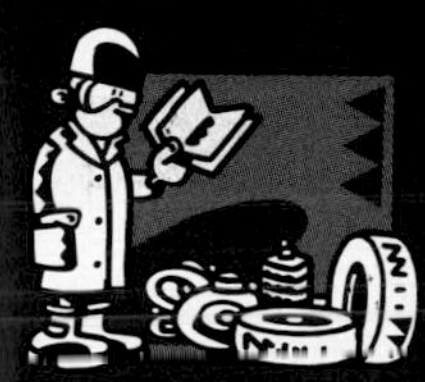

6. Musculoskeletal Problems

Disorders of the musculoskeletal system may present in a variety of ways including limp, pain in a limb or joint, or variations in posture.

Presenting symptoms include:

- Limb or joint pain.
- Fever.

Important signs are:

- Limp.
- Altered posture.
- Point tenderness.
- Reduced range of movement.

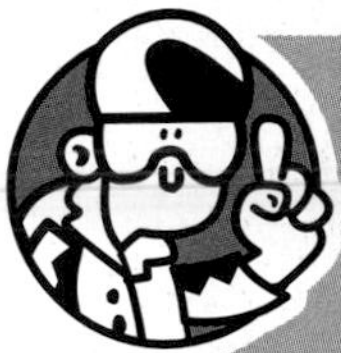

- **The most common cause of an acute limp in a well child is 'irritable hip'.**
- **The diagnosis *not* to miss is septic arthritis or osteomyelitis.**

LIMP

A limp is an abnormality of gait (the term applied to the rhythmic movement of the whole body in walking). It may be painful or painless, and the cause varies with age (Fig. 6.1).

History

The history should establish:

- Duration.
- Any prodromal illness or trauma.
- Presence and location of any pain.

Examination

Physical examination can begin by observing the child walking, if this can be done without distress. Important physical signs include:

- Fever: suggests bone or joint infection.
- Range of movement.
- Point tenderness or signs of inflammation.
- Unequal leg length.
- Spinal abnormality, e.g. hairy patch..
- Neurological signs: check tone, power, and tendon reflexes.

Investigations

Useful investigations may include:

- Imaging—X-rays, ultrasound of hip joint
- Full blood count, acute phase reactants.
- Blood cultures (if febrile).

THE PAINFUL LIMB

Pain in a limb may arise from the bone, joint, or soft tissues. In the lower limbs, it may be associated with a limp (see above). Pain in a joint (arthralgia) is considered separately.

Recurrent limb pain

So-called 'growing pains' are common in the lower limbs. Their features are listed in Fig. 6.2.

Causes of a limp	
Age group	**Cause**
all ages	trauma septic arthritis/osteomyelitis
1–2 years	congenital dislocation of the hip (developmental dysplasia of the hip) cerebral palsy
3–10 years	transient synovitis (irritable hip) Perthes disease rarities: • JCA • leukaemia
11–15 years	slipped upper femoral epiphysis Osgood–Schlatter's disease rarities: • bone tumours • JCA • hysteria

Fig. 6.1 Causes of a limp.

An important *rare* cause of limb pain, especially at night, is malignant deposits in the bone (e.g. leukaemia).

Limb pain of acute onset

In a young infant this may present as pseudoparalysis.

Important causes include:

- Trauma.
- Osteomyelitis.
- Sickle-cell disease ('painful crisis').

Trauma is usually accidental (e.g. sports injury), but non-accidental injury should also be a consideration. Osteomyelitis usually presents with a painful, immobile limb in a febrile child. The long bones around the knee are the most common site of infection.

Septic arthritis is a medical emergency—joint destruction may occur. X-rays are initially normal, but may show widening of the joint space and soft tissue swelling. Aspiration of the joint space is indicated if septic arthritis is suspected. Early treatment is vital.

Growing pains

Features
occur between the age of 7 and 11 years
always affect lower limbs
occur late in the evening and at night
settle with massage and comfort

Growing pains are never
present in the morning
associated with a limp
associated with abnormal signs

Fig. 6.2 Features of growing pains.

THE PAINFUL JOINT

Arthralgia usually reflects inflammation, i.e. arthritis. Diagnostic possibilities depend on whether the presentation is acute or insidious, and whether one or several joints are involved. Causes of an acutely painful joint are shown in Fig. 6.3.

Polyarthritis may have an acute onset, but is more likely to run a chronic and relapsing course. Causes to consider are shown in Fig 6.4.

Causes of acute monoarthralgia

Cause	Features
septic arthritis	systemic febrile illness: acutely tender joint most common <2 years
transient synovitis	irritable hip
haemophilia	traumatic or spontaneous
lyme disease	
JCA	

Fig. 6.3 Causes of acute monoarthralgia.

Causes of polyarthritis

Type	Cause
infection	viral: • rubella • hepatitis • mumps other: • mycoplasma
vasculitis	Henoch–Schönlein purpura
auto-immune	JCA systemic lupus erythematosus rheumatic fever (rare)

Fig. 6.4 Causes of polyarthritis.

NORMAL POSTURAL VARIANTS

These are common and most resolve without treatment (Fig. 6.5). They include:

- Bow legs (genu varum)—common in infants and toddlers up to 2 years.
- Knock knees (genu valgum)—common 2–6 years.
- Flat feet (pes planus)—often present in toddlers.
- Intoeing—metatarsus varus in infants, medial tibial torsion in toddlers, femoral anteversion in children (Fig. 6.6).

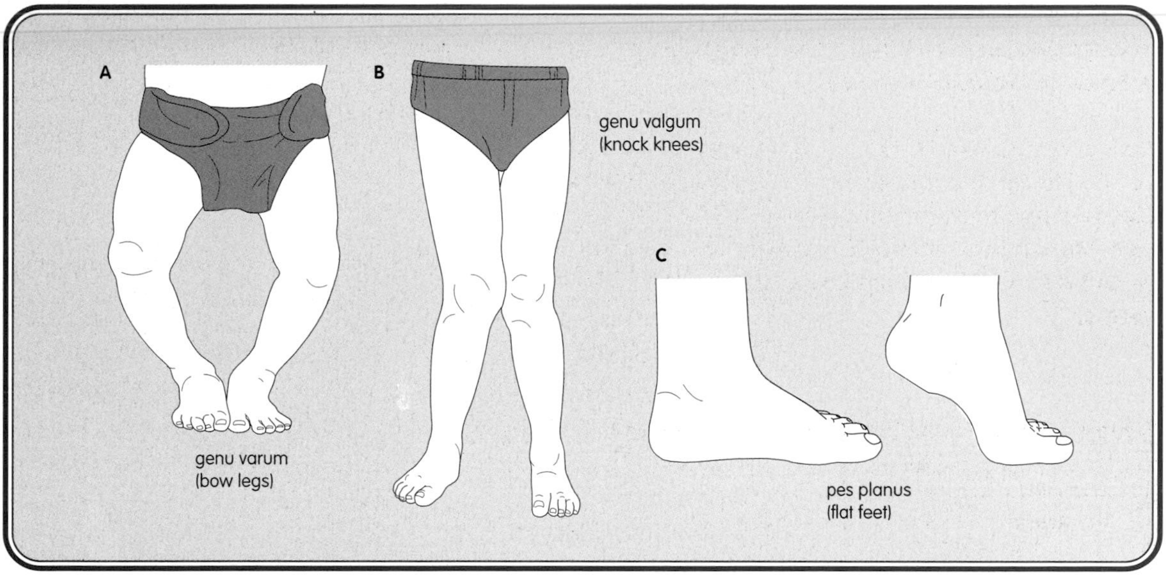

Fig. 6.5 Normal postural variants: (A) genu varum (bow legs), (B) genu valgum (knock knees), (C) pes planus (flat feet). Note the medial longitudinal arch appears when standing on tiptoe.

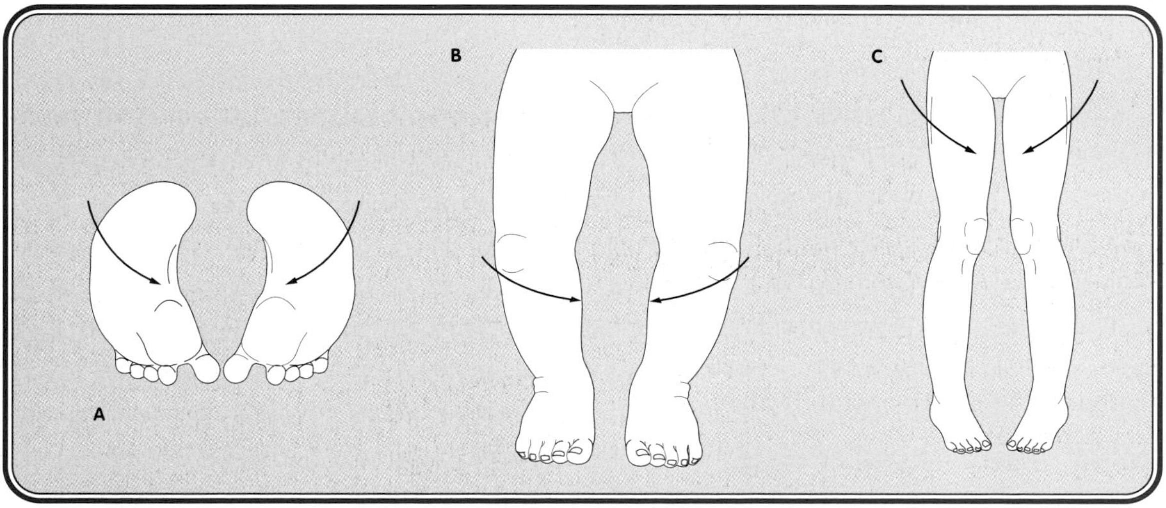

Fig. 6.6 Causes of intoeing: (A) metatarsus varus, (B) medial tibial torsion, (C) femoral anteversion.

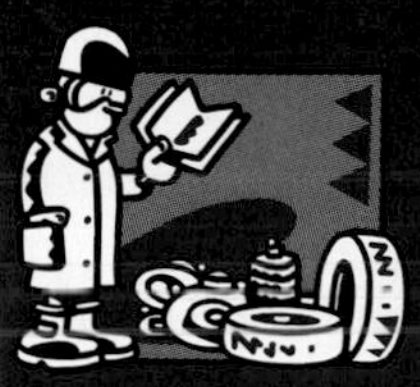

7. Pallor, Bleeding, or Lymphadenopathy

In childhood, disorders of the blood or bone marrow often present with striking physical signs rather than complex symptomatology. The pallor of anaemia is the most common sign, but abnormal bruising or bleeding, enlargement of the spleen or liver, or a propensity to infection may all reflect an underlying haematological problem.

PALLOR

A reduction in circulating haemoglobin concentration is an important but not the sole determinant of skin colour in caucasians. It is very important to inspect the mucous membranes. Vasoconstriction in the skin causes the striking pallor that accompanies circulatory failure (shock). It is easy to miss mild degrees of anaemia especially in those patients with pigmented skin.

Anaemia

The history and physical examination will often provide a good idea of the likely cause (Fig. 7.1).

Causes of anaemia in infants and children	
Cause	**Type**
decreased red cell production iron deficiency anaemia	nutritional occult blood loss (Meckel's diverticulum) malabsorption (coeliac disease)
haemoglobinopathy	β-thalassaemia
marrow replacement	malignant disease—acute leukaemia marrow aplasia
chronic disease	renal failure, inflammatory disorders
reduced red cell life span (haemolytic anaemia) intrinsic red cell defects	abnormal membrane—spherocytosis abnormal haemoglobin—sickle cell disease, thalassaemia enzyme deficiencies—G6PD (X-linked), pyruvate kinas
extrinsic disorders	immune-mediated: • ABO, rhesus incompatibility • auto-immune diseases • bacterial infections • malaria microangiopathy—haemolytic uraemic syndrome hypersplenism
excessive blood loss gastrointestinal	hookworm infestation Meckel's diverticulum
iatrogenic	excessive venesection in babies
epistaxis	recurrent, severe
menstruation	

Fig. 7.1 Causes of anaemia in infants and children.

History

This should include enquiry concerning:

- Dietary history—adequate iron intake?
- Family history—relatives with inherited disorders such as sickle cell disease, thalassaemia, or hereditary spherocytosis?

Examination

Age and ethnic group

Causes of anaemia are very age-dependent and inherited anaemias show a striking increased incidence in certain racial groups:

- Afro-Caribbean: sickle cell disease.
- Mediterranean, Asian: thalassaemia.

Associated signs

The associated signs include:

- Jaundice—suggests acute haemolysis.
- Petechiae or bruising—suggests marrow failure.
- Splenomegaly—suggests haemolysis or haemoglobinopathy.

Investigation

The most important initial investigation is examination of the peripheral blood (full blood count) to confirm reduced haemoglobin concentration and document red cell indices (Fig 7.2).

Additional valuable information from the full blood count (FBC) includes:

- Reticulocytes—an increase suggests haemolytic anaemia; a decrease suggests marrow aplasia.
- Pancytopenia—a reduction in all cell types suggests marrow failure or hypersplenism.

Red cell indices and film
MCV (mean corpuscular volume): • microcytic anaemia suggests iron deficiency, thalassaemia • macrocytic anaemia (normal in neonates) suggests folate, vitamin B_{12} deficiency (rare)
MCHC (mean corpuscular haemoglobin concentration): • hypochromic anaemia suggests iron deficiency, thalassaemia
The film may reveal: • sickle cells—sickle-cell disease • microcytic, hypochromic cells—iron deficiency • spherocytes—hereditary spherocytosis

Fig. 7.2 Red cell indices and film.

Depending on the initial results further investigations to clarify the cause may include:

- Serum iron, ferritin and total iron-binding capacity.
- Red cell folate, vitamin B_{12}.
- Haemoglobin electrophoresis.
- Red cell enzyme estimation—G6PD, pyruvate kinase.
- Bone marrow aspiration.

BLEEDING DISORDERS

Normal haemostatic mechanisms prevent blood loss from intact vessels and stop excessive bleeding from severed vessels. These involve a complex interaction between vessels, platelets, and coagulation factors. Both inherited and acquired disorders of these three components occur in childhood. The site and type of abnormal bleeding provides an important clue to the probable mechanism (see Hints & Tips). A mild defect may be unmasked by local factors (e.g. trauma). A severe defect will cause excessive bleeding spontaneously.

Clinical evaluation

The history and examination should answer the following questions:

- Is there a generalized haemostatic problem?
- Is it inherited or acquired?
- What is the likely mechanism: vascular, platelets, coagulation, or a combination?

Investigations will be required to establish the precise nature of the underlying abnormality.

History

Find out the following:

- Age of onset—inherited disorders usually present in infancy, but if mild may not be unmasked until adulthood.
- Response to previous operations or trauma (e.g. circumcision, tonsillectomy, appendectomy).
- Family history—a positive family history may be very helpful in diagnosis, but a negative history does not exclude an inherited disorder (e.g. haemophilia is X-linked—only males are affected.)

Examination

The most usual clinical manifestation is excessive bleeding into the skin, but other sites of spontaneous

- **Bleeding into skin and mucous membranes: platelet or vascular disorder.**
- **Bleeding into muscles or joints: coagulation disorder.**

bleeding include the nasal mucosa (epistaxis), gums, joints (haemarthrosis), and the genitourinary tract (haematuria). Spontaneous bleeding from multiple sites suggests a generalized haemostatic disorder.

Manifestation of skin bleeding

The terms used vary with the size of lesion. Test small lesions using a transparent glass to see if they blanch. Failure to blanch indicates extravasated blood.

The terms used when desribing manifestations of skin bleeding are:

- Petechiae—small red spots the size of a pinhead.
- Purpura—confluent petechiae.
- Ecchymosis—a large area of extravasated blood (a synonym for a bruise).
- Haematoma—extravasated blood that has infiltrated subcutaneous tissue or muscle to produce a deformity.

An important differential diagnosis of excessive bruising is non-accidental injury. There are some very important causes of a petechial/purpuric rash (see Chapter 1).

Investigations

Laboratory investigation of a suspected bleeding disorder initially includes:

- Platelet count: normal is 150–450 x 10^9/L (spontaneous bleeding may occur at counts below 30 x 10^9/L).
- Coagulation screen (Fig. 7.3).

Causes of bleeding disorders

The causes are set out in Fig. 7.4 and arranged according to the underlying basic mechanism. Most causes are acquired.

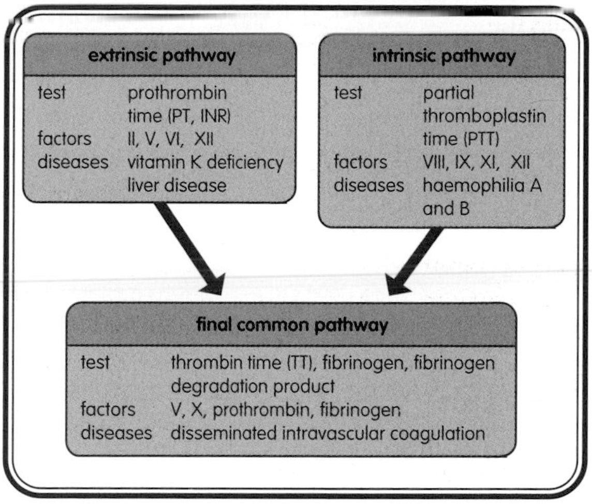

extrinsic pathway
test prothrombin time (PT, INR)
factors II, V, VI, XII
diseases vitamin K deficiency liver disease
intrinsic pathway
test partial thromboplastin time (PTT)
factors VIII, IX, XI, XII
diseases haemophilia A and B
final common pathway
test thrombin time (TT), fibrinogen, fibrinogen degradation product
factors V, X, prothrombin, fibrinogen
diseases disseminated intravascular coagulation

Fig. 7.3 Coagulation cascade: tests and defects.

The most common vascular problem encountered is Henoch–Schönlein purpura. The characteristic distribution of petechiae (buttocks, lower limbs) and associated features usually allow a clinical diagnosis.

Excessive bruising with thrombocytopenia in a well child is most commonly due to idiopathic thrombocytopenic purpura.

Inherited coagulation disorders are not common but haemophilia must be considered in a male infant or child with a bleeding tendency.

Haemostatic failure due to liver disease or disseminated intravascular coagulation occurs as a well-recognized complication of severe disease.

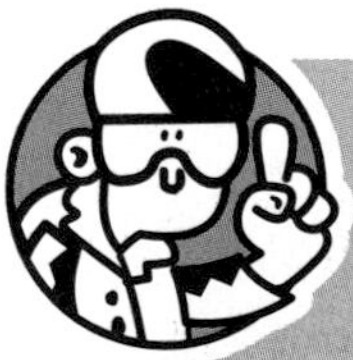

Bruising—normal and abnormal:

- **Mobile toddlers commonly have multiple bruises on shins.**
- **Bruises in a baby always require explanation.**
- **Platelet count to exclude idiopathic thrombocytopenic purpura should be done before ascribing excessive bruising in a child to non-accidental injury (NAI).**

Bleeding disorders in chidhood		
Defect	**Inherited**	**Acquired**
vascular defects	hereditary haemorrhagic telangiectasia (rare) Ehlers–Danlos syndrome (rare)	Henoch–Schönlein purpura scurvy (vitamin C deficiency) Cushing's disease Meningococcal septicaemia
platelet defects • thrombocytopenia	rare	immune-mediated: • idiopathic thrombocytopenic purpura (most common) peripheral consumption: • disseminated intravascular coagulation (DIC) • haemolytic–uraemic syndrome marrow failure: • aplastic anaemia • acute leukaemia
• abnormal function	rare	drug-induced, e.g. aspirin, dipyridamole
coagulation defects	haemophilia A (factor VIII) haemophilia B (factor IX, Christmas disease) von Willebrand disease	vitamin K deficiency: • haemorrhagic disease of newborn • malabsorption • liver disease
		drugs—anti-coagulant therapy with warfarin, heparin

Fig. 7.4 Bleeding disorders in childhood.

SPLENOMEGALY

In infants, the spleen may just be palpable below the left costal margin. The spleen may enlarge during acute infections and splenomegaly is a feature of a number of haematological diseases. Enlargement of both liver and spleen together suggests a different aetiology from that associated with isolated splenomegaly (Figs 7.5 and 7.6).

History

- Systems review—may elicit symptoms related to the many infective causes.
- Family history—inherited anaemias, storage disorders, e.g. Gaucher's disease.

Examination

Note co-existent lymphadenopathy, hepatomegaly, pallor (anaemia), fever, or rash.

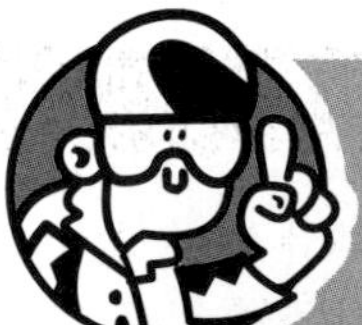

Differential diagnosis of a left-sided abdominal mass:

- **Splenomegaly.**
- **Renal masses: Wilms' tumour, hydronephrosis.**
- **Neoplasia: neuroblastoma (non-renal), lymphoma.**

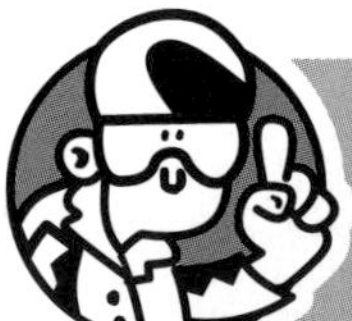

In sickle-cell disease:

- **Splenomegaly is present in early life but splenic infarction subsequently reduces the spleen in size.**
- **The immunological function of the spleen is always impaired regardless of size.**

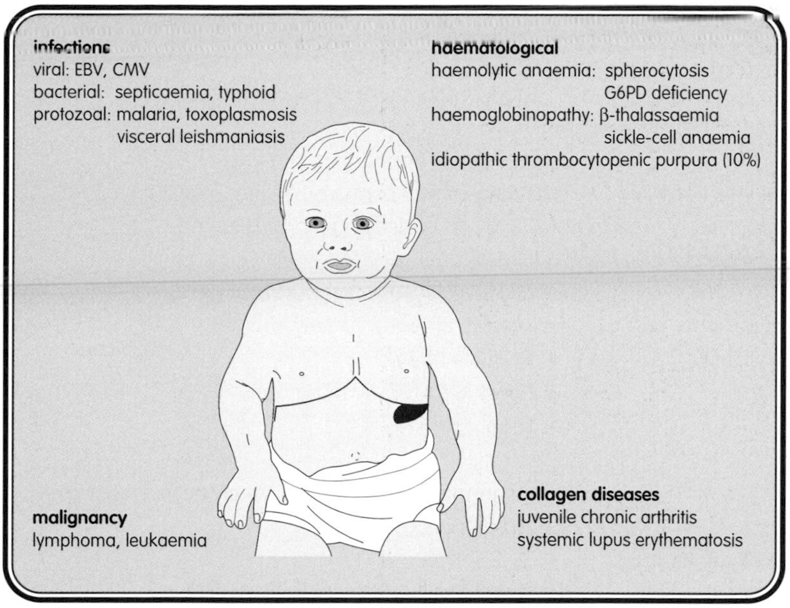

infections
viral: EBV, CMV
bacterial: septicaemia, typhoid
protozoal: malaria, toxoplasmosis
visceral leishmaniasis
haematological
haemolytic anaemia: spherocytosis
G6PD deficiency
haemoglobinopathy: β-thalassaemia
sickle-cell anaemia
idiopathic thrombocytopenic purpura (10%)
malignancy
lymphoma, leukaemia
collagen diseases
juvenile chronic arthritis
systemic lupus erythematosis

Fig. 7.5 Causes of splenomegaly.

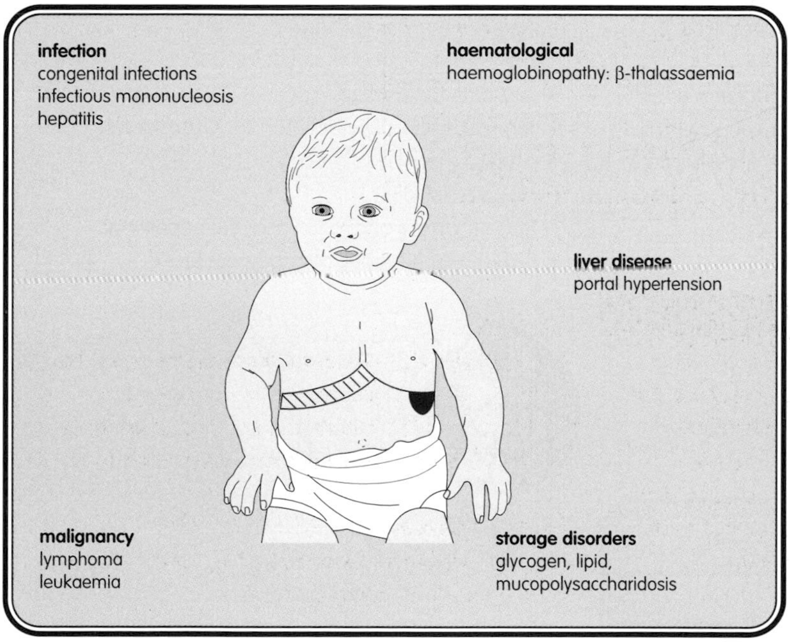

Fig. 7.6 Causes of hepatosplenomegaly.

Investigations

Investigate as follows:

- Abdominal ultrasound scan (USS).
- Infections—monospot, blood cultures, film for malaria parasites.
- Haematological—FBC, blood film, reticulocyte count.
- Malignancy—bone marrow aspiration.
- Liver disease—liver function tests (LFTs), hepatitis serology.

LYMPHADENOPATHY

Lymph node enlargement, particularly in the cervical region, is a common clinical problem in children. Cervical lymph nodes are normally palpable in many children, and the first problem is to distinguish this from pathological enlargement.

Local infection is the most common cause of transient regional lymphadenopathy but uncommon sinister causes of persistent or progressive lymphadenopathy do exist (Figs 7.7 and 7.8).

History

The history should establish:

- Duration—less than 4 weeks in most infections; more than 1 year less likely to be neoplastic.
- Constitutional symptoms—e.g. weight loss, fever, night sweats.
- Rash—associated rash suggests viral exanthemata.
- Pets—cat-scratch fever.
- Family history of TB.
- Drugs—phenytoin, carbamazepine.

Examination

Palpate all nodal sites: look for regional or generalized lymphadenopathy. Examine the nodes:

- Size: greater than 1 cm diameter is more likely to be significant. Small, mobile nodes are less likely to be significant than large, firm, fixed nodes.
- Erythema and tenderness suggest bacterial adenitis.
- Drainage region—ENT and scalp for cervical nodes.
- Skin—infective lesions, eczema, and exanthemata.
- Abdomen—hepatosplenomegaly?

Investigations

In most children with lymphadenopathy, the diagnosis is apparent and further investigations to establish the cause are unnecessary. This includes the following common clinical situations:

- Transient node enlargement with local infection.
- Lymphadenopathy in the context of diagnosed systemic illnesses such as rubella, Epstein–Barr virus, atopic eczema, and Kawasaki disease.

In contrast, lymphadenopathy presenting in the following clinical contexts requires investigation to establish an underlying diagnosis.

Persistent significant cervical lymphadenopathy

Initial tests are:

- FBC (infection).
- Chest X-ray (TB, lymphoma).
- Tuberculin skin test.

If malignancy is suspected a lymph node biopsy may be indicated.

Generalized lymphadenopathy

Constitutional symptoms and hepatosplenomegaly may or may not be present.

Initial tests:

- FBC plus differential.
- Monospot and Epstein–Barr IgM antibodies.
- Chest X-ray.
- Abdominal USS.
- Bone marrow aspiration may be necessary.
- Lymph node biopsy may be necessary.

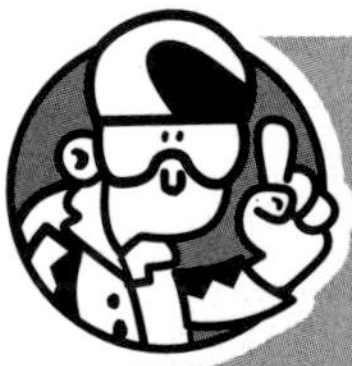

Cervical nodes are quick to enlarge but are slow to resolve with local infection. Consider TB or malignancy in persistent and progressive cervical lymphadenopathy.

Causes of generalized lymphadenopathy	
Cause	**Example**
infection	infectious mononucleosis rubella toxoplasmosis cytomegalovirus HIV infection
malignancy	acute leukaemia lymphoma
immunological	JCA sarcoidosis (rare) Kawasaki disease atopic eczema

Fig. 7.7 Causes of generalized lymphadenopathy.

Causes of cervical lymphadenopathy	
Type	**Features**
acute, short duration	reactive and secondary to local infection in throat or scalp: cervical adenitis—bacterial infection in gland
persistent, non-inflamed	reactive and secondary to local infection: • tuberculous adenitis—TB, atypical mycobacteri • neoplasia—lymphoma, neuroblastoma

Fig. 7.8 Causes of cervical lymphadenopathy.

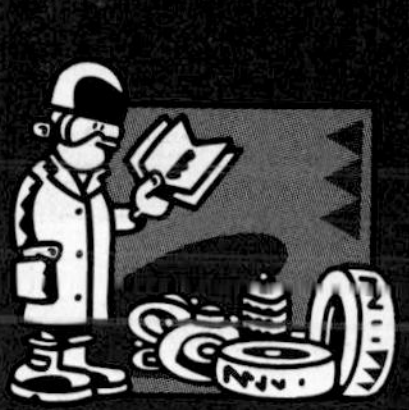

8. Short Stature or Developmental Delay

MPH =
~~HAGHt~~ FHt + MHt / 2

Male, ♂ → add 7 cm
♀ subtract 7cm

centile nearest to MPH
± 10 ♂
± 8.5 ♀

GROWTH

Growth is assessed by mea…
parameters:
- Height (or length in childre…
- Weight.
- Head circumference.

Centile charts are available wh… range of values for these from … (see Part II). Problems with inad… ('failure to thrive') and abnormal … (microcephaly and macrocephal… …ered elsewhere. An approach to the evaluation of 'short stature' is presented here.

Short stature

A pragmatic definition of short stature requiring further evaluation is:
- A height below the 0.4 centile for age.
- A predicted height less than the midparental target height.
- An abnormal growth velocity as indicated by the height changing by more than the width of one centile band over 1–2 years.

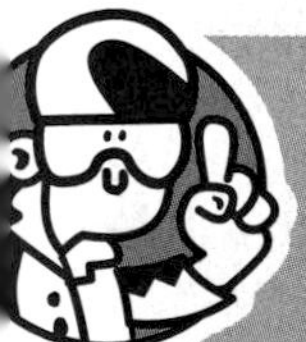

To estimate the adult height potential calculate the midparental height (MPH):
- **Father's height plus mother's height divided by 2.**
- **Then adjust for the sex of the child:**
  Boys—add 7 cm
  Girls—subtract 7 cm.
- **Identify the midparental centile, i.e. centile nearest to MPH.**
- **Target centile range (TCR) is encompassed by MPH:**
  ± 10 cm—boys
  ± 8.5 cm—girls.

…should be monitored …12 months in response …tal concern …s of current centile.

… short stature has triggered …either familial short stature …bertal growth spurt. The … short stature are shown in Fig. 8.1.

History

This should elicit information about:
- Pregnancy and birth—size at birth.
- Parental height—the genetic height potential is estimated by calculating the target centile range (TCR) from the midparental height (MPH).
- Family history—inherited skeletal dysplasias.

Causes of short stature
familial short stature
constitutional delay of pubertal growth spurt
endocrine disorders: • growth hormone deficiency • hypopituitarism • hypothyroidism • Cushing syndrome/steroid excess
chromosomal disorders/syndromes: • Turner syndrome • Silver–Russell syndrome
skeletal dysplasias: • achondroplasia
emotional/psychosocial deprivation
chronic illness: • congenital heart disease • cystic fibrosis • cerebral palsy • chronic renal failure

Fig. 8.1 Causes of short stature.

Examination

Examine the following:

- Height—measure accurately with a wall-mounted, calibrated stadiometer.
- Growth velocity—a minimum of two measurements, 6 months apart is required. Adjust to cm/year and plot at midpoint in time.
- Dysmorphic features—these may identify a syndrome (see Hints & Tips).
- Weight (see Hints & Tips).
- Visual fields and fundi—may indicate pituitary tumour.
- Stage of puberty.

An approach to the evaluation of short stature is shown in Fig. 8.2.

Investigations

Investigations that may be of value include the following:

- Bone age—estimated from X-rays of the left wrist (delayed skeletal maturity in constitutional pubertal delay).
- Karyotype—chromosomal analysis to identify Turner syndrome (45, X0) in short girls.
- Skeletal survey—in disproportion (skeletal dysplasias).
- Endocrine investigations—thyroid function tests (T4, TSH) and growth hormone (secretion is pulsatile so a provocation test, e.g. exercise or insulin-induced hypoglycaemia, is necessary to identify deficiency).
- Skull X-ray—for suspected craniopharyngioma.

Syndromes associated with short stature:

- **Turner syndrome—neck-webbing, wide-spaced nipples, low hairline in a girl.**
- **Prader–Willi syndrome—obesity, hypotonia and in boys, small genitals.**
- **Skeletal dysplasias—disproportionate limbs and trunk: Short limbs—achondroplasia. Short trunk—mucopolysaccharidosis (MPS).**

Endocrine causes of short stature are often associated with increased weight, e.g.

- **Hypothyroidism.**
- **Growth hormone deficiency.**
- **Steroid excess.**

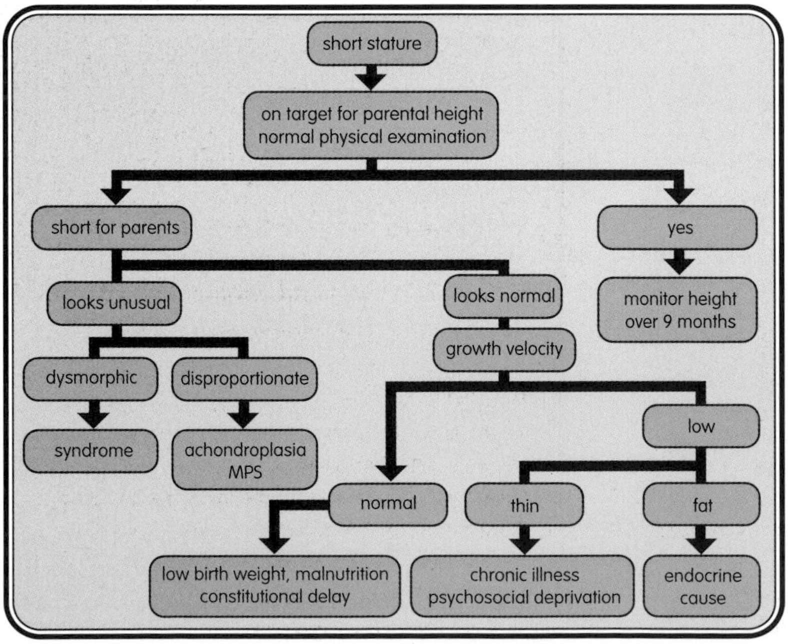

Fig. 8.2 Short stature algorithm.

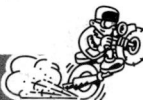

DEVELOPMENTAL DELAY

Normal development depends on genetic potential and environment—nature and nurture. There is a wide variation in normal rates of development in all spheres. Delay may be global or specific. Normal development is described in Part II.

Delay may present through:

- Parental concern.
- Routine surveillance.
- Concern of teacher, health visitor, etc.

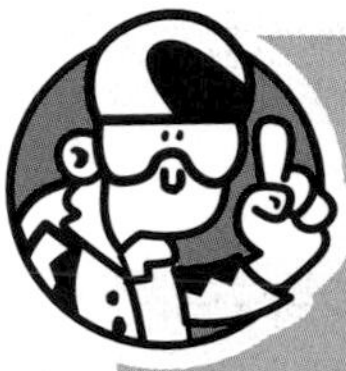

Development is assessed in four main areas:

- **Gross motor.**
- **Vision and fine motor.**
- **Hearing and speech.**
- **Social behaviour.**

Warning signs of developmental delay by age	
Year	**Sign**
First 8 weeks	not smiling in response poor eye contact head lag silent baby—no coos, gurgles
8 months	poor interaction not sitting with support not babbling
Second 18 months	not recognizing own name not walking three steps alone not using first words
24 months	not giving/receiving affection unable to build a three-brick tower not linking two words
Third	unable to play unsteady gait not using more than 50 words

Fig. 8.3 Warning signs of developmental delay by age.

A list of warning signs shown in developmental delay by age is given in Fig. 8.3.

Global delay

An explanation and diagnosis is found in about 30% of children with moderate delay and 60% of those with severe delay. An intellectually impaired child is delayed in all aspects of development, but not all children with general delay are intellectually impaired.

History

This should encompass:

- Birth history—details of pregnancy and birth including prematurity and hypoxia.
- Family history—of learning disability.
- Developmental milestones.
- Social history—risk factors, e.g. psychosocial deprivation.

Examination

You should examine the following:

- Developmental assessment.
- Appearance—dysmorphic features in syndromes associated with delay, e.g. Down syndrome, Williams syndrome, fragile X syndrome.
- Head circumference—microcephaly.

Causes of global developmental delay	
Type	**Cause**
genetic disorders	Down syndrome fragile X syndrome William syndrome phenylketonuria (now detected on neonatal screening)
psychological disorders	autism attention-deficit hyperactivity disord
CNS insult	perinatal hypoxia–ischaemia intracranial infections congenital infections head injury
emotional deprivation	non-stimulating environment
idiopathic	–

Fig. 8.4 Causes of global developmental delay.

Investigations

These are directed towards identifying a specific aetiology (Fig. 8.4) and may include:

- Karyotype—Down syndrome, fragile X syndrome.
- Thyroid function tests.
- Congenital infection screen.
- Plasma and urine amino acids.
- Brain imaging—MR spectroscopy.

It is important to distinguish developmental delay from actual regression. Loss of previously acquired skills suggests a serious inherited neurodegenerative disorder.

Specific developmental delay

Two common and important examples of delayed development in specific areas are walking and speech.

Delayed walking

The percentage of children who are walking unsupported is:

- 50% by 12 months.
- 90% by 15 months.

Further assessment is indicated if a child is not walking unsupported by age 18 months. Many will be normal late walkers, especially if a 'bottom shuffler', but a small percentage will have an underlying problem (Fig. 8.5).

Examination

- Hips—signs of dislocation (waddling gait, leg length discrepancy, limited abduction).
- Tone, power, and tendon reflexes in all limbs.
- Locomotion—'commando crawler' or 'bottom shuffler'?

Investigations

If indicated:

- X-ray hips.
- Creatine kinase for Duchenne muscular dystrophy.

Speech and language delay

The development of normal speech and language requires:

- Adequate hearing.
- Cognitive development.
- Coordinated sound production.

Speech refers to the meaningful sounds that are made, whereas language encompasses the complex rules governing the use of these sounds for communication. Language can be further divided into language comprehension and language expression, and independent delays may occur in either aspect. As might be expected, the development of language is highly dependent on general intellectual development.

The causes of delay in speech and language development include:

- Hearing impairment.
- Environmental factors—lack of stimulus.
- Global delay.
- Psychiatric disorders—autism.
- Familial.

It is worth distinguishing between delay and actual disorders of speech and language such as stammering, dysarthria due to mechanical problems (e.g. cleft palate), or neuromuscular problems (e.g. cerebral palsy).

Causes of late walking	
Normal variants	**Organic causes**
familial 'bottom shuffler' 'commando crawler'	cerebral palsy congenital dislocation of the hip Duchenne muscular dystrophy (boys)

Fig. 8.5 Causes of late walking.

Normal speech and language development:

- **6 months: babbles.**
- **12 months: says 'mama' or 'dada', understands simple commands and responds to name.**
- **18 months: single words with meaning.**
- **2 years: speaks in phrases.**
- **4 years: conversation.**

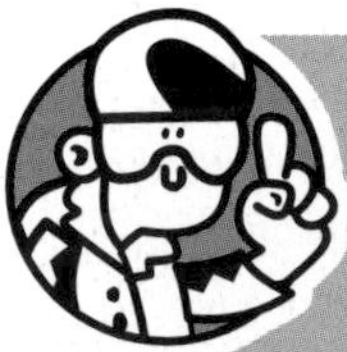

Check the hearing in any child with delayed speech.

9. Neonatal Problems

Important presenting problems in the term newborn infant include:

- Feeding difficulties.
- Vomiting.
- Jaundice.
- Breathing difficulties.
- Seizures.
- Congenital malformations.
- Ambiguous genitalia.

FEEDING DIFFICULTIES

Difficulties in establishing feeding may occur with both breast and bottle-fed newborn infants.

Breastfeeding

Breastfeeding should be encouraged by antenatal education and then supported until it is established. Problems, which may occur, include:

- Latching on—chin forward and head tilted back (the baby's, not the mother's!). The areola should be in the baby's mouth as this encourages successful feeding and avoids damage to the nipple.
- Cracked nipple—occurs commonly and is more likely if the baby does not latch on well.
- Breast engorgement—prevented by demand feeding and alleviated by expression after feeding.
- Intestinal hurry—frequent loose stools are common on day four or five when the supply of milk is plentiful.

Bottle-feeding

Problems, which may occur, include:

- Teat hole too small—excessive air swallowing.
- Teat hole too large—excessive air swallowing as infant gulps to avoid choking.

Drops should follow each other quickly from the inverted bottle but not form a continuous stream.

VOMITING

Babies often regurgitate (posset) small amounts of milk during and between feeds. This is of no pathological significance and should not be confused with vomiting (the forceful expulsion of gastric contents through the mouth).

Vomiting in the newborn may reflect systemic disease or intestinal obstruction. It is important to establish whether the vomit is:

- Milk.
- Bile-stained.
- Blood-stained.
- Frothy, mucoid.

Important causes are listed in Fig. 9.1. Bile-stained vomit suggests intestinal obstruction. Blood in the vomit may be of maternal or infant origin (see Hints & Tips box below).

Plain abdominal X-ray is the most useful investigation (supine and lateral decubitus views [Fig. 9.2]).

◦ Full-term infants should regain their birthweight by day 7–10.
◦ Reluctance to feed in an infant who has previously fed normally may indicate severe disease.

Blood-stained vomit in the newborn may be due to:

◦ Swallowed maternal blood—predelivery or from a cracked nipple.
◦ Trauma from a feeding tube.
◦ Haemorrhagic disease of the newborn—vitamin K deficiency.

Vomiting in the newborn	
Cause	**Features/examples**
intestinal obstruction	small bowel: • duodenal atresia/stenosis (30% have Down syndrome) • malrotation with volvulus • meconium ileus (cystic fibrosis) large bowel: • Hirschsprung's disease • rectal atresia
tracheo-oesophageal fistula	frothy mucoid vomiting occurs if a feed is given
infections: • gastroenteritis • urinary tract infection • septicaemia • meningitis	–
necrotizing enterocolitis	
raised intracranial pressure	bulging fontanelle
congenital adrenal hyperplasia	ambiguous genitalia in a female infant

Fig. 9.1 Vomiting in the newborn.

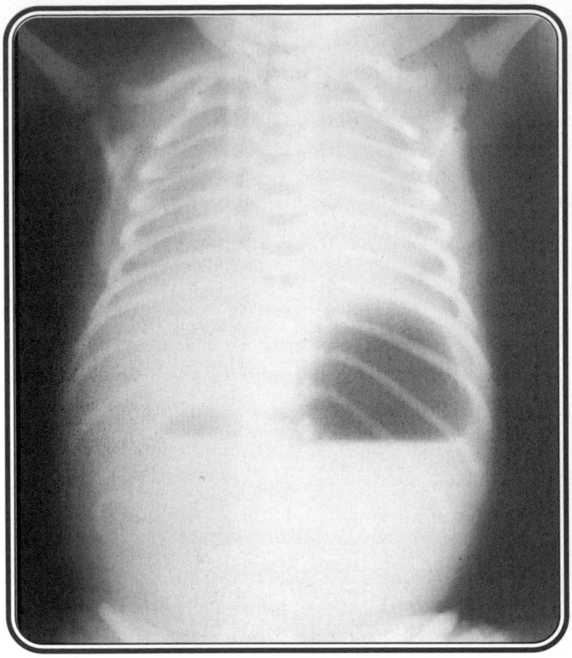

Fig. 9.2 Abdominal X-ray in duodenal atresia showing a 'double bubble' from distension of the stomach and duodenum. Air is absent distally.

NEONATAL JAUNDICE

Physiological jaundice occurs in many newborn infants, especially if born preterm. A combination of increased red cell breakdown and immaturity of the hepatic enzymes causes unconjugated hyperbilirubinaemia. It is exacerbated by dehydration, which may occur if establishment of feeding is delayed.

Onset of jaundice in the first 24 hours of life is always pathological, the causes are listed in Fig. 9.3. Recognition and treatment of severe neonatal unconjugated hyperbilirubinaemia is important to avoid kernicterus (brain damage due to deposition of bilirubin in the basal ganglia). Evaluation of persistent conjugated hyperbilirubinaemia is important to allow early (less than 6 weeks) diagnosis and treatment of biliary atresia.

- **Onset of jaundice in the first 24 hours of life is always pathological.**
- **Consider biliary atresia in an infant with persistent neonatal jaundice due to conjugated hyperbilirubinaemia and pale stools (rare but treatable).**

Definition of physiological jaundice:

- **Onset after 24 hours of birth.**
- **Resolves within 2 weeks.**
- **More than 85% unconjugated.**
- **Total bilirubin <350 μmol/L.**

BREATHING DIFFICULTIES

In the newborn, breathing difficulties are referred to as respiratory distress. The signs of respiratory distress are:

- Tachypnoea—respiratory rate over 60/min.
- Recession—subcostal or intercostal.

Causes of neonatal jaundice	
Onset	**Cause**
less than 24 hours old	excess haemolysis: • immune-mediated—rhesus or ABO incompatibility • intrinsic RBC defects—G6PD, pyruvate kinase deficiency, or hereditary spherocytosis congenital infections
between 24 hours and 2 weeks old	physiological jaundice breast milk jaundice infection, e.g. UTI excess haemolysis, bruising, or polycythaemia
persistent jaundice after 2 weeks old	unconjugated: • breast milk jaundice • infections, e.g. UTI • excess haemolysis, e.g. ABO incompatibility, G6PD deficiency • hypothyroidism (screened for in newborn) • galactosaemia conjugated (>15% of total bilirubin): • biliary atresia • neonatal hepatitis

Fig. 9.3 Causes of neonatal jaundice.

- Nasal flaring.
- Expiratory grunting.
- Cyanosis.

Common breathing difficulties

The most common cause of breathing difficulties in the newborn is the respiratory distress syndrome due to surfactant deficiency, a condition largely confined to preterm infants. The major causes of respiratory distress in term infants are shown in Fig. 9.4.

Causes of respiratory distress in term infants	
Pulmonary	**Non-pulmonary**
common: • transient tachypnoea of the newborn • meconium aspiration • pneumonia • milk aspiration • persistent fetal circulation uncommon: • diaphragmatic hernia • choanal stenosis/atresia • respiratory distress syndrome • pneumothorax rare: • primary ciliary dyskinesia	congenital heart disease severe anaemia metabolic acidosis group B septicaemia

Fig. 9.4 Causes of respiratory distress in term infants.

Transient tachypnoea of the newborn (TTN)

This is believed to be caused by a delay in the normal reabsorption of the lung fluid at birth and is more common after caesarean section. The chest X-ray (CXR) may show a streaky appearance with fluid in the horizontal fissure. This usually resolves within 48 hours.

Meconium aspiration

The percentage of babies passing meconium before birth increases with gestational age. Meconium should be cleared from the oropharynx and airway at delivery. If the infant inhales meconium into the airways, severe respiratory distress may ensue caused by bronchial obstruction and collapse, chemical pneumonitis, and secondary infection. There is a high incidence of air-leak (pneumothorax, pneumomediastinum) and persistent fetal circulation.

Pneumonia

Risk factors include premature labour and prolonged rupture of the membranes (over 24 hours). Group B streptococcal infection is an important cause of early onset pneumonia.

Pneumothorax

Pneumothorax may occur spontaneously in term infants (rare).

Persistent fetal circulation

High pulmonary vascular resistance causes right to left shunting at both atrial and ductal levels with severe cyanosis. It may occur as a primary disorder, but more commonly as a complication of birth asphyxia, meconium aspiration, or respiratory distress syndrome. A CXR may show pulmonary oligaemia.

Diaphragmatic hernia

In this uncommon malformation (1:4000 births), a hole in the diaphragm (usually on the left) allows the abdominal contents to herniate into the chest. Most are diagnosed on antenatal ultrasound scan. Initial resuscitation involves early intubation and nasogastric aspiration (to avoid inflation of the bowel). Surgical repair is then undertaken. If not diagnosed on antenatal ultrasound, it usually presents with failure to respond to resuscitation at birth. The apex beat and heart sounds are displaced to the right with poor air entry on the left. The relatively high mortality is accounted for by the inevitable pulmonary hypoplasia due to compression of the fetal lung.

A CXR in diaphragmatic hernia is shown in Fig. 9.5.

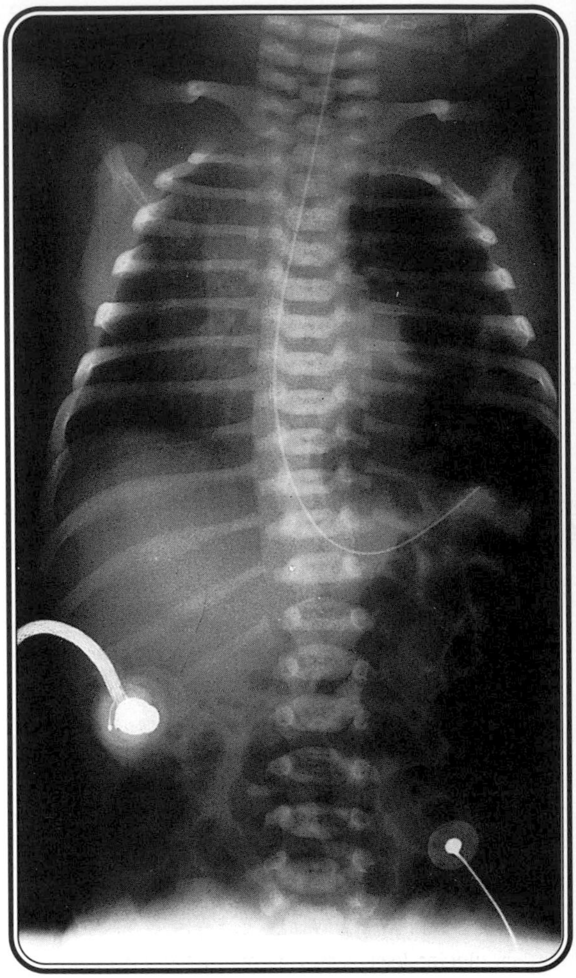

Fig. 9.5 Chest X-ray of congenital diaphragmatic hernia showing loops of bowel in the chest and mediastinal displacement. A nasogastric tube is *in situ*.

NEONATAL SEIZURES

Seizures are a common problem in the newborn period. Their manifestations are rather different from those in older children and it can be difficult to distinguish true seizures from normal baby movements (see Hints & Tips).

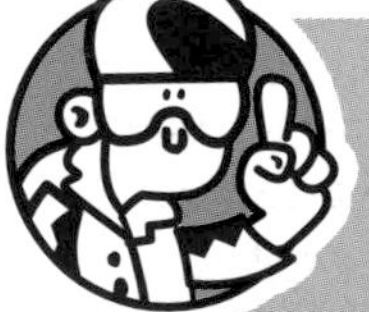

Neonatal episodes which are *not* seizures:

- **Jitteriness: the movement is a tremor—rhythmic movements of equal rate and amplitude (in seizures, clonic movements have a fast and slow component). There are no ocular phenomena. It is sensitive to external stimuli and is stopped by holding.**
- **Benign myoclonus—fragmentary jerks when asleep.**
- **Stretching, sucking movements.**

The main types of seizure that occur include:

- Subtle seizures—eye deviation, apnoeas, pedalling, or boxing movements.
- Clonic seizures—focal or multifocal.
- Myoclonic seizures—focal, multifocal, or generalized.
- Tonic seizures—generalized.

The perinatal and birth history together with clinical examination will often indicate the cause. Further investigations may include:

Initial investigations:

- Blood glucose, electrolytes, Ca^{2+}, Mg^{2+}.
- Cerebrospinal fluid (CSF) analysis.
- Cranial ultrasonography.

As indicated:

- Inborn error of metabolism?
  —Blood ammonia, lactate, and amino acids.
  —Urine amino acids, organic acids.
  —IV pyridoxine test.
- Congenital infection screen.
- Cranial imaging—computed tomography (CT) or magnetic resonance imaging (MRI) (more sensitive).

A detectable cause is present in the majority and varies with the time of onset (Fig. 9.6). The most common cause is hypoxic–ischaemic encephalopathy, which tends to cause seizures within the first 48 hours of life.

CONGENITAL MALFORMATIONS

Up to 70% of major congenital malformations can now be detected antenatally using ultrasound.

Congenital malformations may affect any of the major organ systems. Some of the most important are described below.

Craniofacial disorders

Cleft lip and palate

This affects about 1:1000 babies. A cleft lip may be unilateral or bilateral. Inheritance is polygenic but some are associated with maternal anticonvulsant therapy. Some affected infants can be breast fed and special long teats or other feeding devices may help bottle fed infants. Surgical repair is carried out at several months of age on the palate, and either early (first week) or late (3 months) on the lip.

Causes of neonatal seizures

hypoxic–ischaemic encephalopathy
metabolic:
- hypoglycaemia
- ↓ Na^+, Ca^{2+}, Mg^{2+}
- pyridoxine dependency
- inborn errors of metabolism

drug withdrawal, e.g. maternal opiates
periventricular haemorrhage (preterm infants)
infection:
- meningitis
- congenital infections

kernicterus (hyperbilirubinaemia)
cerebral malformations (rare)
benign familial neonatal convulsions (rare)

Fig. 9.6 Causes of neonatal seizures.

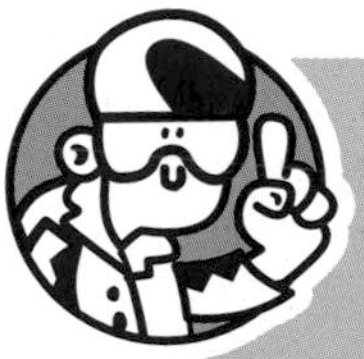

'Congenital' refers to any condition present at birth. The cause may be genetic, environmental, infectious, or idiopathic.

Pierre Robin anomaly

This is an association of micrognathia, posterior displacement of the tongue, and midline cleft of the soft palate.

Gastrointestinal disorders

Oesophageal atresia

The incidence is 1:3500 live births. A tracheo–oesophageal fistula (TOF) is usually present (Fig. 9.7). As the fetus is unable to swallow during intrauterine life, there is associated polyhydramnios. Diagnosis should be established before the first feed by attempting to pass a feeding tube into the stomach and checking its location by X-ray. Forty per cent of cases have other associated abnormalities, e.g. as part of the VACTERL association:

- Vertebral.
- Anorectal.
- Cardiac.
- Tracheo–oEsophageal.
- Renal.
- Limb (radial).

Abdominal wall defects

Gastroschisis (1:5000)

The bowel protrudes without any covering sac through a defect in the anterior abdominal wall adjacent to the umbilicus. This is usually an isolated anomaly.

Exomphalos (1:2500)

The abdominal contents herniate through the umbilical ring and are covered with a sac formed by the peritoneum and amniotic membrane. It is often associated with other major congenital abnormalities.

Neural tube defects

These arise from failure of fusion of the neural plate in the first 28 days postconception. The incidence in the UK has fallen dramatically in the last 25 years. This is probably because of improved maternal nutrition and

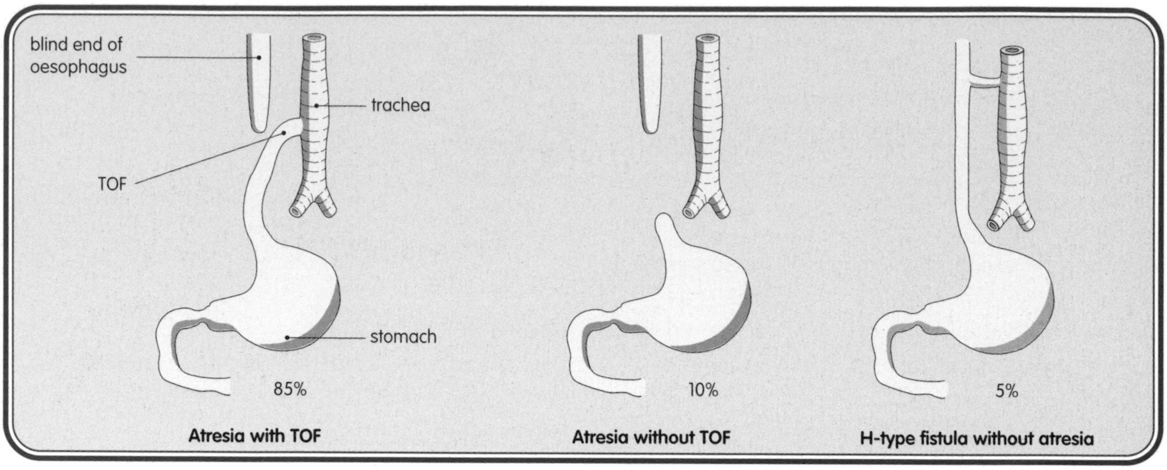

Fig. 9.7 Oesophageal atresia and tracheo-oesophageal fistula (TOF).

supplementation of low folic acid levels (both before conception and in early pregnancy). Antenatal screening and subsequent elective termination have also reduced the incidence of this problem.

There are three main types:

- Spina bifida occulta.
- Meningocele.
- Myelomeningocele.

They are usually in the lumbosacral region (Fig. 9.8).

Spina bifida occulta

The vertebral arch fails to fuse. There may be an overlying skin lesion such as a tuft of hair or small dermal sinus. Tethering of the cord (diastomyelia) may cause neurological deficits with growth.

Meningocele

This is uncommon (5% of cases). The smooth, intact, skin covered cystic swelling is filled with CSF. There is no neurological deficit and excision and closure of the defect is undertaken after 3 months.

Folic acid supplements should ideally be taken preconception and all pregnant women are advised to take them during the first trimester.

Myelomeningocele

This accounts for more than 90% of overt spina bifida. These are usually open, with the unfused neural plate, and meninges exposed, and leaking CSF. Neurological deficits are always present and may include:

- Motor and sensory loss in the lower limbs.
- Neuropathic bladder and bowel

In addition, there is often scoliosis and associated hydrocephalus due to the Arnold–Chiari malformation (herniation of the cerebellar tonsils through the foramen magnum).

Congenital talipes equinovarus (club foot)

The entire foot is fixed in an inverted and supinated position (Fig. 9.9).

It should be distinguished from 'positional talipes' in which the deformity is mild and can be corrected with passive manipulation.

Features of talipes equinovarus:

- **1.5 per 1000 live births.**
- **Male to female ratio 2:1.**
- **50% bilateral.**
- **Multifactorial inheritance.**
- **Associated with oligohydramnios, congenital hip dislocation, and neuromuscular disorders, e.g. spina bifida.**

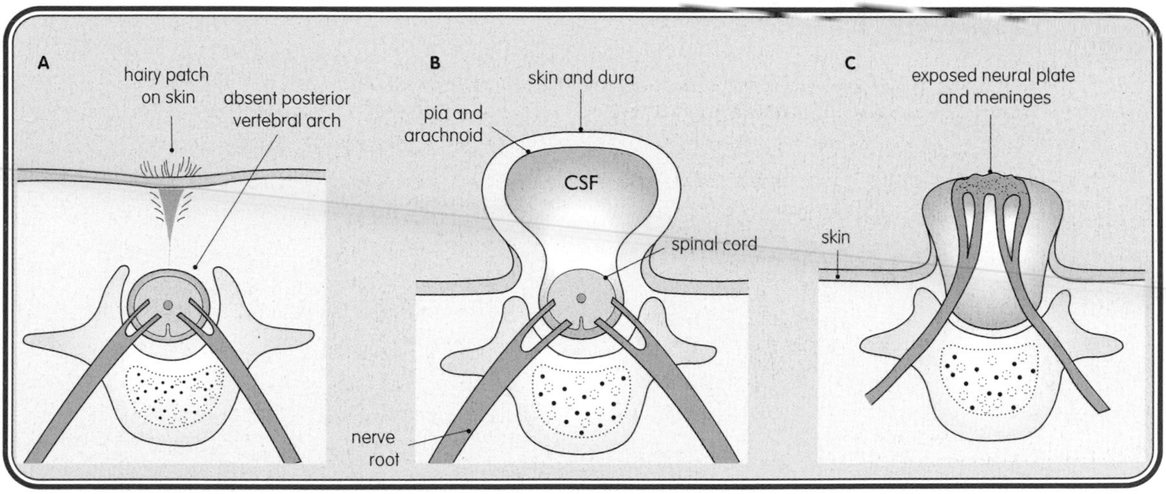

Fig. 9.8 Neural tube defects. Spina bifida occulta (A); meningocele (B); myelomeninigocele (C).

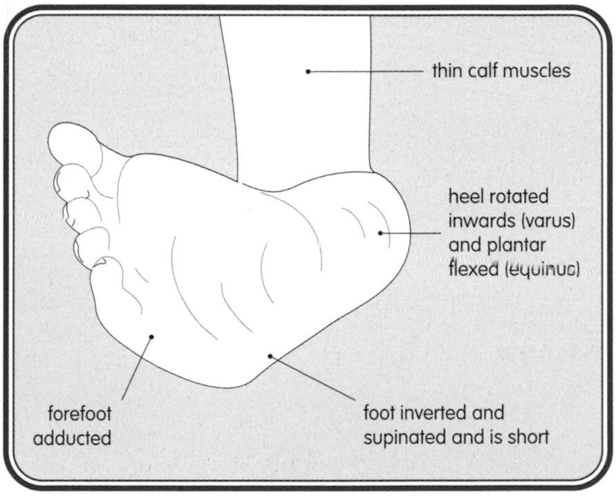

Fig. 9.9 Talipes equinovarus (club foot).

AMBIGUOUS GENITALIA

On occasion, it is not possible to give an immediate answer to the question: "Is it a boy or a girl?" The most common cause of ambiguous external genitalia is congenital adrenal hyperplasia (CAH) leading to a virilized female (see Chapter 23).

Establishing the definitive cause of ambiguous genitalia takes time, and it is important *not* to attempt to guess the future sex of rearing. Expert counselling is required.

Examination should include measurement of the BP (adrenal problem).

Investigations will include:

- Chromosomal analysis—karyotype.
- Ultrasound imaging of pelvic organs and adrenal glands.
- Endocrine investigations (17hydroxyprogesterone is increased in CAH).

The chromosomal sex does not necessarily determine the sex of rearing. In many intersex conditions, it is preferable to raise the child as a female as it is easier to fashion female external genitalia than to create a functioning penis.

- **Congenital adrenal hyperplasia (CAH) leading to virilization of a female infant is the most common cause of ambiguous genitalia.**
- **In two-thirds of children with CAH a life-threatening, salt-losing adrenal crisis occurs at 1–3 weeks of age requiring urgent IV treatment with saline and glucose. This may be the first indication in boys.**

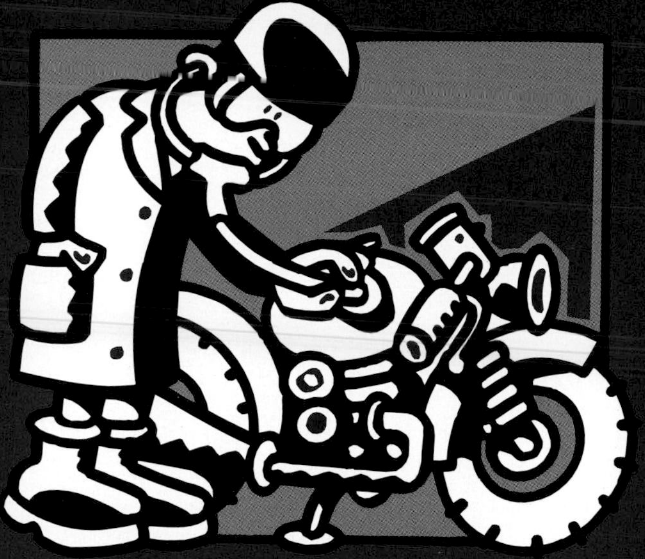

HISTORY, EXAMINATION, AND INVESTIGATIONS

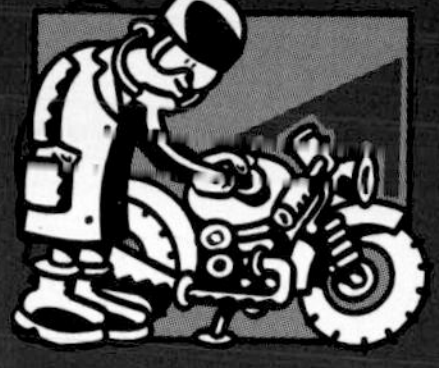

10. History and Examination

Paediatrics encompasses a wide spectrum of patients from the unborn child to the adolescent verging on adulthood. Clearly, a uniform approach to clinical evaluation is not applicable.

It is useful to distinguish the following age groups:

- Fetus: *in utero*.
- Neonate: birth to 28 days.
- Infant: birth to 1 year.
- Toddler: 1–3 years.
- Preschool: 3–5 years.
- School child: 5–16 years.
- Adolescent: 12–18 years.

A clinical approach for two important categories of paediatric patient is set out in this chapter:

- The toddler and preschool child aged 1–5 years.
- The newborn infant.

During the history taking:

- **Remember parents, especially mothers, observe their children very closely.**
- ***Never* ignore or dismiss parental observations.**
- **Listen carefully: the diagnosis is often apparent in the history.**
- **Avoid leading questions.**

CHILDREN (1–5 YEARS)

Taking a history

For the majority of paediatric patients the history will be mainly from a parent, usually the mother. The general format is the same as that in adult medicine, but with some very important differences in emphasis. Set out below is a scheme for paediatric history taking.

Introductions

On meeting the patient:

- Introduce yourself (it is only polite), e.g. 'Hello, I'm Hippocrates, a student doctor.'
- Identify the patient (find out name, age and sex in advance), e.g. 'Is this Billy? How old is he?'
- Confirm the relationship of the accompanying adult, e.g. 'Are you his mother?' (it could be the au pair, older sister, social worker, etc.).

Presenting complaint

Give a prompt to allow the parent to have their say, e.g. 'What has been the main worry as far as you're concerned?'

Listen carefully and patiently and then follow up with specific questions to elicit the full details of presenting symptoms:

- Establish the onset and duration of illness, e.g. 'When did the vomiting start?'
- Clarify the exact meaning of terms, e.g. 'Does the milk shoot out, or just dribble down his chin?'
- Obtain relevant extra detail, e.g. 'Is there any blood or green staining in the vomit?'
- Enquire about related symptoms, e.g. 'Has there been any diarrhoea?'
- Ask about any treatment, e.g. 'Has he been given any medicines?'
- Enquire about foreign travel (if relevant), e.g. 'Have you been abroad recently?'

Previous history

This must include:

- Birth history: 'Where was he born? Was the pregnancy and delivery normal? Was he early or late? What did he weigh? Were there any problems in the newborn period?'
- Immunizations: 'Has he had all his immunizations?'
- Medical: 'Any hospital admissions or operations?'

Developmental history

- 'What age did he smile in response, sit unsupported, walk, talk, etc.?' Vision? Hearing?

Family history

- Age and sex of siblings, parental consanguinity? 'Do you have other children?'
- Family illness, e.g. TB, asthma, epilepsy? 'Do any illnesses run in the family?'

Social history

- Build up a picture of the family circumstances. Identify socio-economic deprivation. 'Are you or your partner working at present? Any problems with your housing? Does anyone help to look after him? How is he getting on at school?'

Systems review

This is a set of questions used to identify key symptoms in all systems, with the emphasis on the system implicated by the presenting complaint:

- Respiratory system: cough or breathing difficulties?
- Cardiovascular system: syncope, breathlessness, or cyanotic episodes?
- Gastrointestinal system: appetite, vomiting, bowel habit, or abdominal pain?
- Genito-urinary tract: excessive thirst, polyuria, or dysuria?
- Central nervous system: headache, paroxysmal episodes, or regression (loss of skills)?

On taking a history be comprehensive: if you don't ask, they won't tell. Formulate a differential diagnosis by the end of the history. Examine the patient with your diagnosis in mind.

Examination

Young infants and school-age children are relatively easy to examine, but the most commonly encountered patient in general paediatric practice is a frightened, tired, and uncooperative toddler in the 1–3 year age group. In this group particularly, the following dos and don'ts apply.

Do:

- Be friendly and cheerful: try to smile and keep up some idle chatter (unless of course the child is acutely and severely ill). A silent, gloomy doctor inspires fear.
- Be gentle: rapport is lost if you cause pain or discomfort.
- Be opportunistic: if asleep—auscultate the chest; if screaming—inspect the tonsils.
- Explain or demonstrate what you are about to do: auscultate a doll or teddy.
- Leave unpleasant procedures until last: examination of ears, nose, and throat, rectal examination (rarely necessary), blood pressure measurement.

Don't:

- Tower over the child.
- Stare at the child: avoid looking too intently at toddlers.
- Separate the child from the mother: a toddler is best examined sitting on his mother's lap.
- Undress the child: ask the mother to take off outer layers while the history is taken, but don't strip the child naked—a certain way to make toddlers cry is to undress them and lie them on a couch.

The following approach is suitable for routine examination of a child in the age range of about 9 months to 5 years:

- Inspection.
- Look at hands.
- Palpate for cervical lymphadenopathy.
- Check pulses.
- Chest.
- Abdomen.
- CNS.
- ENT.
- Measure blood pressure (if necessary).
- Rectal examination (if necessary).

Inspection

Careful initial observation should be made to assess:

- Severity of illness: is the child well, unwell, or ill?
- Growth: is the child well grown and well nourished? Height, weight, and head circumference should be entered on the centile chart.

Look hard but unobtrusively before you touch. Careful observation is the key to success. Vital information is available just from *looking*.

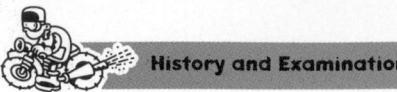

- Appearance: are there any dysmorphic features? Is the child clean and well kempt?
- Fever or rash: infection?
- Major signs relating to specific systems: level of consciousness, pallor or bruising, cyanosis, tachypnoea, or jaundice.

Hands/neck/pulse

The first touch on the hands is non-threatening, as is palpation of the neck for cervical lymphadenopathy. The radial or brachial pulse can be palpated for rate, rhythm, and volume.

Chest

This will encompass examination of the cardiovascular and respiratory systems. Important signs common to both will have been noted on initial inspection:

- Cyanosis.
- Tachypnoea (Fig. 10.1).
- Clubbing (rare).

Respiratory system

Listen for:

- Cough.
- Stridor, which is noise caused by narrowing of the extrathoracic airways.
- Wheeze, which is noise caused by narrowing of the intrathoracic airways.

Look for:

- Intercostal or subcostal recession.
- Nasal flaring.
- Use of accessory muscles, especially sternomastoids.
- Chest shape and movement specifically hyperexpansion (or an increase in AP diameter), Harrison sulcus, and asymmetrical movements.

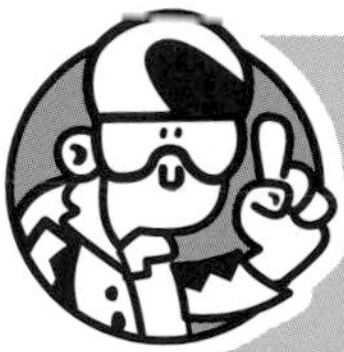

Upper airways noises are readily transmitted to the upper chest in infants. They can be difficult to distinguish from coarse rhonchi.

Percuss (but this is seldom helpful in very young infants).

Auscultate and note:

- Breath sounds—these may be vesicular or bronchial.
- Added sounds—such as wheeze (indicates distal airway narrowing) and crackles (indicates opening of bronchioles).

Cardiovascular system

Check the pulse:

- Palpate radial, brachial, and femoral pulses.
- Note the rate, rhythm, and volume (Fig. 10.2).

Examine the precordium (Fig. 10.3):

- Inspect for bulge or visible ventricular impulse.
- Palpate for thrill (palpable murmur) and abnormal cardiac impulse: a normal apex beat is within the fourth intercostal space at the midclavicular line.

Sinus tachycardia in children occurs with fever, exercise, and stress (maximum rate 180/min). A heart rate >200/min suggests an arrhythmia, most commonly a supraventricular tachycardia.

Upper limit of respiratory rate

Age	Tachypnoea (breaths/minute)
neonate	>60
infant	>50
young child	>40
older child	>30

Fig. 10.1 Upper limits of respiratory rate.

Normal heart rates in children

Age	Beats/minute
<1 year	110–160
2–5 years	95–140
5–12 years	80–120
>12 years	60–100

Fig. 10.2 Normal heart rates in children.

Auscultate and listen for:

- Heart sounds I and II.
- Murmurs—note the timing (systolic/diastolic), loudness (grade 1–6), site (valve areas), and radiation (to neck in aortic stenosis, to back in coarctation of the aorta).

Detailed evaluation will include:

- Measuring blood pressure: use a cuff covering two-thirds of the upper arm.
- Checking for hepatomegaly: this is an important sign of cardiac failure in infants.

Abdomen

Check for:

- Jaundice.
- Clubbing.

Look for:

- Distension, which may indicate ascites (e.g. nephrotic syndrome) or intestinal obstruction.
- Masses (Fig. 10.4).
- Peristalsis, which is a useful sign in pyloric stenosis.
- Inguinal region and genitalia (hernia, hydrocele, testicular torsion).

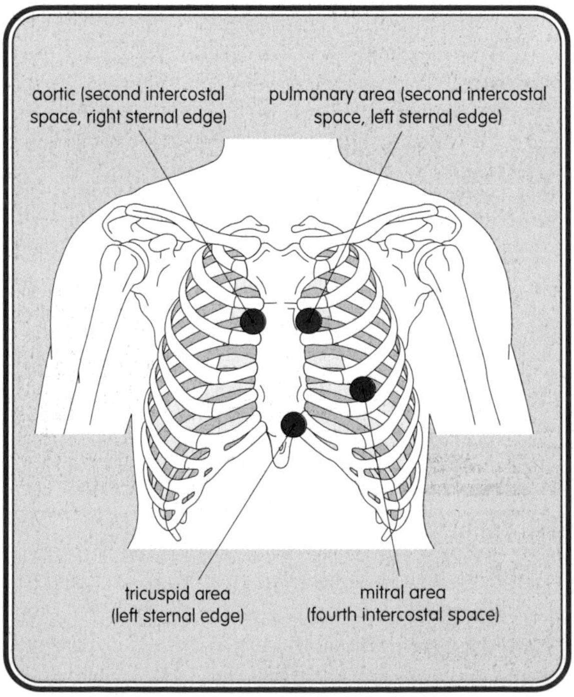

Fig. 10.3 The precordium.

Watch a child's face for grimaces as you palpate the abdomen.
Putting the child's hand under yours may enhance cooperation.

Palpate, with the flat of the hand, for:

- Tenderness or guarding.
- Masses.
- Organomegaly—liver, spleen, kidneys.

Percuss over the liver or spleen to confirm enlargement. Ascites may be associated with shifting dullness.

Auscultate—listen to the bowel sounds, which are:

- Increased in obstruction and acute diarrhoea.
- Reduced in ileus.
- Absent in peritonitis.

Rectal examination may be indicated in suspected appendicitis or intussusception.

Nervous system

Important signs noted on inspection include:

- Level of consciousness.
- Higher mental functions: consider the patient's speech, language, and social interaction.
- Vision and hearing.
- Motor function: note the patient's gait, coordination, and posture.

In infants, it is important to:

- Measure occipitofrontal head circumference (Fig. 10.5) (cranial volume is an important indicator of neurological disease).

Causes of an abdominal mass
Wilms tumour
neuroblastoma
intussusception—right lower or upper quadrant
faecal mass
appendix mass

Fig. 10.4 Causes of an abdominal mass.

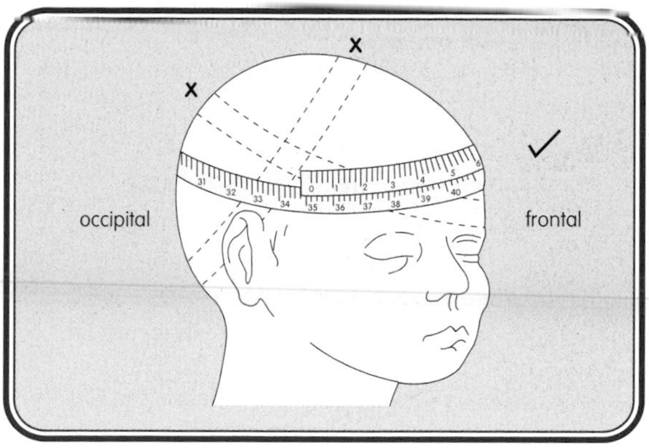

Fig. 10.5 Measuring head circumference.

- Palpate the anterior fontanelle: this is a window in the skull that allows assessment of intracranial pressure. It closes at about 12 months.

If indicated, more detailed evaluation may include:
- Tone in trunk and limbs: note whether it is increased (cerebral palsy) or decreased (Down syndrome), and whether symmetrical or asymmetrical.
- Tendon reflexes.
- Eyes: look for movements, squint, and nystagmus. Use ophthalmoscope to look for the red reflex (absent with cataract, retinoblastoma) and examine the fundus (choroidoretinitis, haemorrhages).
- Meningism: evaluate if meningitis suspected.
- Cranial nerves (Fig. 10.6).

Ears and throat

Usually left to the last, as their examination is not enjoyed by toddlers. The key to success is parental help in holding the child. The child should be seated on the mother's lap and held firmly by her with one hand on the forehead and one around the trunk and both arms (Fig. 10.7).

Examine the:
- Ears first.
- Throat last: the occasional child will cooperate by 'opening wide'; in some cases it is necessary to insert a wooden spatula between clenched teeth on to the tongue.

Cranial nerves—quick examination

II, III	pupils: reaction to light and accommodation
II	fundoscopy (may require dilatation)
III, IV, VI	external ocular movements
V	clench teeth and waggle jaw • ask about chewing • corneal reflex distressing—sensory problems rare in isolation
VII	smile, show teeth, and screw up eyes
IX, X	say "aagh" and inspect palatal movement • ask about swallowing
XI	shrug shoulders, turn head against resistance
XII	put out tongue and move from side to side

Fig. 10.6 Cranial nerves—quick examination.

THE NEWBORN INFANT

History

Before examining the infant, details of the mother's health, the pregnancy, and labour should be ascertained.

Maternal health

Conditions that may affect the baby

Ask about:
- Diabetes mellitus type I.
- Auto-immune disorders, e.g. hyperthyroidism, systemic lupus erythematosus.

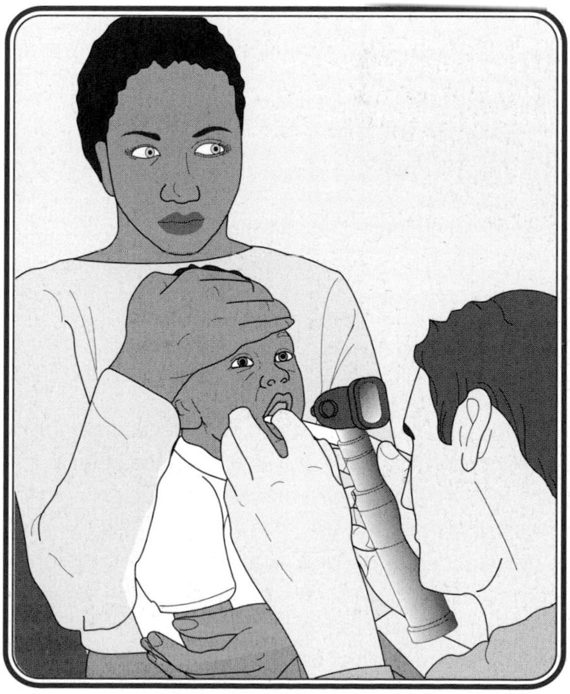

Fig. 10.7 Throat examination.

Maternal drugs

Find out about medication, e.g.

- Anti-epilepsy drugs, e.g. phenytoin.
- Warfarin.
- Androgens.
- Cytotoxic agents.

Check any past drug abuse:

- Alcohol, smoking.
- Opiates, cocaine.

Maternal infections

Infections that may affect the fetus include:

- Rubella.
- Cytomegalovirus.
- *Toxoplasma gondii.*
- Varicella zoster.
- *Listeria monocytogenes.*
- *Treponema pallidum (syphilis).*
- HIV.

Pregnancy

Ask about:

- Length of gestation.
- Complications, e.g. pre-eclamptic toxaemia, intrauterine growth retardation.
- Antenatal diagnoses.

Birth

Ask about:

- Mode of delivery.
- Intrapartum complications.

The mother should be encouraged to express any concerns or questions about her infant. Enquire about the mode of feeding.

Examination

Routine examination

As soon as a baby is born, the midwife (obstetrician or paediatrician if present) will check that the baby is pink, breathing normally, and has no major congenital malformations. Obviously, if the infant is of low birthweight (<2500g) or ill (e.g. after birth asphyxia), admission to a special care baby unit will be required.

About 95% of babies are born at term and appear healthy. However, they all need a full medical examination within the first 24 hours of life.

The purpose of this is:

- To give the parents a chance to ask any questions about their baby.
- To identify any problems anticipated as a result of maternal disease or familial disorders, e.g. congenital infection, maternal diabetes mellitus.
- To detect congenital abnormalities, which may not be immediately obvious at birth, e.g. cataract, cleft palate, heart murmur, undescended testes, dislocatable hip.

A scheme for the routine examination of the normal term infant is shown in Fig. 10.8. The various skin lesions that may be found are listed in Fig. 10.10.

Neonatal screening

On day six of life, at which time feeding has been established, all babies have a blood sample from a heel prick taken on to a card (the Guthrie test). This is analysed to detect two inborn errors of metabolism:

- Phenylketonuria: 1:6000 births.
- Hypothyroidism: 1:3000 births.

In the first 24 hours, many babies have a quiet systolic 'flow' murmur. Features suggesting a significant murmur:

- **Loud murmur.**
- **Diastolic murmur.**
- **Associated cardiac signs.**
- **These should be investigated with CXR, ECG, and echocardiogram.**

To test for congenital dislocation of the hip, use the:

- **Barlow manoeuvre—the hip is dislocated posteriorly out of the acetabulum.**
- **Ortolani manoeuvre—the dislocated hip is relocated back into the acetabulum.**

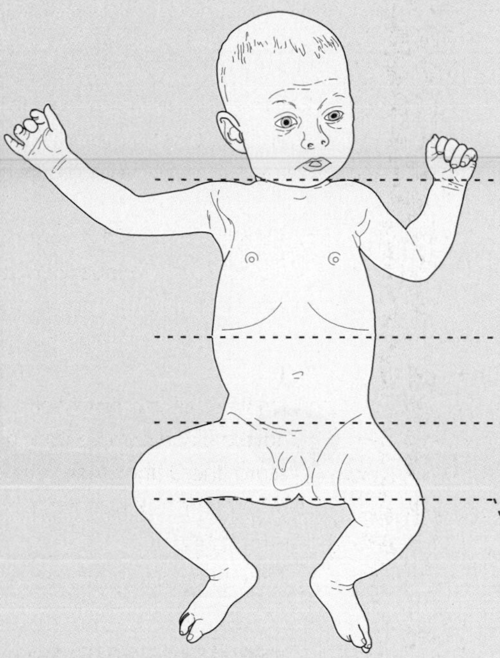

- birth weight and centile
- colour (Fig. 10.9)
- skin lesions (Fig. 10.10)
- palpate fontanelle and sutures
- measure occipito–frontal head circumference
- check eyes for cataract, red reflex
- examine facies for dysmorphic features
  –Down syndrome
- check palate

- observe breathing rate and chest wall movement
- palpate precordium
- auscultate the heart
  –count heart rate
  –heart murmurs (see Hints & Tips)

- palpate abdomen
  liver 1–2cms. Spleen tip may be palpable
- inspect the umbilical cord

- palpate the femoral pulses
- inspect genitalia for
  –inguinal herniae
  –hypospadies
  –undescended testes and anus for patency
- check hips for congenital dislocation (see Hints & Tips)

- assess muscle tone
  pick up the baby and hold in ventral suspension
- inspect back and spine for midline defects
- Moro reflex

Fig. 10.8 Routine newborn examination

Colour guide for newborn babies

• red-plethora	- polycythaemia check (PCV)
• blue-cyanosis	- hands and feet only: normal peripheral cyanosis
	- central: cardiac or respiratory disease
• white-anaemia	- e.g. placental abruption
• grey-circulatory collapse	- e.g. asphyxia, septicaemia
• yellow-jaundice	- hyperbilirubinaemia

Fig. 10.9 Colour of newborn babies.

Skin lesions in newborn babies

- capillary haemangiomata/"stork bites": pink macules on upper eyelids/forehead and nape of neck where stork holds infant in its beak!
- milia: white pimples on nose and cheeks from retained keratin
- erythema neonatorum: white pin-point papules on red base usually on trunk
- mongolian blue spots: blue-black macular discolouration at base of spine and buttocks, most common in Afro-Carribean and Asian infants
- port wine stain: vascular malformation of capillaries in the dermis
- strawberry naevus: capillary haemangioma: usually appear after birth during first month of life, increase in size during first year, then regress, 90% disappear by age of 7 years

Fig. 10.10 Skin lesions in newborn babies

MEDICAL SAMPLE CLERKING

A sample medical clerking is shown below. It illustrates some of the points discussed earlier in this chapter.

CHECKLIST	EXAMPLE
Name:	A. Baby
Date:	1st January 2000
Time:	2030 hrs
Place:	Accident & Emergency
Age:	6 weeks
Sex:	male
Referred by:	General Practitioner

PC (presenting complaint)

Vomiting

HPC (history of presenting complaint)

Gradual onset over previous five days of intermittent vomiting. Usually occurs in period after a feed.
Vomit is milk only—no bile or blood staining.
Forceful vomiting—milk clears mother's lap.
Infant appears hungry and eager to feed. Breast fed.
Stool frequency reduced. No diarrhoea.

PMH (past medical history)

Born at ST Elsewhere's Hospital.
Full term normal delivery (FTND). Birth Weight 3650g.
Mild jaundice days 3–5.
No significant perinatal problems.

Developmental history

Smiles in response.

FH (family history)

Siblings	1 brother age 4 years—mild asthma.
	1 sister age 2 years—VSD. Under review.
Mother	Age 31 years. Well.
Operated on for 'bowel obstruction' at age 4 weeks.	
Father	Age 33 years. Asthmatic.

SH (social history)

Father electrician. Mother a Nurse (not working).
Live in own flat.

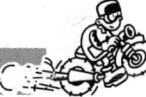

S/E (systems enquiry)

CVS
No cyanotic episodes.

RS
Episodes of shallow breathing.

GIT
Breast fed. No 'possetting'. Stool frequency previously x5 per 24 hours.

GU
Good urinary stream.

Medication
Nil.

O/E (on examination)

General
Well infant.
Mild jaundice. Dehydration 5%.
Oral thrush.
ENT: NAD.

CVS
Heart rate 110/min. Peripheral pulses present. BP—95/70 mmHg.
Cardiac impulse—normal.
Heart sounds I & II. No murmurs.

RS
Respiratory rate 35/min.
No recession.
Breath sounds vesicular. No added sounds.

Abdomen
Not distended. No visible veins.
Visible peristalsis—intermittent.
Soft. No masses.
No hepatomegaly. No splenomegaly.
Hernial orifices—NAD.
PR—not done.

CNS
Alert. Vigorous.
Anterior fontanelle—soft, slightly depressed.
Tone: normal and symmetrical.
Movements symmetrical.
Relexes: not examined.

SUMMARY

6 week old infant boy with a five day history of projectile vomiting, non bile stained. Family history of possible pyloric stenosis and visible peristalsis on examination.

Diagnosis: Pyloric Stenosis (PS)

Plan: Organise 'test feed'.
Investigations: Urea and elecyrolytes including serum HCO_3^-.
Abdominal USS (if 'test feed' equivocal).
Inform paediactrics surgical team.
Nursing plan: Nasogastric tube.
Fluid balance chart.
Daily weight.

Site IV line. Intravenous rehydration.
IF PS diagnosis confimed, nil by mouth and schedule for Ramstedt's pyloromyotomy in 24–28 hours when rehydrated and metabolic alkalosis corrected.

Signed Dr X Cellent
Paediatric SHO

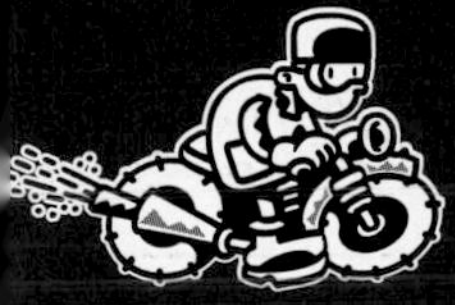

11. Developmental Assessment

INTRODUCTION

Growing up involves the acquisition of new abilities and skills as well as physical growth. The process by which an immobile, incontinent, and speechless baby develops into a mobile, communicating, socially interactive, and (hopefully!) well-behaved child involves a complex interaction between genes (nature) and environment (nurture).

Much study over many years has established the average rate and pattern of development and identified a very wide range of normal variation. A child may be far from average but still normal. A major challenge is to distinguish such normal variation from a significant problem requiring active intervention.

Developmental screening is offered routinely to all children in the UK. It is one component of child health surveillance, which also encompasses physical health and growth.

Surveillance and screening are a vital component of child health promotion.

The aim is to identify developmental problems at an early stage to allow appropriate intervention. Any delay may be global or specific (see Chapter 8), but it is important to bear in mind the close inter-relationships involved, e.g. hearing impairment may cause delay in speech and language with consequent disruption of social interaction and behaviour.

Clinical assessment of a child's developmental status is based on a thorough history, physical examination, and observation of the child's performance.

HISTORY

Certain aspects of the history clearly assume special importance in assessing development. In particular, it is important to enquire about and document 'risk factors' that contribute to vulnerability and poor outcome (Fig. 11.1).

Risk factors

prenatal insults, e.g. maternal alcohol
perinatal insults, e.g. hypoxia
chronic disease, e.g. cystic fibrosis
specific developmental problems
- visual impairment
- sensorineural deafness

maternal depression
psychosocial deprivation

Fig. 11.1 Risk factors for development.

The history should therefore include inquiry into:

- Pregnancy and birth.
- Developmental milestones—depending on age.
- Family circumstances.
- Specific parental concerns
- Parent held personal child health record.

EXAMINATION

Four aspects of development are routinely assessed:

- Gross motor.
- Fine motor and vision.
- Hearing and speech.
- Social behaviour.

Routine surveillance is carried out during well-recognized stages of development:

- Newborn.
- Supine infant (6 weeks).
- Sitting infant (8–9 months).
- Mobile toddler (18–24 months).
- Communicating child (3–4 years).
- School-age child (5 years).

The milestones for each area in each of the above age groups are considered below.

Newborn

Gross motor

- Symmetrical movements in all four limbs.
- Normal muscle tone.

Milestones reflect the average age that a child acquires a particular ability:

- **Motor problems often manifest in the first year.**
- **Talking and coordination problems often manifest in the second year.**
- **Behavioural and social problems often manifest in the third year.**

Fine motor and vision:

- Fixes on mother's face and follows through 90°.

Hearing and speech

- Cries.

Social

- Responds to being picked up.

Six weeks

Gross motor

- Good head control when pulled up to sitting (Fig. 11.2).
- When held in ventral suspension holds head transiently in horizontal plane (Fig. 11.3).
- Presence of the Moro response (Fig. 11.4).

The Moro response consists of extension of the arms, then brisk adduction towards the chest when the infant is startled or the baby's head allowed to drop back slightly (see Fig. 11.4). It should be symmetrical and should have disappeared by 6 months. Persistence of this or any of the primitive reflexes beyond 6 months may indicate a cerebral disorder.

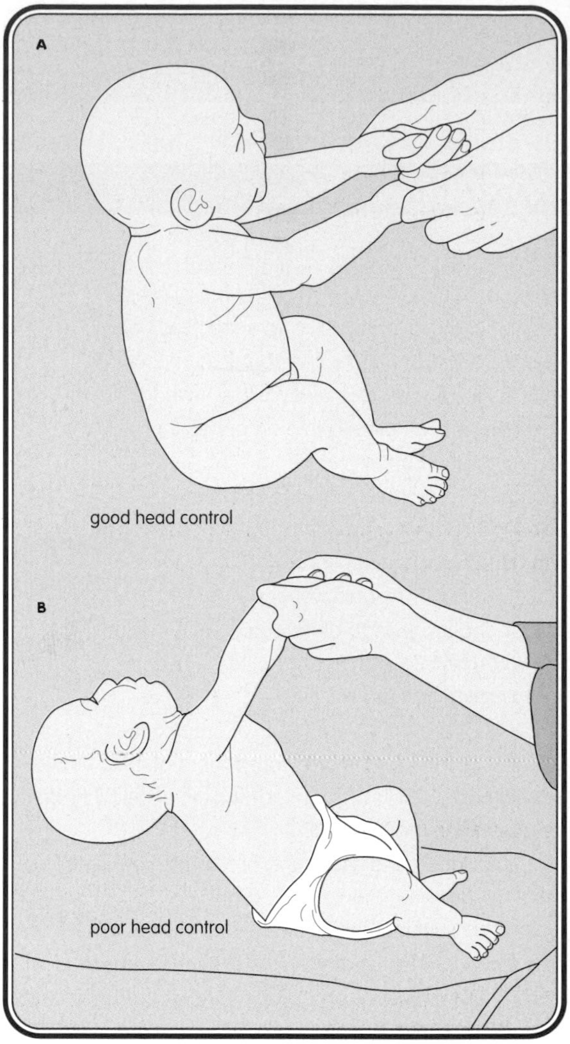

Fig. 11.2 (A) Good head control compared with (B) poor head control at 6 weeks.

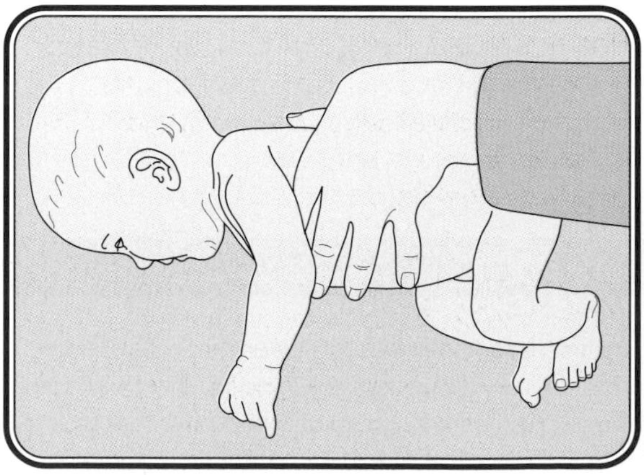

Fig. 11.3 Ventral suspension at 6 weeks.

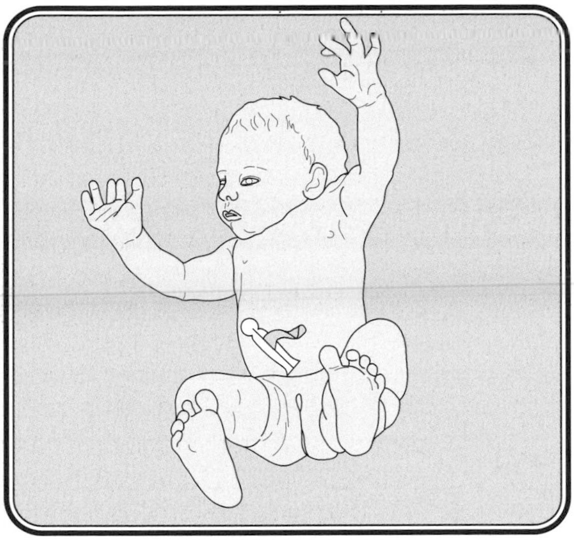

Fig. 11.4 The Moro response.

Fine motor and vision

- Stares at and follows mother's face.

Hearing and speech

- Coos.
- Startles to loud noises.

Social

- Smiles in response.

Eight months

Gross motor

- Sits unsupported.
- Weight bears on legs.
- Rolls. Starting to crawl.

Fine motor and vision

- Reaches out for toys and has a palmar grasp.
- Transfers objects hand to hand or hand to mouth.
- Follows fallen toys (and points).
- Fixes on small objects.

Hearing and speech

- Babbles, e.g. 'dada'.
- Responds to own name.
- Distraction test (turns to sound) (Fig. 11.5).

Social

- Puts objects into mouth.
- Hand and foot regard.
- Plays peekaboo.
- Stranger awareness.
- Separation anxiety.

Eighteen months

Gross motor

- Walking.
- Climbs stairs two feet to a step.
- Climbs onto and sits on a chair.

Fine motor and vision

- Pincer grip (Fig. 11.6).
- Turns pages.
- Builds a three-brick tower.
- Picks up 100s and 1000s.

Hearing and speech

- Uses three or more words.
- Points to parts of body or named objects.
- Understands simple instructions.

Social

- Uses a spoon.
- Domestic mimicry.
- Takes off socks and shoes.
- Developing toilet awareness.

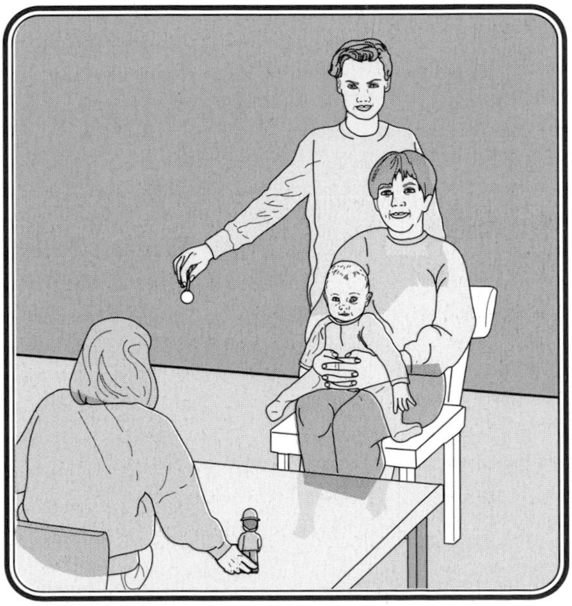

Fig. 11.5 Distraction test.

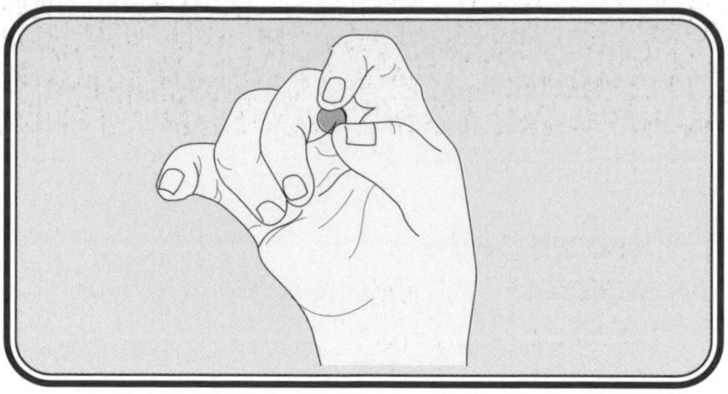

Fig. 11.6 Pincer grip.

Three years

Gross motor

- Runs, jumps.
- Throws and kicks a ball.
- Pedals a tricycle.
- Climbs stairs (like an adult).

Fine motor and vision

- Threads beads on a string.
- Builds an eight-brick tower.
- Copies a line and a circle.
- Letter matching using charts.

Speech and language

- Short sentences—using and understanding prepositions, e.g. 'on'.

Social

- Toilet trained—dry by day.
- Dresses with supervision.
- Plays with other children.
- Matches two colours.

Five years

Gross motor

- Skips.
- Catches a ball.
- Heel–toe walking.

Fine motor and vision

- Draws a man with all features.
- Copies alphabet letters.
- Snellen's chart test (by name or matching).

Hearing and speech

Comprehensive speech.

Social

- Plays games.
- Learning to read.
- Can tell the time.

DEVELOPMENTAL 'LIMIT AGES'

Fig. 11.7 lists the worrying signs at the ages given.

Worrying signs	
Age	**Developmental sign**
6–8 weeks	asymmetrical Moro excess head lag no visual fixation/following no startle or quietening to sound no responsive smiling
8 months	persisting primitive reflexes not weight bearing on legs not reaching out for toys not fixing on small objects not vocalizing
10 months	unable to sit unsupported
1 year	showing a hand preference not responding to own name
18 months	not walking no pincer grip persistence of casting
3 years	inaccurate use of a spoon not speaking in sentences unable to understand simple commands unable to use the toilet alone not interacting with other children

Fig. 11.7 Worrying signs at various ages.

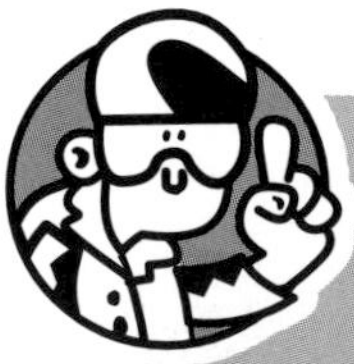

Management options for concern over development:

- **Reassure if within normal range.**
- **Review again**
- **Refer for expert assessment.**

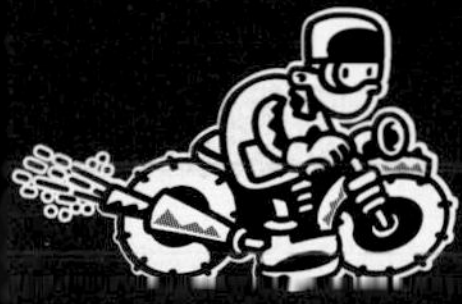

12. Investigations

INTRODUCTION

Special investigations are often used to confirm, or refute, a diagnosis that is uncertain clinically, and to monitor the progress of a disease or its treatment. They should be performed only when there are specific indications, not as a 'routine'. In all cases, the potential benefits must be weighed against any associated pain or discomfort.

In this chapter, the indications for and interpretation of the following common and important special investigations are considered.

Imaging:

- Ionising radiation—chest X-rays (CXR), abdominal X-rays (AXR), skull X-rays (SXR), computed tomography (CT) and radionuclide scanning.
- Ultrasound—antenatal ultrasound, cranial ultrasound (newborn), and abdominal and renal ultrasound.
- Magnetic resonance imaging (MRI).

Blood tests:

- Haematological tests—full blood count (FBC), peripheral blood film, sickle test, haemoglobin electrophoresis, coagulation studies.
- Biochemical tests—urea and electrolytes, creatinine, liver function tests, albumin, glucose, calcium and phosphate, magnesium, blood gases, and acid–base status.
- Immunology tests—tests for immunodeficiency, auto-antibodies, diagnostic serology, and acute phase reactants.
- Microbiology tests—blood culture.

Urine tests:

- Dipstick for protein, blood, glucose, and ketones.
- Microscopy and culture.

'Routine' investigation is rarely good practice. Tests should be done for the benefit of the patient, not the doctor.

Cerebrospinal fluid:

- Microscopy and culture.
- Protein and glucose levels.
- Virology.

IMAGING

All the major imaging methods are used in paediatric practice:

- Ionizing radiation—X-rays: simple or computed X-ray tomography and nuclear medicine.
- Ultrasound.
- MRI.

The main circumstances in which each of these tests may be used are described in the following sections.

X-rays

Most commonly requested are:

- CXR.
- Plain AXR.
- SXR.
- CT.

Chest X-ray

When inspecting a CXR, adopt a systematic approach for viewing and presentation:

- Check patient name, date, L/R orientation, posterior–anterior (PA), or anterior–posterior (AP).
- Note any striking abnormalities.
- Heart and mediastinum.
- Lung fields and pulmonary vessels.
- Diaphragm and subdiaphragmatic areas.
- Bony thorax.
- Soft tissues.

Cardiac size can not be reliably estimated on an AP film because the heart is relatively more magnified compared with the chest wall dimensions.

Indications for doing a CXR

Acute:

- Pneumonia.
- Severe bronchiolitis.
- Asthma—severe or first presentation.
- Cardiac failure.
- Foreign body inhalation.
- Non-accidental injury (fractures).

Non-urgent investigation of:

- Cervical lymphadenopathy.
- TB.
- Cystic fibrosis.
- Cardiac disease.
- Malignant disease.

Abdominal X-ray

Supine AP is the standard plain film. An erect AP (or decubitus) or erect CXR should be ordered in cases of possible obstruction or perforation to look for fluid levels and free gas. There is wide variation in the normal appearance of these X-rays.

The checklist for an AXR includes:

- Check patient name, date, erect, or supine.
- Note striking abnormalities.
- Hollow organs: stomach, bowel, and bladder.
- Solid organs: liver, spleen, and kidneys.
- Diaphragm.
- Bones.

Skull X-ray

The most common indication for skull radiography is head trauma. However, even with the advent of cranial imaging by CT and MRI, SXRs may still prove useful in a variety of clinical contexts.

The standard views are lateral and AP. An example of a normal SXR is shown in Fig. 12.1.

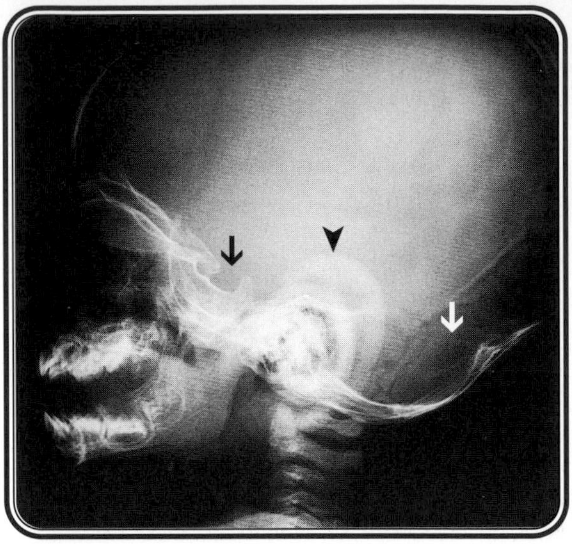

Fig. 12.1 Normal skull X-ray. Note: pituitary fossa (black arrow), soft tissue of ears (arrow heads), and lamboid suture (white arrow).

Indications for SXR include:

- Head trauma.
- Investigation of possible pituitary tumour or craniopharyngioma (which may calcify).
- Microcephaly—craniosynostosis (premature fusion of a suture).

SXR in head trauma

Although the role of skull radiography in severe head trauma has decreased with the advent of CT scanning, it remains a useful first investigation in the following circumstances:

- Suspected penetrating injury.
- 'Boggy' scalp haematoma.
- Suspected non-accidental injury.
- All but the most minor injuries in infants.
- All moderate head injuries.

The presence of a skull fracture and/or neurological signs increases the likelihood of intracranial damage, but there may be severe brain injury with no fracture or a fracture with no neurological damage.

The main problem is distinguishing fractures from the normal lucent linear markings in the skull (due to sutures and vascular markings). The characteristic features of these are:

- Sutures—constant position.
- Vascular markings—tortuous, branching pattern, variable position, taper as they pass upwards.
- Fractures—linear and usually non-branching, very lucent (i.e. black), rarely cross sutures.

Computed tomography

CT scanning uses multidirectional X-rays which, instead of falling onto film, are quantified by a detector and fed into a computer. Different readings are produced as the X-ray beam rotates round the body and the information is then presented as a two-dimensional image.

CT is a useful and widely available imaging modality for evaluating brain, chest, and abdominal disorders. These include:

- Brain—intracranial haemorrhage (e.g. head injury), tumours, intracranial calcification (e.g. tuberose sclerosis).
- Chest—mediastinal masses (e.g. lymphoma), lungs (e.g. bronchiectasis).
- Abdomen—masses (e.g. neuroblastoma or Wilms), injury (e.g. splenic rupture).

CT accurately assesses the nature of a mass, e.g. fluid, fat, necrosis, or calcification. Disadvantages include a disappointing lack of contrast between different organs. Intravenous contrast enhances the resolution between tissue planes.

The axial sections of a CT scan are viewed as if the observer is at the patient's feet and looking up towards the head.

Ultrasound

Ultrasound scanning (USS) uses ultra-high frequency sound waves to provide cross-sectional images of the body. In addition, Doppler ultrasound can be used for estimating the direction and velocity of blood flow.

The advantages of USS include:

- Non-invasive—no ionizing radiation involved.
- Portable equipment.

Body tissues reflect sound waves to different degrees and are therefore said to be of different echogenicity:

- Hyperechoic tissues appear white (e.g. fat).
- Hypoechoic tissues appear dark (e.g. fluid).

Ultrasound does not penetrate gas or bone and is therefore less useful for assessment of bony lesions. Intracranial contents are only accessible to ultrasound examination in young infants in whom the anterior fontanelle is still open.

The main applications include:

- Antenatal ultrasound.
- Cranial ultrasound in the neonate.
- Abdominal and renal ultrasound.
- Hip ultrasound.

Antenatal ultrasound

Initial ultrasound screening is carried out at 12 weeks (in some units) with a detailed scan at 18–20 weeks gestation. Antenatal USS allows:

- Estimation of gestational age (less than 20 weeks).
- Identification of multiple pregnancies.
- Monitoring of fetal growth.
- Detection of structural malformations.
- Amniotic fluid volume estimation.

Neonatal cranial ultrasound

This is useful for the detection and evaluation of intracranial pathology (Fig. 12.2) including:

- Intracranial haemorrhage, e.g. intraventricular haemorrhage (IVH).
- Periventricular leucomalacia.
- Hydrocephalus.
- Hypoxic–ischaemic encephalopathy.

Abdominal and renal ultrasound

Abdominal ultrasound

This may be useful in the evaluation of:

- Abdominal pain—acute (e.g. identification of appendix abscess).
- Vomiting infant—pyloric stenosis may be demonstrable on USS.
- Liver disease—provides information on size and consistency of both the liver and spleen. The gall bladder and extrahepatic bile ducts can be visualized.

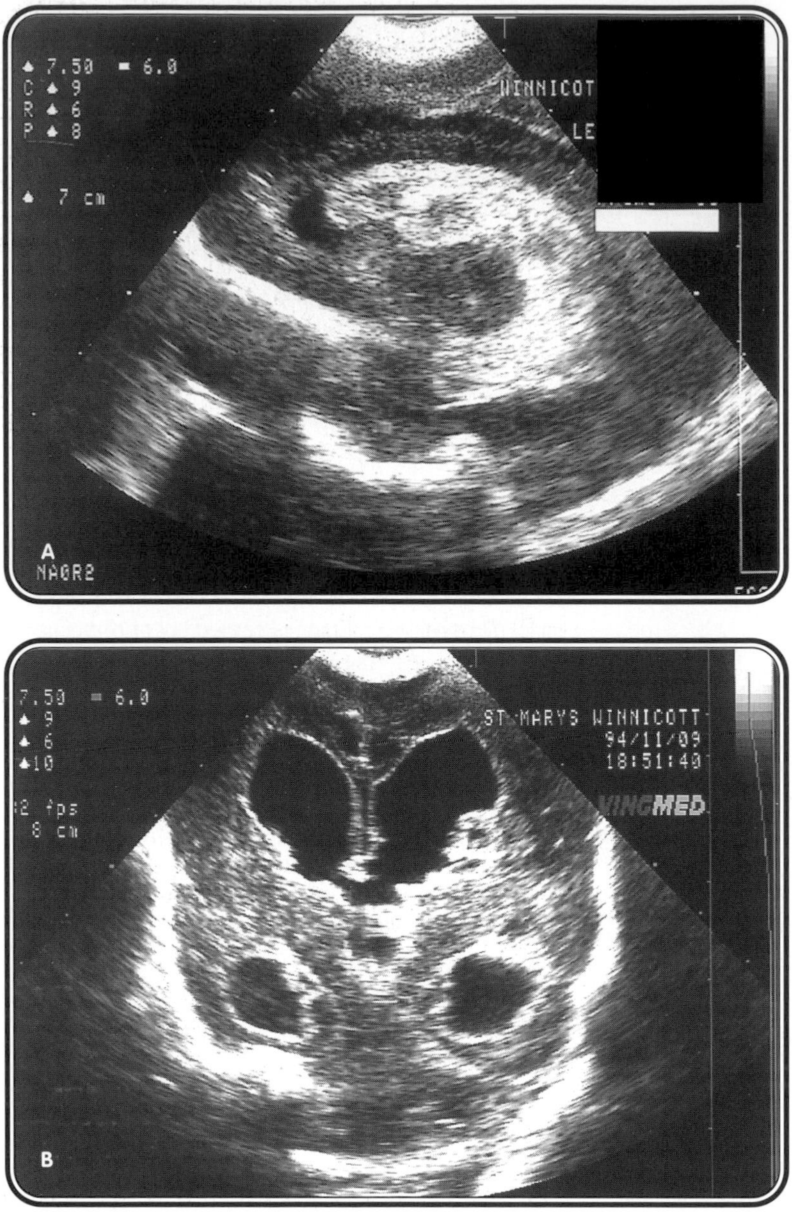

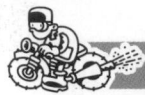

Fig. 12.2 (A) A parasagittal neonatal cranial ultrasound scan showing extensive intraventricular haemorrhage. (B) Coronal ultrasound scan of a neonatal brain with hydrocephalus.

Renal ultrasound

Ultrasound is very useful in the investigation of disorders of the genitourinary tract (Fig. 12.3). It provides information on:

- Kidney size.
- Structural abnormalities of the urinary tract, e.g. hydronephrosis, hydroureter, or increased bladder size.
- Gross renal scarring.
- Renal calculi.
- Tumours (e.g. Wilms).

All infants and young children should have a renal USS after a confirmed UTI. Its main role is to reveal structural abnormalities and it does not reliably detect vesicoureteric reflux or minor renal scars.

Hip ultrasound

Ultrasound is a useful modality for the investigation of hip disease. It is the imaging method of choice for assessing neonatal hip instability, and is more reliable than plain radiography up to the age of 6 months. It allows evaluation of:

- Acetabular morphology.
- The degree to which the acetabulum covers the femoral head.

Ultrasound is also useful in the investigation of suspected hip pathology in young children. Even small effusions can be detected, and needle aspiration can be carried out under ultrasound guidance.

Magnetic resonance imaging

Magnetic resonance imaging (MRI) has several distinctive features that confer a number of useful advantages:

- No ionizing radiation.
- Images can be obtained in any plane.
- Excellent soft tissue contrast.

It is the imaging modality of choice for many disorders of the brain and spine (in which sagittal views are particularly useful). MRI is also helpful in the evaluation of musculoskeletal disorders. It has not replaced other approaches, such as CT or ultrasound, in the imaging of many thoracic and abdominal disorders.

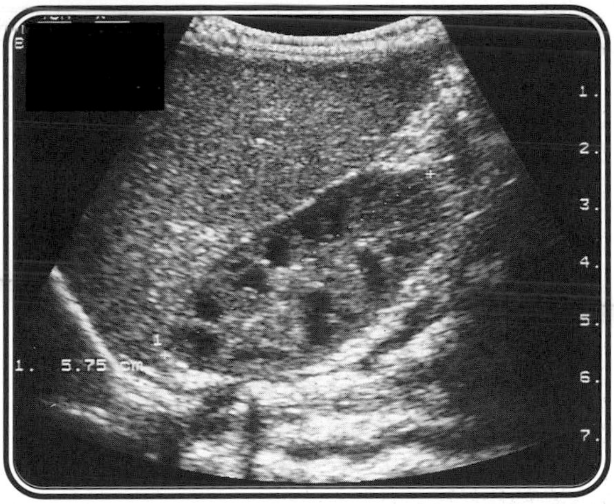

Fig. 12.3 Normal renal ultrascound. Normal prominent pyramids are demonstrated.

BLOOD TESTS

Venous or capillary blood is usually satisfactory and may be obtained by venepuncture or capillary sampling. Arterial blood sampling is only occasionally necessary for blood gas analysis or estimation of acid–base status. (Pulse oximetry has rendered arterial sampling for determination of oxygenation rarely necessary). With experience, skill, and local anaesthetic cream, blood can be obtained quickly and with minimal discomfort from most infants and children.

Blood tests fall into the following general categories. See Fig. 12.4 for clinical chemistry reference values.

Haematology

Full blood count

This provides information on:

- Haemoglobin, Hb (g/dL).
- Total white cell count, WBC (x 10^9/L).
- Platelet count (x 10^9/L).

It can also provide:

- Red cell indices—MCV (fl), MCH (pg), MCHC (%).
- Reticulocytes (%).
- Differential white cell count—neutrophils, lymphocytes, eosinophils, monocytes (% or 10^9/L).

The examination of the film allows evaluation of:

- Red cell morphology (Fig. 12.5).
- Differential white cell count.
- Platelet numbers and morphology.
- Presence or absence of abnormal cells (e.g. blast cells).

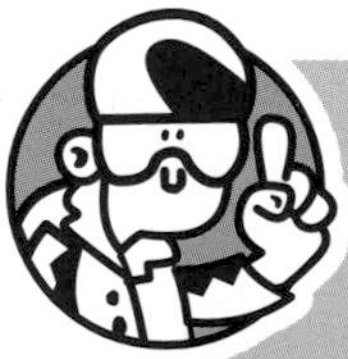

Haemoglobin concentration and white cell counts must be interpreted in relation to age:
Hb concentration is high at birth (15–19g/dl) and falls to a nadir at 3 months (9–13g/dl).
The total white cell count is high at birth and rapidly falls to normal adult levels. There is a relative lymphocytosis during the first 4 years of life after the neonatal period.

Clinical chemistry			
Test	**Normal range (plasma or serum)**		
sodium		133–145 mmol/L	
potassium	infant	3.5–6.0 mmol/L	
	child	3.3–5.0 mmol/L	
urea	neonate	1.0–5.0 mmol/L	
	infant	2.5–8.0 mmol/L	
	child	2.5–6.5 mmol/L	
creatinine	infant	20–65 µmol/L	
	1–10 years	20–80 µmol/L	
osmolality		275–295 mosm/kg	
calcium (total)	24–48 h	1.8–3.0 mmol/L	
	child	2.15–2.60 mmol/L	
calcium (ionized)	24–48 h	1.00–1.17 mmol/L	
	child	1.18–1.32 mmol/L	
phosphate	neonate	1.4–2.6 mmol/L	
	infant	1.3–2.1 mmol/L	
	child	1.0–1.8 mmol/L	
alkaline phosphatase	neonate	150–700 U/L	
	1–12 months	250–1000 U/L	
	2–9 years	250–850 U/L	
	years	females	males
	10–11	250–950 U/L	250–730 U/L
	14–15	170–460 U/L	170–970 U/L
	>18	60–250 U/L	50–200 U/L
albumin	neonate	25–35 g/L	
	child	35–55 g/L	
creatine kinase	infant/child	60–300 U/L	
glucose	I day	2.2–3.3 mmol/L	
	>I day	2.6–5.5 mmol/L	
	child	3.0–6.0 mmol/L	
iron	infant	5–25 µmol/L	
	child	10–30 µmol/L	
ferritin	child	<150 µg/L	
C-reactive protein		<10 mg/L	
blood gas (arterial, not preterm)	pH	7.35–7.45	
	pO_2	11–14 kPa (82–105 mmHg)	
	pCO_2	4.5–6.0 kPa (32–45 mmHg)	
	bicarbonate	18–25 mmol/L	
	base excess	–4 to +4 mmol/L	

Fig. 12.4 Normal ranges for blood tests (normal range for some tests varies between laboratories and must be checked with the local laboratory).

Also see Fig. 12.6 which shows important abnormalities that may be identified from a FBC.

Sickle test

This is a screening test for the sickle cell trait or disease. Sickle cells are seen when the blood is deoxygenated with Na_2HPO_4.

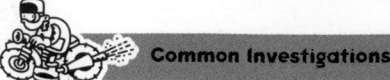

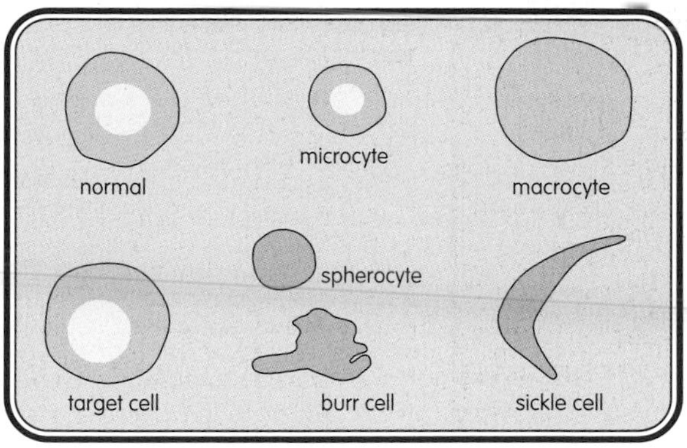

Fig. 12.5 Red cell morphology.

Important problems identifiable on a full blood count
anaemia, e.g. iron deficiency
thrombocytopenia, e.g. idiopathic thrombocytopenic purpura
neutropenia, e.g. immunosuppression
pancytopenia, e.g. bone marrow failure
neutrophil leucocytosis, e.g. bacterial infection
lymphocytosis, e.g. *Bordetella pertussis*

Fig. 12.6 Important problems identifiable on FBC.

Haemoglobin electrophoresis

The pattern of haemoglobin electrophoresis at different ages (birth and adult) and in different haemoglobinopathies is shown in Fig. 12.7.

Coagulation studies

Basic screening tests include:

- Prothrombin time—PT (usually expressed as 'international normalized ratio': INR).
- (Activated) Partial thromboplastin time—APTT.
- Thrombin time—TT.

The evaluation of a bleeding disorder also requires an estimation of platelet numbers, morphology, and function.

Common patterns of abnormality include:

- PT prolonged—liver disease.
- APTT prolonged—haemophilia (Factor VIII), Christmas disease (Factor IX).
- PT and APTT prolonged—vitamin K deficiency, liver disease.
- PT, APTT, TT prolonged—disseminated intravascular coagulation (DIC).

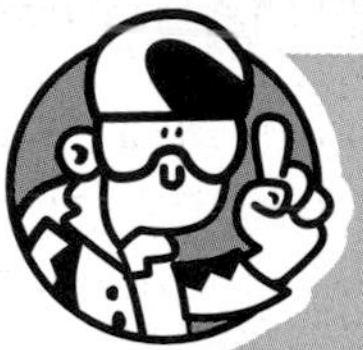

Structure of haemoglobin:
Foetal haemoglobin HbF $\alpha_2 \gamma_2$
Adult haemoglobin HbA $\alpha_2 \beta_2$
HbA$_2$ $\alpha_2 \delta_2$
Sickle haemoglobin HbS $\alpha_2 \beta_2^S$

von Willebrand's disease (VWD)

This is a heterogeneous group of inherited disorders with a defect in the von Willebrand factor (which is important in platelet adhesion and as a carrier molecule for factor VIII). Bleeding time and APTT are prolonged. VWF levels can be measured directly.

Disseminated intravascular coagulation (DIC)

Uncontrolled activation of coagulation causes:

- Widespread intravascular fibrin deposition.
- Consumption of coagulation factors and platelets.
- Accelerated degradation of fibrin and fibrinogen.

In DIC the constellation of laboratory findings includes:

- Prolonged PT, APTT, TT.
- Low fibrinogen.
- Elevated fibrinogen degradation products (FDPs) or D-dimers.
- Low platelets.
- Red cell fragmentation.

Further detailed investigations may be required, e.g. when clinical evidence indicates a bleeding disorder but screening tests are normal. These tests may include:

- Assays of individual factors (e.g. Factor XIII).
- Tests for presence of endogenous anticoagulants.

Biochemical analysis

Most biochemical analyses are carried out on plasma rather than serum (the sample must be placed in a bottle containing anticoagulant). This is heparin in most cases—glucose estimations are a notable exception and should be in fluoride oxalate.

Capillary blood samples can be used for many estimations but, if badly collected, they are subject to artefactual errors due to red cell lysis and tissue fluid dilution.

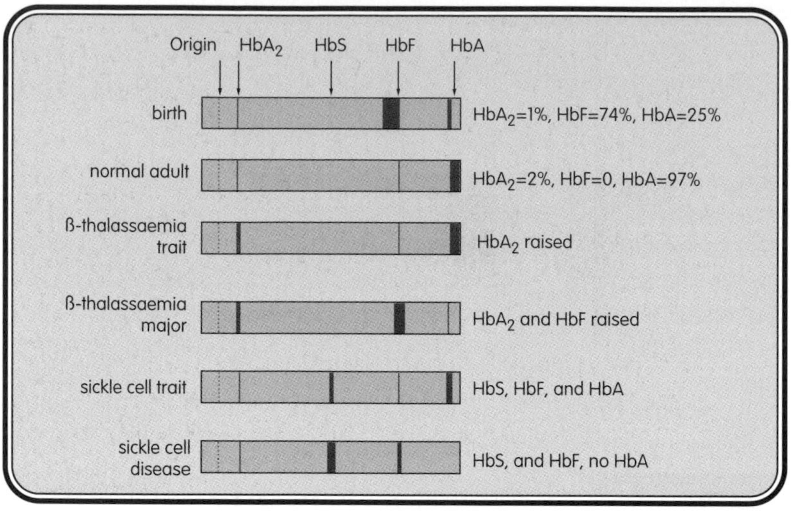

Fig. 12.7 Haemoglobin (Hb) electrophoresis.

Urea and electrolytes

U&Es (urea, Na^+, K^+, Cl^-) are the most commonly requested biochemical analysis and may be useful in a host of circumstances including:

- Dehydration—diarrhoea, vomiting.
- Patients on IV fluids—monitoring electrolyte status.
- Diabetic ketoacidosis.
- Renal disease.
- Diuretic therapy.

Urea

Urea is a major metabolite of protein catabolism. It is synthesized in the liver and excreted by the kidneys. The plasma concentration is influenced by:

- State of hydration.
- Protein intake.
- Catabolism.
- Glomerular filtration rate (GFR).

The creatinine concentration is a more reliable indicator of renal function. The most commonly encountered cause of a raised plasma urea is dehydration.

Sodium (Na^+)

Changes in the plasma sodium concentration may reflect changes in either the sodium or water balance. Causes are shown in Figs 12.8 and 12.9.

Potassium (K^+)

This is a predominantly intracellular cation. Plasma concentration is therefore influenced by exchange with the intracellular compartment as well as the whole-body potassium status.

The causes of changes in plasma potassium are shown in Figs 12.10 and 12.11.

Causes of hyponatraemia (Na^+ <130 mmol/L)

Mechanism	Cause
water excess	iatrogenic: excess hypotonic IV fluids water retention due to inappropriate ADH secretion, e.g. postoperative, meningitis, head injury
sodium depletion	diarrhoea diuretics adrenal insufficiency (rare) cystic fibrosis/sweating (rare)

Fig. 12.8 Causes of hyponatraemia (Na^+ <130 mmol/L).

Causes of hypernatraemia (Na^+ >150 mmol/L)

Mechanism	Cause
water deficit	diarrhoea diabetes insipidus excessive insensible water loss, e.g. overhead heater
sodium excess	high solute intake iatrogenic: excess hypertonic IV fluids child abuse: salt poisoning (rare)

Fig. 12.9 Causes of hypernatraemia (Na^+ >150 mmol/L).

Concerning plasma sodium:

- **Artefactually low plasma sodium concentration may occur with hyperlipidaemia, e.g. in diabetic ketoacidosis, parenteral feeding.**
- **A normal plasma sodium concentration may be found in salt depletion or overload if associated parallel changes in body water has occurred.**
- **Rapid falls in plasma Na^+ cause brain swelling.**

Concerning plasma potassium:

- **The intracellular K^+ concentration is very high: >100 mmol/L.**
- **Acidosis brings K^+ out of cells in exchange for H^+.**
- **Haemolysis releases K^+ from red cells and causes artefactual hyperkalaemia.**
- **ECG changes reflect plasma K^+ concentration.**

Causes of hypokalaemia (K^+ <3.4 mmol/L)	
Mechanism	**Cause**
potassium depletion	diarrhoea diuretics
inadequate intake	daily need 2–3 mmol/kg
redistribution	metabolic alkalosis glucose and insulin

Fig. 12.10 Causes of hypokalaemia (K^+ <3.4 mmol/L).

Causes of hyperkalaemia (K^+ >5.5 mmol/L)	
Mechanism	**Cause**
failure of renal excretion	renal failure adrenocortical insufficiency
redistribution	metabolic acidosis, e.g. diabetic ketoacidosis
excess intake	iatrogenic
tissue injury	hypoxia, catabolism
artefact	haemolyzed specimen

Fig. 12.11 Causes of hyperkalaemia (K^+ >5·5 mmol/L).

Chloride (Cl^-)

Hypochloraemia is seen particularly in vomiting associated with pyloric stenosis and leads to a metabolic alkalosis.

Creatinine

Creatinine is a naturally occurring substance which is formed in muscles. The normal plasma concentration increases with age as muscle mass increases with growth. The plasma concentration of creatinine is a useful indirect measure of the glomerular filtration rate (GFR). In renal failure, the creatinine concentration increases steadily by more than 30 mmol/L/day.

Liver function tests

The basic biochemical tests of liver function include bilirubin, enzymes, and albumin and are outlined below.

Plasma K^+ in diabetic ketoacidosis:

- **Whole body K^+ is always depleted.**
- **Plasma K^+ concentration may be normal, high or low depending on the balance between acidosis and diuresis.**
- **Plasma K^+ falls with treatment as redistribution into cells occurs.**

Bilirubin:
- Conjugated and unconjugated.

Enzymes:
- Aspartate transaminase (AST).
- Alanine transaminase (ALT).
- Alkaline phosphatase (ALP).
- γ-glutamyltranspeptidase (γGT).

Additional investigations, which are useful for evaluating hepatic function (and are deranged in liver failure), include:
- Coagulation tests—PT, PTT.
- Ammonia.
- Glucose.

Bilirubin
Clinical evaluation of the severity of jaundice is unreliable, so it is important to document plasma levels of unconjugated and conjugated bilirubin. The normal proportion of conjugated bilirubin should not exceed 15% in infants. The causes of hyperbilirubinaemia are considered elsewhere (see Chapter 9).

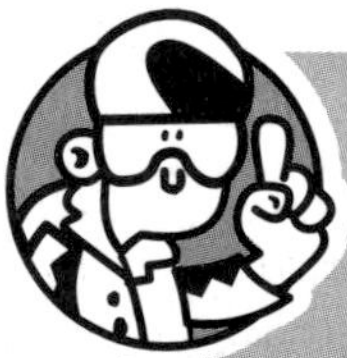

Excess conjugated hyperbilirubinaemia is a worrying sign in young infants as it may indicate biliary atresia.

Liver enzymes
Transaminases (aminotransferases)
These intracellular enzymes occur in many tissues including the liver, heart, and skeletal muscle. Normal plasma activity reflects release of enzymes during cell turnover, and increases occur with tissue injury. Elevated serum aminotransferase activity is therefore primarily seen in hepatocyte damage, e.g. hepatitis (infection, drugs).

However, elevation is not a specific marker of primary hepatocellular disease as it occurs in other forms of hepatobiliary disease (e.g. biliary atresia, cholecystitis) and also in non-hepatic conditions such as myocarditis and pancreatitis.

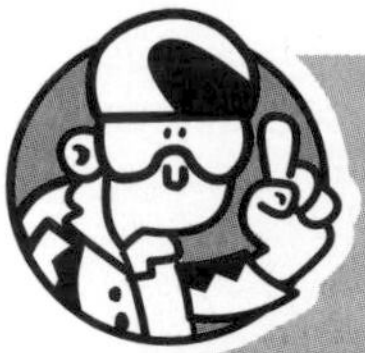

Raised transaminases indicate hepatocellular damage.
Raised alkaline phosphatase suggests biliary obstruction (cholestasis).

AST is the more sensitive indicator of liver injury, but ALT is more specific.

Alkaline phosphatase
Isoenzymes of alkaline phosphatase are widely distributed in many organs including liver and bone. Normal activity levels change markedly throughout childhood and reference ranges are both age and method-dependent.

Activity is increased in:
- Biliary obstruction—intrahepatic or extrahepatic.
- Hepatocellular damage.
- Increased osteoblastic activity—e.g. rickets.
- Normal growth and pubertal growth spurt.

γ-glutamyltranspeptidase
Serum activity is commonly raised in liver disease especially when there is cholestasis. It may also be raised in the absence of liver disease in patients taking certain drugs, e.g. phenytoin, phenobarbitone, and rifampicin (as a result of enzyme induction).

Albumin
Albumin is synthesized in the liver and is the main contributor to plasma oncotic pressure. It also has an important role as the protein to which many circulating substances are bound such as:
- Bilirubin.
- Calcium.
- Drugs.
- Hormones.

Albumin has a long half-life of about 20 days.

Plasma albumin levels are a useful indicator of hepatic function. Low levels occur in several important clinical contexts (Fig. 12.12).

Prolonged hypoalbuminaemia (e.g. in nephrotic

syndrome) is associated with oedema because fluid leaks into the extravascular space and hypovolaemia triggers renal salt and water retention.

Glucose

Blood glucose concentrations are normally maintained within fairly narrow limits, which are lower in the newborn. Blood glucose can be estimated very rapidly at the bedside using test sticks, but values should be verified by laboratory investigation.

The only common cause of hyperglycaemia in children is insulin-dependent type 1 diabetes mellitus. There are, however, many causes of hypoglycaemia (Fig. 12.13).

Causes of hypoalbuminaemia (<30 g/L)

Type	Cause
decreased synthesis	chronic liver disease malnutrition (protein–energy malnutrition) malabsorption
increased losses	nephrotic syndrome burns protein-losing enteropathy

Fig. 12.12 Causes of hypoalbuminaemia (<30 g/L).

Causes of hyperglycaemia and hypoglycaemia

Hyperglycaemia	Hypoglycaemia
diabetes mellitus • IDDM (most common) • secondary—pancreatic disease, Cushing syndrome stress-related, e.g. postconvulsive iatrogenic • drugs, e.g. corticosteroids • total parenteral nutrition	neonatal • infant of diabetic mother • small for gestational age postneonatal • ketotic hypoglycaemia • hyperinsulinaemia—known diabetic, pancreatic tumour (rare) • ↓GH, ACTH, cortisol—hypopituitarism (rare), adrenal failure (rare)

Fig. 12.13 Causes of hyperglycaemia and hypoglycaemia.

Calcium and phosphate

Disorders of calcium and phosphate metabolism in childhood are uncommon and usually reflect abnormalities in the major controlling hormones, vitamin D and parathormone. Laboratory estimations provide a measure of both total and ionized calcium. Changes in plasma albumin concentration affect total calcium levels independently of ionized calcium, leading to misinterpretation if serum albumin is outside the normal range. Therefore, the total calcium concentration needs to be corrected to give the expected value if albumin were in the normal range. Major causes of hypercalcaemia and hypocalcaemia are shown in Fig. 12.14.

Causes of hypercalcaemia and hypocalcaemia

Hypocalcaemia	Hypercalcaemia
rickets (low phosphate, high alkaline phosphatase) hypoparathyroidism, e.g. DiGeorge syndrome hypoalbuminaemia	hyperparathyroidism syndromic (Williams syndrome) vitamin D excess

Fig. 12.14 Causes of hypocalcaemia and.hypercalcaemia.

Always measure the blood glucose urgently in a fitting or unconscious child.

Calcium (and magnesium) levels should be measured in infants with seizures.

Blood gases and acid–base metabolism

Metabolism generates acid, which is eliminated via the lungs as carbon dioxide and via the kidneys as hydrogen ions. Acidosis, from whatever cause, is a much more common problem than alkalosis. Ideally, estimations of blood gas and acid–base status are made on an arterial sample from an indwelling catheter, but capillary or venous blood can be useful for pH and pCO_2 measurements.

Where the main concern is oxygenation, non-invasive pulse oximetry is a valuable alternative to arterial blood gas analysis.

The pattern of changes seen in different forms of acidosis and alkalosis are shown in Fig. 12.15.

Common clinical contexts in which these disturbances occur include:

- Respiratory acidosis—hypoventilation (e.g. respiratory distress syndrome, severe asthma, neuromuscular diseases).
- Metabolic acidosis—diabetic ketoacidosis, hypoxia, circulatory failure.
- Respiratory alkalosis—hyperventilation, e.g. hysterical (rare in children), iatrogenic (ventilated patients).
- Metabolic alkalosis—pyloric stenosis.

Immunology

Tests of the immune system carried out on the blood may be required in the following clinical contexts:

- Immunodeficiency.
- Auto-immune disease.
- Infection—diagnostic serology, acute phase reactants.

Tests for immunodeficiency

Immunodeficiencies may be primary or secondary. The inherited primary deficiencies are rare. Secondary causes are far more common (Fig. 12.16).

Immunodeficiency should be suspected in the following clinical circumstances:

- Recurrent severe infections.
- Infections with atypical organisms.
- Common infections with a severe or atypical clinical course.
- Failure to thrive.

Basic screening tests of immune function should include:

- Immunoglobulins.
- FBC including differential WCC and lymphocyte subsets.

Immunoglobulins

Serum immunoglobulin levels vary with age. Maternally transferred IgG is present at high levels at birth, but has mostly disappeared by 6 months of age. This decline occurs before endogenous synthesis has fully developed, creating a physiological trough between 3–6 months of age. This is shown in Fig. 12.17.

IgG is the major immunoglobulin in normal human serum accounting for about 70% of the total pool. There are four distinct subclasses (IgG 1–4) which have different functions. Specific IgM changes are very useful in the diagnosis of viral infections, e.g. rubella.

Differential white cell count

Immunodeficiency caused by marrow-suppressive cytotoxic or immunosuppressive therapy is related to the absolute neutrophil count. Patients with absolute neutrophil counts below 1.0×10^9/L are at increased risk of Gram-negative septicaemia.

Lymphocyte subsets

Lymphocytes are further subdivided into T cells and B cells. T cells are categorized into:

Acid–base disturbances			
	pH	$PaCO_2$	HCO_3^-
Acidosis			
respiratory	low	high	normal or high (compensation)
metabolic	low	normal or low (compensation)	low
Alkalosis			
respiratory	high	low	normal or low (compensation)
metabolic	high	normal or high (compensation)	high

Fig. 12.15 Acid–base disturbances.

Causes of immunodeficiency

Primary
primary antibody deficiencies:
- common variable immune deficiency
- X-linked antibody deficiency
- IgG subclass deficiency
- specific antibody deficiency
- selective IgA deficiency

severe combined immunodeficiency
chronic granulomatous disease

Secondary
malnutrition
infections, e.g. HIV, measles
immunosuppressive therapy, e.g. steroids, cytotoxic drugs
hyposplenism, e.g. sickle cell disease, splenectomy

Fig. 12.16 Causes of immunodeficiency.

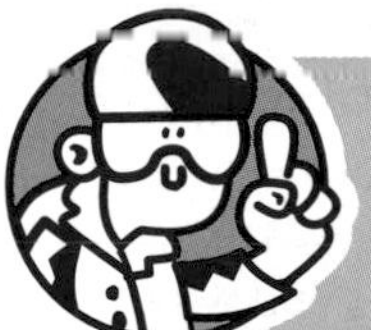

Immunoglobulins:

- **IgG_2 is the most common subclass deficiency and may be associated with IgA deficiency. The total IgG level may be normal. It causes recurrent respiratory infections, e.g. sinusitis, pneumonia.**
- **Selective IgA deficiency is common (1:700 population) and may cause no symptoms.**

- Cytotoxic T cells (Tc), which are mostly $CD8^+$.
- Helper T cells (TH), which are mostly $CD4^+$.

Cytotoxic T cells recognize infected target cells and lyse them. Helper T cells secrete regulatory molecules (lymphokines) which affect both other T cells and cells of various lineages.

Monitoring absolute numbers of $CD4^+$ helper cells is useful in monitoring the progression of HIV-related diseases.

Auto-antibodies

Auto-immune disease is uncommon in childhood, but includes such entities as juvenile chronic arthritis (JCA), systemic lupus erythematosus (SLE), and auto-immune thyroiditis causing juvenile hypothyroidism.

The following tests may be of value.

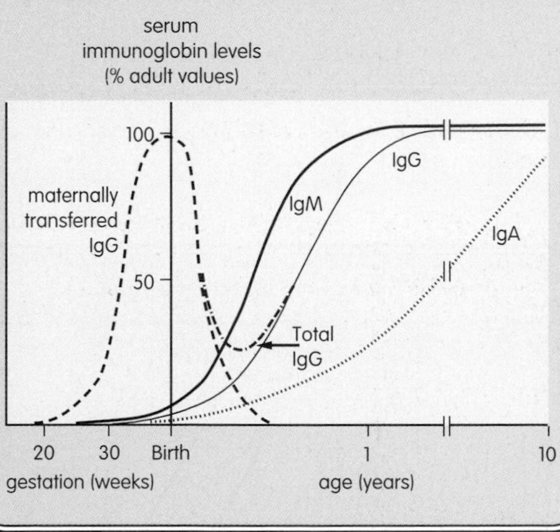

Fig. 12.17 Serum immunoglobulin (Ig) levels in fetus and infant.

Antinuclear antibodies (ANA)

A broad group of antibodies present in 5% of normal children and induced by a wide spectrum of inflammatory conditions.

- High titres of ANA occur in 95% of SLE patients.
- Presence of ANA in subgroups of JCA is a risk factor for chronic anterior uveitis.

SLE is associated with antibodies against specific nuclear antigens such as double-stranded DNA.

Rheumatoid factors

These are IgM autoantibodies against IgG. They should not be used to screen for JCA, as they are neither sensitive nor specific. The majority of children with JCA are rheumatoid factor negative. Rheumatoid factors may be useful as a prognostic indicator in polyarticular JCA (their persistent presence is a poor prognostic factor).

Thyroid antibodies

Thyroid microsomal (peroxisomal) and thyroglobulin titres should be measured in suspected auto-immune thyroiditis.

Diagnostic serology

This is most widely used in the diagnosis of viral infections, but is also of value in certain specific non-viral infections such as *Mycoplasma pneumoniae*, group A β-haemolytic streptococci and *Salmonella spp*.

Viral antibody tests
Serological diagnosis depends on the detection of virus antibody. Diagnosis of recent infection requires the demonstration of a rising titre of specific IgM between the acute phase and convalescence. Methods used include:
- Immunofluorescence.
- Enzyme-linked immunoabsorbent assay (ELISA).
- Radio-immune assay (RIA).

Epstein–Barr virus (EBV)
Specific EBV serology is the most reliable diagnostic test. Antibodies to viral capsid antigen (VCA) are detected. IgG anti-VCA merely indicates a past infection. A positive IgM to VCA is diagnostic and is found early in the disease.

Tests for heterophile antibody, which agglutinates sheep red blood cells, are the basis of slide agglutination tests (monospot and Paul–Bunnell). However, this antibody does not appear until the second week or even later, and may not be produced at all in young children.

Mycoplasma pneumoniae
Diagnosis of infection with *Mycoplasma pneumoniae* is most quickly established by serology: a four-fold rise in complement-fixing antibodies is diagnostic.

Antistreptolysin O titre (ASOT)
Estimation of antibody to streptolysin O is a useful means of retrospectively diagnosing infection by group A β-haemolytic streptococci. The ASOT is a valuable investigation in the evaluation of:
- Suspected acute nephritis.
- Rheumatic fever.
- Scarlet fever.
- Kawasaki disease.

Acute-phase reactants
An inflammatory stimulus provokes the production of proteins in the liver known as the acute-phase response. This response is documented by the measurement of:
- C-reactive protein (CRP).
- Erythrocyte sedimentation rate (ESR).

The response is non-specific and does not help in identifying aetiology. However, if acute phase reactants are elevated at the onset of disease, serial measurements are useful for monitoring progress.

The response times vary:
- CRP—elevated within 6 hours.
- ESR—peaks at 3–4 days.

Microbiology
Blood is normally sterile. Transient asymptomatic bacteraemia may occur after dental treatment, or invasive procedures such as catheterization. However, bacteraemia leading to septicaemia and shock may accompany a number of important childhood diseases such as pneumonia, meningitis, and typhoid fever.

Blood culture should be taken under the following circumstances:
- Pyrexia of unknown origin.
- Clinical signs of septicaemia.
- Febrile illness—in an immunodeficient child (e.g. sickle-cell disease, nephrotic syndrome, neutropenia) or in patients with a central catheter.
- Investigation of specific infections—meningitis, pneumonia, pyelonephritis, enteric fever.

The most common pathogens recovered from the blood are shown in Figs 12.18 and 12.19. Most significant isolates will be obtained within 48–72 hours of inoculation.

Common causes of septicaemia in children after the newborn period
Streptococcus pneumoniae *Neisseria meningitidis* *Staphylococcus aureus* *Salmonella spp.* *Haemophilus influenzae* type B

Fig. 12.18 Common causes of septicaemia in children after the newborn period.

Common causes of septicaemia in the newborn
group B streptococcus *Staphylococcus aureus* coagulase-negative staphylococci coliforms • enterococcus • *E. coli* • *Klebsiella*

Fig. 12.19 Common causes of septicaemia in the newborn.

Lipitor
atorvastatin calcium
HELPS MORE PATIENTS TO TARGET
Parke-Davis

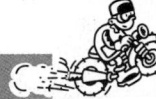

s:
in,
tes,
ntified
e

In certain clinical contexts, urine testing by dipstick is mandatory. These include:

- History of polyuria, polydipsia—diabetes mellitus?
- Generalized oedema—nephrotic syndrome?

Microscopy and culture

Microscopy is required to look for casts and red cells in suspected glomerular disease, and is combined with culture in the investigation of suspected urinary tract infection (UTI).

Collection of an uncontaminated urine sample presents a problem in infants and young children. Alternative methods for collection in babies include:

- A clean-catch sample into a sterile pot.
- An adhesive plastic bag applied to the perineum after careful washing ('bag' urine).
- Suprapubic aspiration SPA—appropriate in a severely ill infant less than 1 year old requiring urgent diagnosis.

The urine should be examined microscopically and cultured immediately, or refrigerated (to prevent overgrowth of contaminants) if there is unavoidable delay.

In UTI, pus cells and bacteria may be seen on microscopy. However, pyuria may occur with fever in the absence of UTI, and cell lysis may obscure pyuria if the sample is not examined immediately. The urine white cell count is not therefore a reliable feature in the diagnosis of UTI.

A mixed growth in the absence of pyuria usually represents contamination. Confident diagnosis of a UTI requires a bacterial culture of more than 10^8/L colony-forming units of a single species in a properly collected specimen.

CEREBROSPINAL FLUID

Cerebrospinal fluid (CSF) is usually obtained by lumbar puncture. This is the critical investigation for the diagnosis of meningitis. The CSF can be evaluated in several ways including (Fig. 12.20):

- Appearance.
- Pressure.
- Microbiology—microscopy [white cell count/mm^3, organisms (Gram stain or acid-fast)], culture, and sensitivity.
- Biochemistry—protein (g/L), glucose (mmol/L).
- Rapid diagnostic techniques—countercurrent immunoelectrophoresis, latex agglutination, polymerase chain reaction.

Appearance

Normal CSF is clear. If the cell count increases to more than 500 cells/mm/^{3}, it becomes turbid. Typically, this occurs in bacterial meningitis.

Microbiology

Microscopy

Normally, a few (<5/mm^3) white cells may be found in CSF. The presence of polymorphs is always abnormal except in the neonatal period when up to 30/mm^3 white cells may be physiological. In the early stages of meningitis, white cells may not be detectable but classically very high counts are found.

Spun CSF is routinely Gram stained:

- Gram-negative cocci—*Neisseria meningitidis.*
- Gram-positive cocci—*Streptococcus pneumoniae.*
- Gram-negative coccobacilli—*Haemophilus influenzae.*

Culture and sensitivity

This is always carried out even if the sample is clear and no white cells were detected on microscopy.

Biochemistry

Protein

Protein content of the CSF rises in bacterial meningitis.

Glucose

Normal CSF glucose is approximately two-thirds of the blood glucose level. In bacterial meningitis, it drops to less than 40% of the blood glucose level.

Type	Appearance	WBC (mm^3)	Protein (g/L)	Glucose
normal CSF (not neonatal)	clear	0–5	0.15–0.4	>50% blood glucose
bacterial meningitis	turbid	500–10 000 polymorphs	0.4–3	low
viral meningitis	clear	<1000	<10	normal
TB meningitis	clear/viscous	up to 500 usually <100	>10	low

Fig. 12.20 A summary of the content and appearance of CSF in different types of meningitis.

Rapid diagnostic techniques

Bacterial antigens can now be detected by sensitive and rapid tests including:

- Countercurrent immunoelectrophoresis.
- Latex agglutination.

Sufficient antigen remains present even after treatment with antibiotics has been initiated and when direct culture is no longer possible. Unfortunately, both tests are unreliable at detecting group B meningococcus, which is the most common type in the UK.

Polymerase chain reaction and DNA hybridization

New techniques that detect bacterial DNA, and viral DNA or RNA are becoming available. These tests are useful for detecting herpes simplex virus in CSF in encephalitis.

Concerning meningitis:

- **Infants may have non-specific clinical signs, therefore a high index of suspicion is required and a low threshold for performing a lumbar puncture.**
- **A missed diagnosis can be catastrophic.**

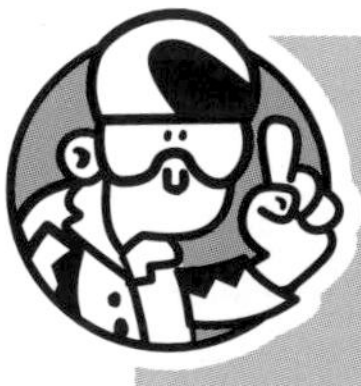

Lumbar puncture is contraindicated in the following circumstances:

- **Signs of raised intracranial pressure.**
- **Focal neurological signs.**
- **Rapidly deteriorating conscious level.**
- **Bradycardia.**
- **A coagulation defect.**
- **Skin infection at the lumbar puncture site.**

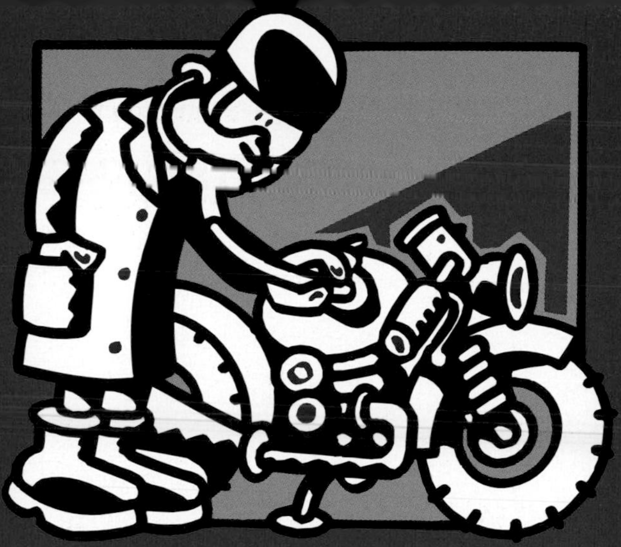

DISEASES AND DISORDERS

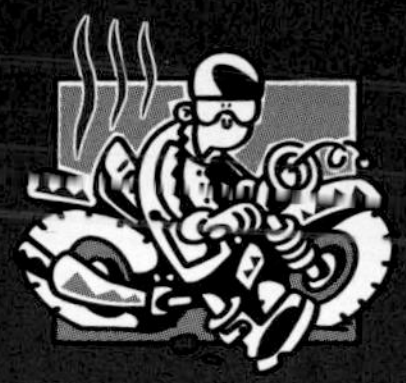

13. Infectious Diseases and Immunodeficiency

Despite the spectacular successes achieved by public health measures and immunization programmes in preventing childhood infectious disease, infections remain a major cause of mortality and morbidity in childhood:

- In the developing world, 12 million children under 5 years of age die each year from the combined effects of malnutrition and infections such as gastroenteritis, pneumonia, measles, and malaria.
- In the developed world, major diseases such as diphtheria and polio have been effectively eliminated, and the infection rates of others such as invasive disease caused by *Haemophilus influenzae* type B, measles, mumps, rubella, and pertussis are greatly reduced.

However, infection remains the most common cause of disease in childhood and the resurgence of TB worldwide, together with the growing impact of human immunodeficiency virus (HIV) infection in childhood, leaves no room for complacency

VIRAL INFECTIONS

Viral exanthems

The term exanthem is applied to diseases in which a rash is a prominent manifestation. Classically, six exanthems with similar rashes were described. They are numbered in the order in which they were described and are listed in Fig. 13.1.

The second disease is of course bacterial in origin and the fourth disease is no longer recognized as an entity.

Measles

Incidence and aetiology

Measles is caused by infection with a single-stranded RNA virus of genus *Morbillivirus*. The incidence in England and Wales declined dramatically after vaccination was introduced (1968), from a pattern of epidemics every 2 years with up to 800 000 cases a year in the 1960s, to 50 to 100 000 cases a year in the 1980s. Following the introduction of MMR (measles, mumps, rubella) vaccination (1988), notifications fell further to just 10 000 cases in 1993.

Clinical features

Fever, cough, coryza, and conjunctivitis are followed by (in some cases) the pathognomonic Koplik's spots on the buccal mucosa, and after 3 or 4 days by an erythematous maculopapular rash. The rash spreads downward from the hairline to the whole body, becomes blotchy and confluent and may desquamate in the second week.

The disease is highly infectious. Transmission is by droplet spread and the incubation period is about 10 days. Children should stay off school for 1 week after appearance of the rash.

Measles is very dangerous in immunocompromised children, such as those in remission from acute leukaemia or with HIV. These children are susceptible to giant cell pneumonia and encephalitis. In developing countries, malnutrition and particularly vitamin A deficiency impairs immunity and renders measles a more severe disease. It is estimated that up to 2 million children die annually from the disease in developing countries.

Complications

Acute complications include febrile convulsions, otitis media, tracheobronchitis, and pneumonia due either to

Viral exanthems		
		Pathogen
first	measles	paramyxovirus
second	scarlet fever	group A β-haemolytic strepococcus
third	rubella	togavirus
fourth	'Duke's disease'	—
fifth	erythema infectiosum	parvovirus B19
sixth	roseola infantum	human herpesvirus 6

Fig. 13.1 Viral exanthems.

the primary virus infection or bacterial superinfection (Fig. 13.2). Rarely, severe encephalitis may occur (1:5000 cases) about 8 days after onset of the illness. The mortality is 15% and severe neurological sequelae occur in 40% of survivors. (Subacute sclerosing panencephalitis, SSPE, is a very rare immune-mediated neurodegenerative disease which may occur 7–10 years after measles.)

Diagnosis
Diagnosis may be confirmed by detection of specific IgM in saliva samples ideally taken from 3 days after the appearance of the rash. The disease is notifiable.

Management
Treatment is symptomatic.

The incomplete coverage with MMR was predicted to lead to an increasing number of susceptible teenagers with a high probability of a major resurgence of measles in the school-age population. Therefore, a highly successful national immunization programme was implemented in 1994, that reached 8 million children aged between 5 and 16 years.

Rubella (German measles)

This mild childhood disease is caused by infection with the Rubivirus. Its importance lies in the devastating effect maternal infection in early gestation has on the fetus.

Clinical features
Infection is subclinical in up to half of infected individuals. After an incubation period of 14–21 days, a low-grade fever is followed by a pink–red maculopapular rash which starts on the face and spreads rapidly over the entire body. The rash is fleeting and may have gone entirely by the third day. Generalized lymphadenopathy, particularly affecting the suboccipital and postauricular nodes, is a prominent feature.

Acute complications of measles
febrile convulsions otitis media tracheobronchitis pneumonia encephalitis

Fig. 13.2 Complications of measles.

Complications
Complications are unusual in childhood but include arthritis (typically affecting the small joints of the hand), encephalitis, and thrombocytopenia.

Diagnosis
Diagnosis is clinical and differentiation from other viral exanthems is often difficult. In circumstances in which it is important, detection of rubella specific IgM in the saliva or serum is necessary to confirm the diagnosis.

Prevention (immunization)
A live, attenuated vaccine has been available for many years. Since 1988, this has been given as part of the MMR vaccine to all children at 13 months of age. Vaccine failure is rare and in most people, it provides lifelong protection. The presence of IgG, specific for rubella, indicates immunity due to prior infection or immunization.

Congenital rubella

Incidence and diagnosis
The risk and extent of fetal damage is mainly determined by its gestational age at the onset of maternal infection. In the first 8–10 weeks the risk is high; beyond 18 weeks' gestation the risk is minimal.

Maternal infection at up to 10 weeks' gestation confers a 90% risk of some degree of damage that is often severe and includes deafness, congenital heart disease, and cataracts. Between 13 and 16 weeks' gestation, there is a 30% risk of hearing impairment. Although congenital rubella is now rare in the UK (14 cases notified in the period 1991–1994), the diagnosis is worth consideration in any growth-retarded newborn or child with unexplained sensorineural deafness.

Clinical features
Clinical features of congenital rubella are shown in Fig. 13.3.

Management
All pregnant women and women contemplating pregnancy should be screened for antirubella IgG. Immigrants to the UK from countries where rubella vaccination is not routine are at particular risk of not being immune. Women found to be seronegative on antenatal screening receive immunization after delivery.

Pregnant women exposed to rubella should be

Clinical features of congenital rubella

growth retardation
hepatosplenomegaly
congenital heart disease
- patent ductus arteriosus
- pulmonary stenosis

eye
- glaucoma
- cataract
- retinopathy

ear
- sensorineural deafness

Fig. 13.3 Clinical features of congenital rubella.

tested for antirubella IgG and IgM regardless of previous history or serological testing. A high likelihood of congenital rubella infection early in pregnancy is an indication for offering termination of the pregnancy.

Erythema infectiosum or slapped cheek disease

This is caused by infection with *Parvovirus B19*, a small DNA virus that is the only parvovirus pathogenic to humans. Transmission may occur via respiratory secretions, from mother to fetus, and by transmission of contaminated blood products.

Clinical features

Asymptomatic infection is common. Erythema infectiosum describes the most common disease pattern of fever followed a week later by a characteristic rash. This starts as a red appearance on the face (hence the name 'slapped-cheek disease') and may progress to a symmetrical lacy rash on the extremities and trunk.

The virus suppresses erythropoiesis for up to 7 days. In children with haemolytic anaemia, such as sickle-cell disease or hereditary spherocytosis, parvovirus infection may cause an aplastic crisis. Maternal infection during pregnancy may be transmitted to the fetus and causes hydrops fetalis (due to fetal anaemia and myocarditis), fetal death, or spontaneous abortion.

Diagnosis and management

Diagnosis is clinical, but if confirmation is important (e.g. in pregnancy), specific IgM can be detected 2 weeks after exposure. Management is symptomatic.

Sixth disease: roseola infantum

Roseola infantum is caused by infection with HHV-6 or HHV-7.

Clinical features and diagnosis

Most children acquire the infection between the age of 3 months and 4 years. There is sudden onset of a high fever with irritability lasting for 3–6 days. Febrile convulsions may occur. The fever then falls abruptly and a widespread macular rash appears.

Diagnosis is clinical and treatment supportive.

Rare complications include aseptic meningitis, encephalitis, and hepatitis.

Herpes infections

There are eight human herpesviruses. They cause a number of common and important diseases in children including chickenpox and glandular fever. A particular hallmark of these viruses is their capacity to become latent with subsequent recurrence, causing, for example, shingles (varicella zoster) and cold sores (HSV1).

The human herpesviruses and their corresponding diseases are shown in Fig. 13.4.

Herpes simplex virus 1 (HSV1, HHV-1)

Clinical features

Most primary infections with HSV1 are asymptomatic. The most common clinical manifestation in childhood is gingivostomatitis. The child (usually a toddler) presents with high fever, misery, and vesicular lesions on the lips, gums, tongue, and hard palate which may progress to painful, extensive ulceration. The illness may last as long as 2 weeks.

Less commonly, infection may involve:

- The eye, causing dendritic ulcers on the cornea.
- Skin, causing eczema herpeticum in children with eczema.
- Fingers causing a herpetic whitlow.
- Brain, causing herpes simplex encephalitis (HSE).

Treatment

Occasionally IV fluid may be required for gingivostomatitis, but in this condition oral aciclovir has only a marginal effect. IV aciclover is used in HSE.

The virus becomes latent in the dorsal root ganglion supplying the trigeminal nerve where subsequent reactivation (by UV light, stress or menstruation) may cause labial herpes (cold sores) in later life.

Human herpesviruses and their diseases

Abbreviation	Virus	Disease
HHV-1	herpes simplex virus 1	stomatitis herpes simplex encephalitis
HHV-2	herpes simplex virus 2	genital herpes neonatal herpes
HHV-3	varicella zoster	chickenpox
HHV-4	Epstein–Barr virus	infectious mononucleosis
HHV-5	cytomegalovirus	congenital infection
HHV-6	—	roseola infantum (sixth disease)

HHV-8 Kaposi sarcoma

Fig. 13.4 Human herpesviruses (HHV) and their diseases.

Herpes simplex virus 2 (HSV2, HHV-2)

Transmission of HSV2 from the genital tract of a mother may result in neonatal herpes infection. This condition has a very high mortality and morbidity. There may be generalized infection with pneumonia, hepatitis, and encephalitis with onset usually in the first week of life.

Elective caesarean section is indicated when a mother with active genital herpes goes into labour.

Varicella zoster (HHV-3, VZV)

Chickenpox is a common childhood disease caused by primary infection with the varicella zoster virus (VZV). It is highly infectious with transmission occurring by droplet infection (the respiratory route), direct contact, or contact with soiled materials. The average incubation period is 14 days.

Clinical features

A brief coryzal period is followed by the eruption of an itchy, vesicular rash. This starts on the scalp or trunk and spreads centrifugally. Crops appear over 3–5 days and the mucous membranes may be involved.

Complications

In immunocompetent children complications are unusual, but may include secondary bacterial infection of the skin with staphylococci or streptococci and an encephalitis (often affecting the cerebellum), which may appear 3–6 days after onset of the rash. It may, however, be a very severe disease (mortality 20%) in the immunosuppressed child (children on systemic steroids) and in the newborn infant if the mother develops chickenpox just before delivery.

Diagnosis

Diagnosis is clinical, but virus isolated from vesicular fluid can be identified by electron microscopy or culture. The period of infectivity is from 2 days before eruption of the rash until all the lesions are encrusted.

Treatment

Treatment is symptomatic. However, the exposed immunosuppressed child should be given varicella zoster immune globulin (VZIG) if known to be seronegative. VZIG should also be given to newborn babies if the mother develops varicella or herpes zoster in the 7 days before or after birth and to any exposed preterm infant. Acyclovir should be given in severe chickenpox or for clinical infection in an immunocompromised child or newborn infant.

A live, attenuated vaccine does exist but is not currently licensed in the UK, and no country has adopted widespread varicella vaccination.

Herpes zoster (shingles)

This is due to reactivation of latent varicella zoster and is uncommon in childhood. A vesicular eruption occurs in the distribution of a sensory dermatome (most commonly in the thoracic region). In contrast to shingles in adults, severe pain is not a feature and neither is underlying malignancy.

Epstein–Barr virus (HHV-4,EBV)

The EBV has a particular tropism for the epithelial cells of the oropharynx and nasopharynx, and for B lymphocytes. It is not only the major cause of the infectious mononucleosis syndrome but is also

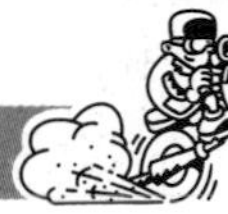

involved in the pathogenesis of Burkitt's lymphoma and nasopharyngeal carcinoma.

Clinical features

Transmission occurs by droplet transmission or directly via saliva ('the kissing disease'). Most people are infected asymptomatically in childhood. Symptomatic infection (infectious mononucleosis or glandular fever) is most common in the adolescent. The incubation period is 30–50 days.

Glandular fever is characterized by fever, malaise, pharyngitis (which may be exudative), and cervical lymphadenopathy. Petechiae may be seen on the palate and a sparse maculopapular rash may occur. Splenomegaly is present in 50% of cases, and hepatomegaly with hepatitis (usually anicteric) in 10%. A florid rash may develop if ampicillin or amoxycillin is given. The infection may persist for up to 3 months.

Diagnosis

Diagnosis is usually clinical. The blood shows atypical lymphocytes (T cells) and a heterophile antibody which is the basis of slide agglutination tests, including monospot and Paul–Bunnell tests. The latter does not appear until the second week and may not be produced in young children. Specific EBV serology—IgM to viral capsid antigen (VCA)—is available and more reliable. The differential diagnosis is from other causes of infectious mononucleosis (CMV, toxoplasmosis) and other causes of pharyngitis.

Management

Management is symptomatic. Rarely, massive pharyngeal swelling may compromise the airway. This is helped by corticosteroid treatment.

Cytomegalovirus (HHV-5, CMV)

Cytomegalovirus (CMV) is a common human pathogen. It is transmitted from mother to fetus via the placenta *in utero*, via the oral or genital routes, and by blood transfusion or organ transplantation.

Incidence

In the UK, about half of all pregnant women are susceptible to CMV, and about 1% of these will have a primary CMV infection during pregnancy. In almost half of these mothers, the infant will be infected, making CMV the most common congenital infection with an incidence of 3:1000 live births. However, most infants with congenital CMV are asymptomatic and develop normally.

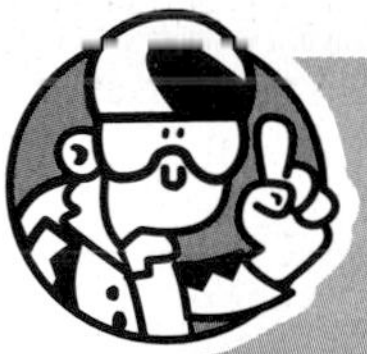

- **CMV is a common congenital infection, but rarely causes severe disease.**
- **CMV is an important cause of sensorineural hearing loss.**
- **CMV-negative blood must be used for transfusion in immunodeficient patients.**

Clinical features

Infection is mild or asymptomatic in adults or children with normal immunity. It can cause a mononucleosis syndrome with pharyngitis and lymphadenopathy.

Severe congenital infection causes:

- Intrauterine growth retardation.
- Hepatosplenomegaly, jaundice, and purpura.
- Microcephaly, intracranial calcification, and chorioretinitis.
- Long-term sequelae may include cerebral palsy, epilepsy, learning disability, and sensorineural hearing loss. Hearing loss may develop later in life without signs of infection in the newborn period.

In the immunocompromised host, CMV can cause severe disease including pneumonitis or encephalitis. It is a particularly important pathogen following organ transplantation.

Diagnosis and treatment

Diagnosis is made by viral isolation, especially from urine or by a strongly positive titre of IgM anti-CMV antibody. To confirm congenital infection, specimens for viral isolation must be taken within 3 weeks of birth.

Treatment with ganciclovir may be effective in immunocompromised patients.

Mumps

Mumps is caused by infection with an RNA virus of the *Paramyxovirus* family. Routine vaccination at 12–15 months, as a component of the MMR vaccine, has markedly reduced the incidence.

Transmission is by droplet spread and the incubation period is 14–21 days.

Clinical features

The clinical manifestations include fever, malaise, and parotitis. Pain and swelling of the parotid gland may be unilateral initially. Parotid gland enlargement is more easily seen than felt. The swelling is between the angle of the mandible and sternomastoid—extending beneath the ear lobe, which is pushed upwards and outwards.

The swelling usually subsides within 7–10 days. Patients are infectious from a few days before salivary gland enlargement and for up to 3 days after the enlargement subsides.

The central nervous system is commonly involved. Before vaccination was introduced, mumps was the most common cause of aseptic meningitis. Up to 50% of patients have lymphocytes in their CSF and 10% have signs of a meningoencephalitis.

Complications

Complications include pancreatitis (abdominal pain and raised serum amylase levels) and epididymo-orchitis. The latter is uncommon in prepubertal males and is usually unilateral. Even when it is bilateral, infertility is very rare. A postinfectious encephalomyelitis occurs in 1 out of 5000 cases.

Diagnosis and treatment

Diagnosis is usually clinical.

Treatment is symptomatic.

Enteroviruses

The human enteroviruses include:

- Coxsackie A and B.
- Echoviruses.
- Poliovirus.

Coxsackie viruses may cause aseptic meningitis, myocarditis, pericarditis, Bornholm disease (pleurodynia), and hand, foot and mouth disease.

Polio

Poliovirus is an enterovirus with antigenic types 1, 2, and 3. Immunization has rendered poliovirus infection uncommon in developed countries, but it remains endemic in parts of the developing world such as Africa and the Indian subcontinent.

Transmission is by the faecal–oral route with an incubation period of 7–21 days.

Clinical features

The clinical features vary:

- Over 90% of cases are asymptomatic.
- 5% have a 'minor illness'—fever, headache, malaise.
- 2% progress to CNS involvement—aseptic meningitis.
- In under 2%, 'paralytic polio' occurs due to the virus attacking the anterior horn cells of the spinal cord.

Diagnosis

In the UK, imported infections, and vaccine-associated infections are seen, but are rare. The differential diagnosis includes other causes of aseptic meningitis and acute paralytic disease such as Guillain–Barré syndrome.

Polio is a notifiable disease.

Viral hepatitis

This may be caused by

- Hepatitis virus A, B, C, D, E, or G.
- Arbovirus—yellow fever.
- Cytomegalovirus, Epstein–Barr virus.

Hepatitis A (HAV)

This is an RNA virus spread by faecal–oral transmission. The incubation period is 2–6 weeks.

Clinical features

In infants and young children, many infections are asymptomatic or present as a non-specific febrile illness without jaundice. Older symptomatic children develop fever, malaise, anorexia, abdominal pain (from a tender enlarged liver), and jaundice. Dark urine (due to urobilinogen) may precede the jaundice.

Diagnosis

Diagnosis is often made on the combination of clinical features and history of exposure, but may be confirmed by measurement of IgM anti-HAV antibody. Serum transaminases and bilirubin levels are elevated.

Treatment

There is no specific treatment. The majority of children have a mild, self-limiting illness and recover within 2–4 weeks. The most serious but rare complication is fulminant hepatic failure.

Active immunization is available and is mostly used

for frequent travellers. Close contacts should be given prophylaxis with intramuscular human normal immunoglobulin (HNIG).

Hepatitis B (HBV)

This is a DNA virus of the Hepadnavirus genus. It is a double-shelled particle with an inner core (HBc) and an outer lipoprotein coat comprising the hepatitis B surface antigen (HBsAg).

Transmission is parenteral via blood and other body fluids. In infants, the most important source of infection is vertical perinatal transmission from infected mothers. Most transmission occurs during or just after birth from exposure to maternal blood. The average incubation period is 20 days.

Serological markers of HBV infection

	HBsAg	Anti-HBs	Anti-HBc IgM	Anti-HBc IgG
acute HBV infection	+	–	+	+
HBV carrier	+	–	+ or –	+
immune: previous infection	–	+ or –	–	+
immune: immunization	–	+	–	–

Fig. 13.5 Serological markers of Hepatitis B (HBV) infection.

Incidence

HBV is an important cause of liver disease worldwide. The prevalence of infection in the population varies globally. In parts of Africa and Asia up to 80% of children are infected by adolescence. In the UK, prevalence is under 2% HBsAg positivity in the indigenous population.

Clinical features

In most children, infection is asymptomatic. Features of acute hepatitis may occur and fulminant hepatic failure occurs in 1% of cases. The most important consequence of infection is the risk of becoming a carrier with subsequent development of cirrhosis or hepatocellular carcinoma. The risk of developing carrier status rises with infection at a young age (reaching 90% in those infected perinatally). Thirty to 50% of carrier children will develop chronic HBV liver disease.

Diagnosis

Diagnosis is dependent on serological testing for antibodies and antigens related to HBV. Acute HBV infection is associated with the presence of HBsAg and IgM antibodies to HBc antigen. Carrier status is defined as HBsAg persisting for more than 6 months. The presence of HBeAg correlates with high infectivity, whereas the presence of antibodies to HBeAg indicates low infectivity (Fig. 13.5).

Management

There is no specific treatment for acute hepatitis B infection at any age. Interferon α treatment is under trial in chronic hepatitis caused by HBV infection.

Prevention

Effective immunization is available and is recommended:

- After perinatal exposure.
- For individuals at risk, e.g. doctors, dentists, or intravenous drug abusers.
- Postexposure, e.g. needlestick injury.

Perinatal exposure

All pregnant women should have antenatal screening for the HBsAg. All babies born to women known to be HBsAg positive should commence a course of hepatitis B vaccine within 24 hours of birth. Unless the mother is known to be anti-HBe positive, the baby should also receive hepatitis B specific immunoglobulin (HBIG).

BACTERIAL INFECTIONS

Staphylococcal infections

The coagulase positive bacterium, *Staphylococcus aureus* is the main pathogen, but coagulase negative bacteria, e.g. *Staphylococcus epidermidis,* are a major problem in Intensive Care Units. Methicillin-resistant *Staphylococcus aureus* (MRSA) causes problems of nosocomial infection (i.e. hospital acquired).

Staphylococcus epidermidis is part of the normal skin flora, and *Staphylococcus aureus* is found in the nares and skin in up to 50% of children. Infections occur when defences are compromised. Many infections are therefore caused by the body's own bacteria, but transmission between individuals occurs with close contact.

Staphylococcus aureus most commonly causes superficial infection such as boils and impetigo, but further invasion and spread leads to deep infections, e.g. of the bones, joints, or lungs (Fig. 13.6). Toxin-producing *Staphylococcus aureus* causes scalded skin syndrome and toxic shock syndrome.

Impetigo
This highly contagious skin infection commonly occurs on the face in infants and young children—especially if there is pre-existing skin disease, e.g. eczema.

Clinical features
Erythematous macules develop into characteristic honey-coloured crusted lesions. Some cases are due to streptococcal infection.

Treatment
Topical antibiotics can be used for mild cases (e.g. mupirocin), but more severe infections require systemic antibiotics (e.g. flucloxacillin). Nasal carriage is an important source of reinfection and can be eradicated by nasal cream containing chlorhexidine and neomycin.

Boils and abscesses
A boil (or furuncle) is an infection of a hair follicle or sweat gland and is usually caused by *Staphylococcus aureus*.

Clinical features
A painful, red, raised, hot lesion develops and usually discharges a purulent exudate heralding spontaneous resolution.

Treatment
Treatment is with systemic antibiotics. Deeper infection may lead to abscess formation in which case incision and drainage are usually required.

Infections caused by *Staphylococcus aureus*	
Direct infection	**Toxin-mediated**
impetigo folliculitis/boils wound infections abscess pneumonia osteomyelitis septic arthritis	toxic shock syndrome scalded skin syndrome food poisoning

Fig. 13.6 Infections caused by *Staphylococcus aureus*.

Osteomyelitis/septic arthritis
See Chapter 20.

Staphylococcal scalded skin syndrome (SSSS)
This is a potentially life-threatening, toxin-mediated manifestation of localized skin infection.

Clinical features
SSSS results from the effect of epidermolytic toxins produced by certain phage types. They cause blistering by disrupting the epidermal granular cell layer. The lesions look like scalds.

Treatment
Management requires attention to fluid balance and treatment with intravenous flucloxacillin.

Streptococcal infections
Streptococci are Gram-positive cocci. Important pathogenic types include:

- Group A β-haemolytic streptococci (*Streptococcus pyogenes*).
- Group B streptococci.
- *Streptococcus pneumoniae* (pneumococcus).

These bacteria are responsible for a number of common and important paediatric diseases which may be caused by:

- Direct infection.
- Toxins.
- Postinfectious immune-mediated mechanisms (acute glomerulonephritis, rheumatic fever).

Infections caused by Streptococci are shown in Fig. 13.7. Most of these are described elsewhere: tonsillitis (see Chapter 16), pneumonia (Chapter 16), meningitis (Chapter 19), glomerulonephritis (Chapter 18), and rheumatic fever (Chapter 15).

Scarlet fever
This occurs in children who have streptococcal pharyngitis. The organism produces a toxin, which causes a characteristic rash.

Clinical features
The clinical features include:

- Tonsillitis.
- Strawberry tongue.
- Palatal petechiae.

Organism	Disease caused
group A Streptococcus	pharyngitis/tonsillitis cellulitis osteomyelitis septicaemia toxin-mediated: • scarlet fever • erysipelas • 'toxic shock-like syndrome'
Streptococcus pneumoniae	otitis media pneumonia meningitis septicaemia
group B Streptococcus	neonatal infection, e.g. pneumonia, meningitis, or septicaemia

Fig. 13.7 Infections caused by Streptococci.

- Rash—a widespread, erythematous rash starting on the trunk that becomes punctate and desquamates on resolution after 7–10 days (flushing of the face is often associated with circumoral pallor).
- Fever.

Diagnosis
Diagnosis is clinical, but can be confirmed by isolation of the streptococcus from a throat swab, and by elevated antistreptolysin 0 titres.

Treatment
Treatment is with penicillin (or erythromycin if the patient has penicillin allergy).

Erysipelas
This intradermal infection is caused by toxin-producing *Streptococcus pyogenes.*

Clinical features
The face or leg is the usual area affected. The skin is dusky and vesicles or bullae may develop.

Diagnosis and treatment
Skin swabs and blood cultures may be negative.

Treatment is with parenteral antibiotics.

Preseptal cellulitis
This presents as unilateral periorbital oedema in a young child usually after an upper respiratory tract infection. Fever may be present. The common pathogens are *Streptococci spp* and *Haemophilus influenzae* (more common in children under 3 years old).

It is important to distinguish this from the less common, but more serious, orbital cellulitis, in which there is proptosis, limitation of ocular movement, and impaired vision.

Treatment is with broad-spectrum antibiotics.

Tuberculosis
Incidence and aetiology
Tuberculosis (TB) remains a major global health problem causing 3–5 million deaths annually. The increasing incidence in patients with HIV, combined with the emergence of multidrug resistant strains of the causative organism, has generated new concern over this age-old public health problem.

Tuberculosis is a disease of the underprivileged and the immunocompromised, and incidence rates in the UK show striking variation between ethnic groups. The highest rate is found in children whose families originated in the Indian subcontinent (India, Pakistan, and Bangladesh), and especially those who were born there.

Tuberculosis is caused by infection with the acid-fast, slow-growing bacillus *Mycobacterium tuberculosis.* Children are usually infected by inhalation of infected droplet nuclei from an adult who is a regular or household contact. Children with the disease (even with active pulmonary disease) are almost always non-infectious.

Clinical features
The clinical features reflect the wide variation in outcomes, which may follow inhalation of the tubercle bacillus, or primary infection. These include the following.

Asymptomatic infection
This is most common. A local inflammatory reaction limits disease progression and the disease becomes latent. Reactivation may subsequently occur.

Symptomatic infection
Multiplication within macrophages occurs at the peripheral alveolar site (the primary or Ghon focus) and the bacilli spread to the regional lymph nodes causing hilar lymphadenopathy. The peripheral lung lesion and

nodes comprise the 'primary or Ghon complex'. Systemic symptoms may then develop including fever, anorexia, weight loss, and cough.

The pulmonary pathology may evolve in several different ways. Bronchial obstruction by enlarged lymph nodes may cause segmental collapse and consolidation. Rarer outcomes include development of a pleural effusion or progressive primary pulmonary TB with cavity formation. Spread in the lymphoid system may lead to cervical, supraclavicular, or axillary lymphadenopathy.

Haematogenous dissemination

In addition to the above intrathoracic events, haematogenous spread probably occurs in most children, although dormant lesions rather than disease occur in these distant sites. Tubercle bacilli may spread to the bones (especially the vertebral column), joints, kidneys, and meninges. Miliary TB is the most severe result of haematogenous spread. It occurs particularly in small infants or immunosuppressed individuals—lesions are found throughout the lungs, liver, spleen, and bone marrow.

Fig. 13.8 shows the clinical course of infection.

Diagnosis

This may be difficult and requires a high index of clinical suspicion supported by tuberculin testing, X-rays, and examination of appropriate specimens by microscopy and culture.

Tuberculin testing

This is done using the Mantoux test in which an intradermal injection of purified protein derivative (PPD) of tuberculin, e.g. 10 units (0.1 ml of 1:1000) is made on the volar aspect of the forearm. The site is read after 48–72 hours by measuring the transverse diameter of indentation in millimetres. A 5 mm diameter reaction is considered positive, especially if risk factors are present. When previous BCG immunization has been carried out, a reaction of 15 mm is indicative of infection.

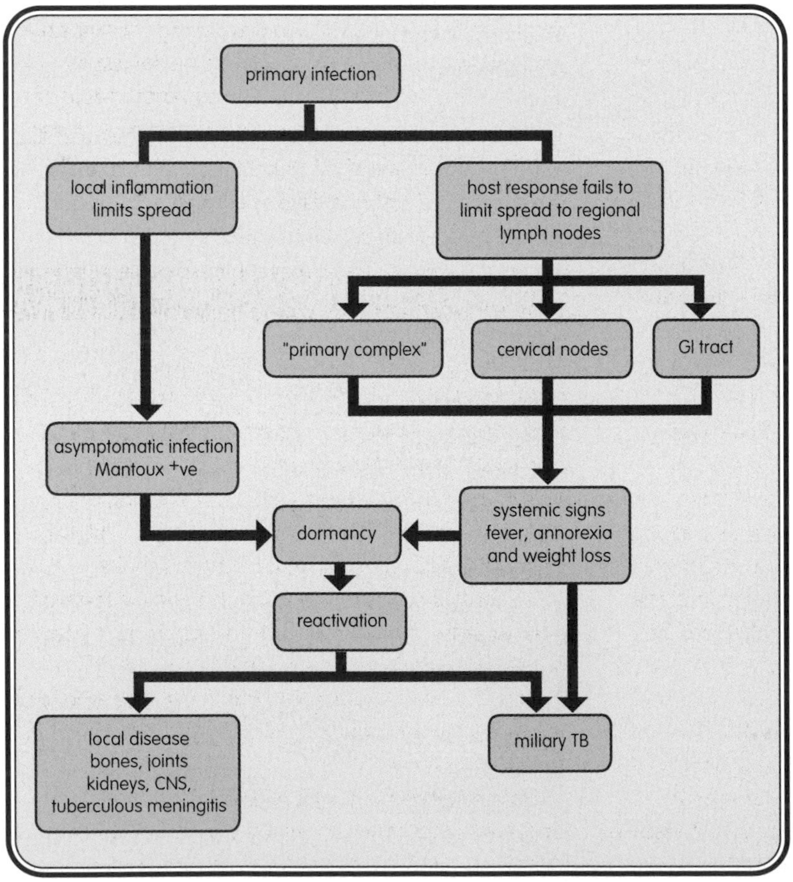

Fig. 13.8 Course of infection in tuberculosis.

Culture and histology
Isolation of *M. tuberculosis* by culture is the 'gold standard', but positive cultures are obtained in a minority of children. Early morning gastric washings on 3 successive days are the best specimens. It takes 6–8 weeks for the bacillus to grow. Microscopy is often negative, but histological examination of a lymph node biopsy may reveal caseating granulomata and acid-fast bacilli.

Radiology
TB is suggested by hilar or mediastinal lymphadenopathy, especially if it is unilateral, or in combination with a 'wedge' of collapse or consolidation. Calcification also suggests TB.

Treatment and prevention
A 6-month triple therapy regimen is most commonly recommended: initially, isoniazid, rifampicin, and pyrazinamide are used. This is usually rationalized to isoniazid and rifampicin after 2 months, by which time antibiotic sensitivities may be known. Resistant strains are still relatively rare in the UK, and it may be possible to predict sensitivities from those of the infecting adult. Asymptomatic at-risk children who are Mantoux positive also require treatment. In this situation, a single agent, e.g. isoniazid may be used.

The most important preventative measures are prompt treatment of infectious cases and thorough contact tracing. Children under 5 years old who are close contacts of a smear-positive adult are at particular risk and should be promptly evaluated with clinical examination, chest X-ray (CXR), and Mantoux test.

The BCG (Bacille–Calmette–Guerin) vaccine has been used in the UK since the 1950s and has been helpful in preventing or modifying TB in the UK. However, its usefulness worldwide is uncertain. BCG is given to infants born into high-risk households, immigrants from countries with high incidence of TB, Mantoux-negative contacts of open TB cases, and tuberculin-negative schoolchildren between 10 and 14 years old. In some areas of the UK, it is recommended for all infants as part of routine vaccination soon after birth or at 1 month.

Typhoid and paratyphoid fever
Typhoid fever is caused by *Salmonella typhi* and paratyphoid by *Salmonella paratyphi*. Both occur worldwide and the main reservoir is humans. These are invasive, systemic infections, in contrast to salmonellosis occurring by infection with *Salmonella enteritidis* or *Salmonella typhimurium*, which usually cause gastroenteritis (food poisoning). Salmonellae are Gram-negative bacilli.

Transmission is by ingestion of food or water contaminated by faeces or urine from an infected person. The incubation period is 1–3 weeks.

Clinical features
The clinical presentation is similar in each case, but paratyphoid fever is milder. Typhoid (enteric) fever is characterized by slow onset of fever, malaise, headache, and constipation. Signs include splenomegaly, relative bradycardia, and a characteristic rash of 'rose spots' on the trunk.

Diagnosis
Diagnosis is made by culture of organisms from the blood (early in the disease) or from stool and urine (after the first week).

Management
Antibiotic treatment is required for at least 14 days. Many organisms acquired in developing countries are resistant to multiple antibiotics but ciprofloxacin is usually effective. Family and close contacts should be screened with stool cultures. Long-term symptomless carriage can occur with a reservoir of infection in the gall bladder and excretion in the faeces.

PARASITIC INFECTIONS

Malaria
Incidence and aetiology
A child under 5 years of age dies of malaria every 12 seconds, most of them in sub-Saharan Africa. With an estimated 40% of humanity at risk of infection and an annual mortality rate of between 1.5 and 2.7 million, malaria remains a major global health problem.

Malaria is caused by infection with any of the four species of the protozoan parasite *Plasmodium*. Most of the several hundred cases of childhood malaria imported to the UK each year are due to *Plasmodium falciparum* which accounts for 85% of malaria seen in travellers to Africa.

Transmission is vector-borne via the female anopheles mosquito. The onset is usually 7–10 days after inoculation but may be delayed by months or even years. The feeding female mosquito injects sporozoites, which pass to the liver via the bloodstream. After asexual multiplication in hepatocytes, they emerge as merozoites, which invade, multiply in, and destroy red cells (some of these form gametocytes which are sucked up by a feeding mosquito). The sexual phase then takes place in the mosquito with formation of a new generation of sporozoites.

Clinical features

Malaria presents with fever, and any child with a fever who has visited a malarious area in the preceding year should be considered to have malaria until proven otherwise. Non-specific symptoms include headache, rigors, abdominal and muscle pains, cough, diarrhoea, and vomiting. Common misdiagnoses include viral influenza, gastroenteritis, or hepatitis.

Apart from the fever, which is rarely periodic, there are no consistent clinical signs. Splenomegaly, anaemia, and jaundice may all occur and a number of signs characterize the severe complication of algid malaria (shock), cerebral malaria (coma, fits), or blackwater fever (haemoglobinuria and renal failure).

Diagnosis

Diagnosis is made by the examination of thick and thin blood films. The former allows rapid scanning of a larger volume of blood per microscopic field. Both the species and the percentage of parasitaemia should be determined. Parasitaemia >2% indicates moderately severe infection. Thrombocytopenia is common.

Management

Children with confirmed or suspected falciparum malaria require hospitalization and treatment with quinine. This is given orally in uncomplicated disease or intravenously if the parasite count is high or complications are present.

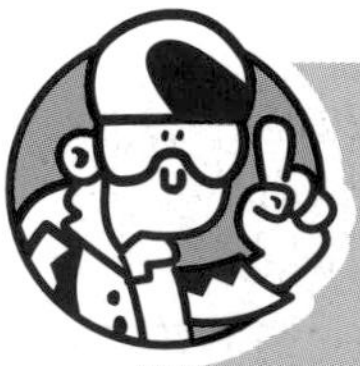

Fever in a child who has been to a malarious area is malaria until proven otherwise:

- **Most cases are falciparum.**
- ***Plasmodium falciparum* requires treatment with quinine.**

G6PD status should be considered because deficiency is a contraindication to some antimalarials.

Worms (nematodes)

There are four important nematodes that infect children:

- *Enterobius vermicularis* (pinworm or threadworm).
- *Ascaris lumbricoides* (roundworm).
- *Ancylostoma duodenale* (hookworm).
- *Toxocara canis.*

Threadworm

This is very common in preschool children. Transmission is via the faecal–oral route. Adult female worms lay their eggs in the perianal area. Scratching results in eggs being carried under the fingernails to the mouth and auto-infection.

Clinical features

Children present with perianal pruritus, vulvovaginitis, irritability, and anorexia.

The worms appear like white cotton threads and may be seen at the anus.

Diagnosis

Diagnosis may be made by applying transparent adhesive tape to the perianal region in the morning and examining the tape for eggs with a magnifying glass.

Management

Treatment is with two doses of piperazine or a single dose of mebendazole (for children over 2 years). Reinfection is common and can be reduced by keeping fingernails short and wearing close-fitting pants. Family members should be treated even if asymptomatic.

Toxocariasis

Human toxocariasis is mainly caused by infection with *Toxocariasis canis,* a common gut parasite of dogs. Toxocara eggs are ingested when a child eats soil, play-pit sand, or unwashed vegetables contaminated with infective dog or cat faeces.

Clinical features

There are two distinct forms of disease:

- Visceral larva migrans (VLM)—characterized by fever, hepatomegaly, wheezing, and eosinophilia.
- Occular larva migrans—a granulomatous reaction in the retina causing a squint or reduced visual acuity.

Management
Treatment is with thiabendazole for VLM and steroids for the eye disease.

Toxocara infection could be prevented by regular de-worming of cats and dogs and avoidance of defecation in public places including sandpits.

KAWASAKI DISEASE

Kawasaki disease (KD) is an uncommon systemic vasculitis is also called mucocutaneous lymph node syndrome. Early diagnosis is important because early treatment may prevent the lethal cardiac complications.

Incidence
It was first described in Japan in 1967 and affects children mainly between the age of 6 months and 4 years (peak at 1 year). It is much more common in children of Asian origin. In the UK the incidence is 3–4 cases per 100 000.

Clinical features
The aetiology is unknown but the disease process is a vasculitis affecting the small and medium vessels including, most importantly, the coronary arteries leading to aneurysm formation. Subsequent scar formation causes vessel narrowing, myocardial ischaemia, or even infarction, and occasionally, sudden death. A bacterial toxin acting as a 'superantigen' may trigger the vasculitis.

Diagnosis
The diagnosis is based on clinical criteria which emerge sequentially. Five out of six are required to make a confident diagnosis (Fig. 13.9).

The differential diagnosis includes measles, scarlet fever, rubella, roseola, and fifth disease.

The following investigations are undertaken if KD is suspected:

- FBC, ESR.
- U&sE, liver function tests.
- Throat swab and ASOT.
- Blood cultures and viral titres.
- Echocardiography.
- ECG.

Thrombocytosis, although common, is a late feature and therefore unhelpful in establishing the diagnosis.

Diagnostic criteria for Kawasaki disease

fever for 5 days or more
bilateral (non-purulent) conjunctival injection
rash—polymorphous
lips—red, dry, or cracked and strawberry tongue
extremities:
- reddening of palms and soles
- indurative oedema of hands and feet
- peeling of skin on hands and feet (convalescent phase)

cervical lymphadenopathy—often unilateral, non-purulent

Fig. 13.9 Diagnostic criteria for Kawasaki disease.

In developed countries, KD is now the most common cause of acquired heart disease in children.

Echocardiography is undertaken to detect coronary artery aneurysm formation. These occur in 30% of cases and typically develop within the first 4–6 weeks of the illness. This investigation is repeated at intervals during the first year.

Treatment
The most effective treatment involves a single dose of IV immunoglobulin (2 g/kg). This reduces both the incidence and severity of coronary artery aneurysm formation if given within the first 10 days.

Aspirin is given concurrently to reduce the risk of thrombosis at a high dose initially (100 mg/kg/day in divided doses) until the pyrexia has resolved. A low dose (3–5 mg/kg/day) is continued for 6–8 weeks.

Further insight into the pathophysiology of the disease is needed before significant advances in management are likely to be made.

Early recognition of Kawasaki disease is vital to reduce the risk of cardiac complications: The fever is often unresponsive to antipyretics. Characteristically, the child is extremely miserable.

IMMUNODEFICIENCY

This can be classified into:

- Primary—in which there is an inherited, intrinsic defect in the immune system.
- Secondary—in which a defect in the immune system has been acquired, as occurs in: malnutrition, infections (e.g. HIV, measles), immunosuppressive therapy (e.g. steroids, cytotoxic drugs), hyposplenism (e.g. sickle-cell disease, splenectomy).

In acquired immunodeficiency, the cause is usually self-evident. Primary immunodeficiency should be suspected in the following clinical circumstances:

- An excess of infections: this is manifest by severe, unusual, or persistent infections, or infections with unusual organisms.
- Unexplained failure to thrive.
- Chronic diarrhoea.

See Hints & Tips for infections associated with immunodeficiency, and Fig. 13.10 for specific susceptibility conferred by particular defects.

Primary immunodeficiencies

These may be inherited as X-linked (affecting boys) or autosomal recessive disorders. Examples are given below.

X-linked agammaglobulinaemia (Bruton's disease)

There is a failure of B cell development and immunoglobulin production. It presents with severe bacterial infections in the first 2 years of life.

Severe combined immunodeficiency (SCID)

A heterogeneous group of disorders with profoundly defective cellular and humoral immunity (hence the name, 'combined'). It presents in the first 6 months of life with failure to thrive, diarrhoea, candidal infections, and recurrent, severe, and unusual infections.

Common variable immunodeficiency (CVID)

This term encompasses a heterogeneous group of patients who have low levels of serum IgG and IgA. Usually present in late childhood with recurrent bacterial infection of sinuses or lungs.

Selective IgA deficiency

This is common (1:700 population). Most people with complete absence of IgA are asymptomatic. It may be associated with autoimmune diseases and IgG subclass deficiency. Children deficient in IgG_2, the subclass providing immunity against polysaccharide antigens, may be susceptible to infection with encapsulated organisms (e.g. *Streptococcus pneumoniae, Haemophilus influenzae* type b).

Chronic granulomatous disease

An inherited disorder, usually X-linked, in which phagocytic cells fail to produce superoxide anion. It presents with repeated bacterial and fungal infections involving the skin, lymph nodes, lungs, liver, and bones. Granulomas and abscesses form in these sites. Diagnosis is confirmed by failure to reduce nitroblue tetrazolium (NBT test).

Management for primary immunodeficiency is outlined in Fig. 13.11.

Immune defects and corresponding susceptibility	
Defect	**Susceptibility**
antibody	bacteria: *Pneumococcus, Staphylococcus, Streptococcus, Haemophilus influenzae* viruses: enteroviruses
cell-mediated	viruses: herpes viruses, measles fungi: *Candida, Aspergillus, Pneumocystis carinii* bacteria: *Mycobacteria, Listeria*
neutrophil function	bacteria: Gram-positive, Gram-negative fungi: *Candida, Aspergillus*

Fig. 13.10 Immune defects and corresponding susceptibility.

Management of primary immunodeficiency

The following treatment options are available:

- antibiotic prophylaxis, e.g. co-trimoxazole, to prevent *Pneumocystis carinii* infection
- vigorous antibiotic therapy for infections
- immunoglobulin replacement therapy—regular IV immunoglobulin can be given for severe defects in antibody production
- bone marrow transplantation
- gene therapy—this has been successfully performed for SCID caused by adenosine deaminase deficiency

Fig. 13.11 Management of primary immunodeficiency.

Secondary immunodeficiency

Immunosuppressive therapy

Therapeutic drugs, which cause immunosuppression, include:

- Cytotoxic agents.
- Steroids.

Cytotoxic chemotherapy for malignant disease (e.g. acute leukaemia) causes immunosuppression due to marrow suppression and neutropenia. Febrile children with neutrophil counts less than 0.5×10^9/L are at risk for serious and potentially fatal bacterial and fungal infection.

Children on high-dose corticosteroids (e.g. for nephrotic syndrome) are particularly at risk for disseminated chickenpox infection. Children with organ transplants are prone to infection with cytomegalovirus.

Infection

Worldwide, the two most important infections, which cause immunodeficiency, are:

- Measles.
- HIV infection.

Paediatric HIV infection

Human immunodeficiency virus Type 1 (HIV-1), the causative agent of acquired immunodeficiency syndrome (AIDS) is transmitted to infants and children by vertical transmission from HIV-infected women or by HIV-contaminated blood or blood products.

Incidence

The WHO estimates that 20 million adults and 1.5 million children have been infected with HIV since the pandemic began.

Transmission

The main route of transmission to children is vertically from mother to child, either intrauterine, intrapartum, or via breastfeeding. Transmission rates vary with geographical area: lower in Europe and higher in Africa.

Diagnosis

All newborns born to HIV-infected women will have circulating maternal HIV antibodies, but only a proportion of these are infected with the virus. Passively acquired antibody disappears at 15–18 months of age so this is not a reliable test for infection under 18 months.

Three approaches exist for diagnosis in children younger than 18 months:

- Detection of viral p24 antigen.
- HIV viral culture—the gold standard, but not widely available.
- Detection of viral genome by polymerase chain reaction.

Clinical manifestations—progression to AIDS

The incubation period from infection to disease varies, but appears to be shorter in perinatally infected children than in adults. There are two patterns reflecting the degree of immunosuppression:

- Up to 25% of infected children progress to AIDS or die in the first year.
- The remainder progress more slowly.

Changes in immune function are shown in Fig. 13.12, and the clinical manifestations in Fig. 13.13.

Management

Cotrimoxazole prophylaxis against *Pneumocystis carinii* pneumonia is given for children with HIV infection. The primary immunization course should be given. BCG should only be considered for uninfected infants born to HIV-positive mothers from countries with high TB prevalence.

Immunological test results in AIDS

- reduced CD4 to CD8 T cell ratio or low CD4 levels for age
- high immunoglobulin levels, especially IgG (although levels are high, antibodies formed are dysfunctional)

Fig. 13.12 Immunological test results in AIDS.

Clinical manifestations of HIV infection in children		
Category	**Severity**	**Manifestation**
category N	asymptomatic	
category A	mild	lymphadenopathy hepatosplenomegaly parotitis
category B	moderate	severe bacterial infection chronic diarrhoea candidiasis lymphocytic interstitial pneumonitis (LIP)
category C	severe (AIDS)	wasting (severe failure to thrive) opportunistic infections, e.g. pneumocystic carinii pneumonia (PCP) encephalopathy severe bacterial infections malignancy (rare)

Fig. 13.13 Clinical manifestations of HIV infection in children.

Antiretroviral treatment with AZT (in combination with didanosine or zalcitabine) is recommended when the child becomes symptomatic or there is a rapid fall in the CD4 count.

Intravenous immunoglobulin is given in some centres to reduce the incidence of bacterial infections, but its efficacy is uncertain.

Coordinated psychological and social support for the whole family is a vital aspect of managing an HIV infected child.

Issues include:

- Telling children their diagnosis.
- Retaining confidentiality.
- Two (mother and child) members of the family may be sick or dying at the same time.
- Social or cultural isolation.
- Stigma of diagnosis.

Prevention

Zidovudine, given to the mother in pregnancy and during delivery and to the neonate for the first 6 weeks of life reduces the risk of vertical transmission of HIV-1. Antenatal HIV testing therefore confers potential benefits. Education campaigns can reduce but not eliminate the spread of HIV. Development of an effective vaccine remains a high priority.

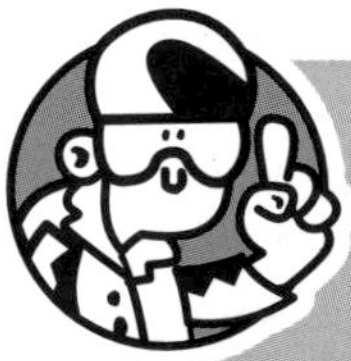

Suspect immunodeficiency in the following circumstances:

- **Recurrent bacterial lower respiratory tract infections.**
- **Bronchiectasis.**
- **Chronic otitis media.**
- **Recurrent or chronic skin infections.**
- **Recurrent or chronic candidal infections.**

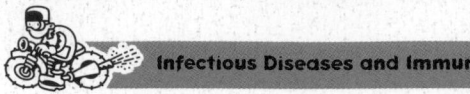

14. Skin Disorders

ECZEMA (DERMATITIS)

The term dermatitis refers to an inflammation of the skin and is synonymous with eczema. (The word 'eczema' literally means to 'to boil over').

Three main varieties occur in infants and children:

- Infantile seborrhoeic eczema.
- Atopic eczema.
- Napkin dermatitis.

Infantile seborrhoeic eczema

This mild condition presents in the first 2 months of life with a scaly, non-itchy rash initially on the scalp ('cradle cap') which may spread to involve the face, flexures, and napkin area (Fig. 14.1).

Treatment is with emollients and mild topical steroids.

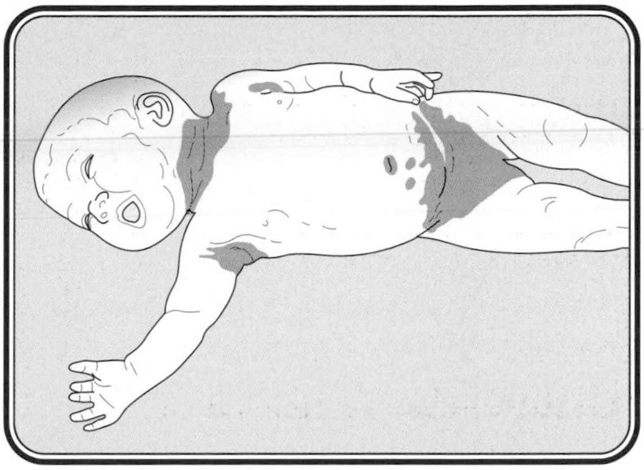

Fig. 14.1 Distribution of infantile seborrhoeic eczema.

Atopic eczema

Atopic eczema is very common and affects 5–10% of children, usually beginning in the first 2 years of life. There is often a family history of atopic disorders (eczema, asthma, and hay fever), reflecting a genetic predisposition that confers an abnormal immune response to environmental allergens.

Clinical features

A dry, red itchy rash occurs which usually starts on, and has a predilection for, the extensor surfaces and face in infants and young children, and the flexures (the antecubital and popliteal fossae) in older children (Fig. 14.2). However, the skin appearance may vary from an acute, weeping papulovesicular eruption to the chronic, dry, scaly, thickened (lichenified) skin that develops, in older children. Itching is the most important and troublesome symptom.

Affected children may have an eosinophilia and raised plasma IgE concentration. Histopathological changes include epidermal oedema and vesicle formation, vascular dilatation, and cellular infiltration.

Diagnosis

The diagnosis is clinical (see Fig. 14.3 for a comparison of atopic and infantile seborrhoeic eczema). Allergy tests (on skin or blood) are unhelpful as multiple positive reactions are usually seen.

Management

This includes:

- Important general measures.
- Topical preparations.
- Specific treatment for complications such as secondary infection.

General measures

Advice should be given on avoiding aggravating factors such as:

- Synthetic or woollen fabrics (cotton clothes are preferable).
- Biological detergents or fabric conditioners.
- Cigarette smoke.
- Dander from furry pets.
- House dust.
- Grass pollen.

Nails should be kept short and excessive heat avoided.

Topical preparations

The mainstays of management are:

- Emollients.
- Topical steroids.

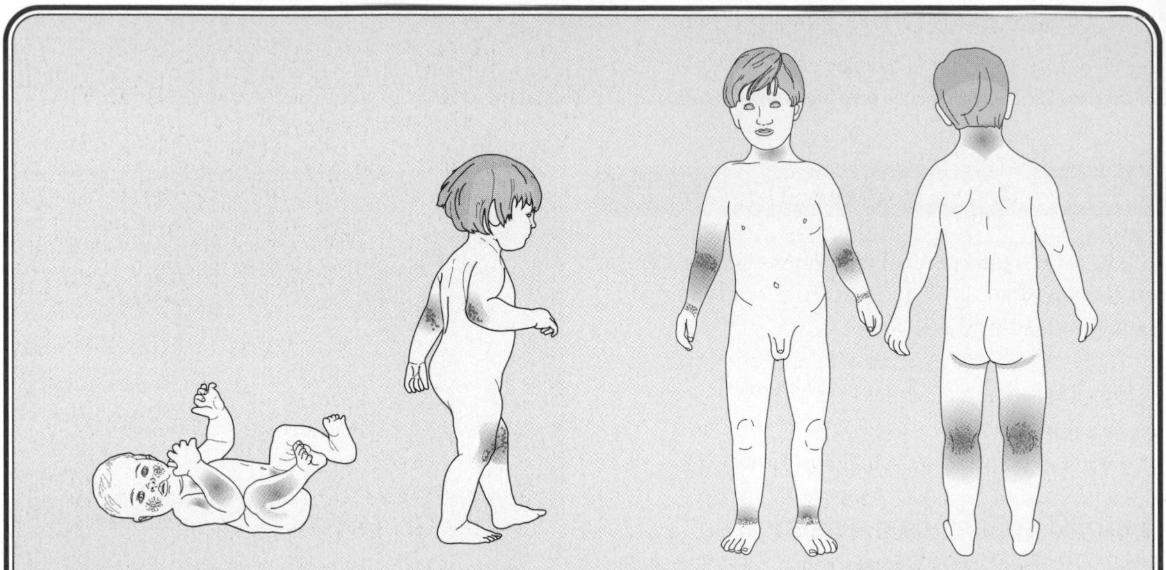

Fig. 14.2 Distribution of atopic eczema.

Emollients moisturise and soften the skin. They are safe and should be used frequently. A daily bath using bath oil and aqueous cream as a soap substitute is advisable, with regular application of an emollient two or three times daily.

Mild topical steroids such as 1% hydrocortisone (ointment rather than cream when the skin is dry) applied to the affected areas twice daily are highly effective. More potent preparations can be used short-term for exacerbations.

Oral antihistamines are useful, especially at night, to reduce itching and help sleep. An exclusion diet (avoidance of dairy products) should be used only in the very young with severe eczema that has proved unresponsive to standard approaches to treatment.

Complications

The most important is secondary infection with either viruses or bacteria. Infection with herpes simplex (eczema herpeticum) is potentially serious and should be treated with aciclovir. Bacterial superinfection is usually caused by staphylococci or streptococci and requires systemic antibiotic treatment.

By the age of 5 years, the eczema in more than half

Differences between infantile seborrhoeic eczema and atopic eczema

	Infantile seborrhoeic eczema	Atopic eczema
age	<3 months (usually)	>3 months (usually)
sleeping	unaffected	disturbed
pruritus	nil	significant
family history of atopy	usually negative	often positive
course	self-limiting	chronic, relapsing

Fig. 14.3 Differences between infantile seborrhoeic eczema and atopic eczema.

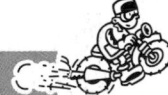

of these children will have resolved. However, a significant proportion will develop other manifestations of atopy such as asthma or hay fever.

Napkin dermatitis

Rashes in the napkin area are common and may be due to:

- An irritant contact dermatitis (nappy rash).
- Candidiasis.
- Seborrhoeic dermatitis.

Clinical features

Nappy rash

Ordinary nappy rash is due to the prolonged contact of urine and faeces with skin. Particular causes include skin wetness, ammonia from the breakdown of urine by faecal enzymes. The skin is red, moist, and may ulcerate. The inguinal folds are spared.

Nappy rash can be prevented by frequent nappy changes (easier with disposable nappies), and barrier creams such as zinc and castor oil cream. Exposure may hasten recovery, but it is impractical to implement this at home.

Candidiasis

Candidiasis is also common and is distinguished by bright red skin with satellite lesions and involvement of the skin folds.

Candidal infection may be treated with an anticandidal and hydrocortisone preparation such as miconazole with hydrocortisone.

INFECTIONS

Bacterial

Bacterial infections of the skin in children include common and important entities such as:

- Impetigo.
- Boils and furuncles.
- Staphylococcal scalded skin syndrome.
- Erysipelas.

These are considered in Chapter 13.

Viral

Viral warts

Hands and feet

The human papilloma virus (HPV) causes viral warts.

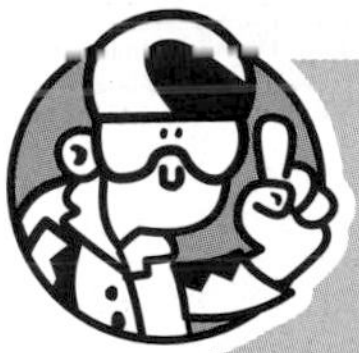

Causes of an 'itchy' rash:

- **Atopic eczema**
- **Scabies**
- **Papular urticaria**
- **Urticaria (hives)**
- **Chickenpox**

Two types are seen:

- Skin warts are common on the fingers and soles in school age children.
- Plantar warts (verrucae) are flat, hyperkeratotic lesions on the soles of the feet.

Most viral warts resolve within a year when immunity develops.

Treatment options include:

- Salicylic and lactic acid paint.
- Cryotherapy with liquid nitrogen.

Repeat treatments over many weeks are required.

Other sites

Viral warts also occur in other locations:

- Laryngeal papillomas are found on the vocal cords.
- Genital warts (condylomata acuminata) are papular or frond-like growths in the perineal area. In young children, these may be a sign of sexual abuse.

Molluscum contagiosum

This common eruption in children is caused by the *Molluscipoxvirus.*

Clinical features

Smooth, pearly papules with an obvious central dimple arise in crops (often on the trunk). They are not irritating and of low infectivity.

Management

They resolve spontaneously without scarring usually within 6 months to 2 years and treatment is not required.

Fungal

These include the dermatophytosis (ringworm) and candidiasis (thrush).

Dermatophytoses (tinea capitis, corporis, pedis, and unguium)

Dermatophytes are filamentous fungi that infect the outer layer of the skin and also the hair and nails. They also affect some animal species (e.g. cattle and cats).

Clinical features

Clinical features vary with the site of infection.

Tinea capitis (scalp ringworm)

On the scalp, tinea causes patchy alopecia and occasionally a boggy inflammatory mass called a kerion.

Tinea corporis (body ringworm)

On the trunk, tinea appears as annular lesions with central clearing and a palpable, erythematous border.

Tinea pedis (athlete's foot)

This presents as itchy, scaling, and cracking of the skin of the feet, especially between the toes.

Diagnosis

Examination under ultraviolet light (Wood's) shows a green–yellow fluorescence of infected hairs with certain fungal species. Diagnosis can be made by microscopic examination of skin scrapings for fungal hyphae. Culture of the organism is definitive.

Treatment

This varies with the severity of infection:

- Mild infections are treated with topical antifungal preparations such as clotrimazole or miconazole.
- Severe infections require systemic treatment with griseofulvin for several weeks.

Candidiasis (thrush, moniliasis)

Candida albicans, a yeast (budding, unicellular organism), is the most common pathogen. The organism colonizes the skin and mucous membranes. Transmission is via person-to-person contact, contaminated feeding bottles, etc.

Clinical features

In infants, candidal infections frequently involve the oral cavity (thrush) or the napkin area. It is acquired from the mother's vaginal flora. It may also affect the nipples of breastfeeding mothers.

Diagnosis

Diagnosis is clinical:

- Oral thrush presents as white plaques on the tongue and buccal mucosa.
- Monilial dermatitis: localized shiny redness typically affecting moist areas and *not* sparing flexural skin creases (this may occur in the absence of oral thrush).

Management

Topical nystatin is first line therapy. Oral treatment should be given as well as direct treatment to lesions in perineal disease.

Prevention requires good hygiene and rigorous disinfection of feeding bottles and dummies.

Chronic or recurrent mucocutaneous candidiasis should raise the suspicion of immunodeficiency.

INFESTATIONS

Papular urticaria

This term describes crops of itchy, erythematous papules or small blisters. They are caused by insect bites, most commonly by the fleas or mites from domestic dogs or cats. Bedbugs may also be the culprits. Secondary infection may occur.

Scabies

Scabies is caused by the mite, *Sarcoptes scabei.* It is transmitted by prolonged skin-to-skin contact. In the first infestation, the incubation period may be up to 8 weeks. The fertilized adult female mite burrows deep in the stratum corneum laying two or three eggs a day until she dies after about 5 weeks. The eggs hatch after a few days and larvae move on to the skin surface, maturing into adults in 10–14 days.

Clinical features

The first symptom is pruritus, worse at night, which is related to hypersensitivity to the mite or its faeces. The presence of burrows is pathognomonic. Common sites for burrows are the interdigital webs and the anterior aspects of the wrists. In infants, the soles of the feet, head and neck are commonly affected.

The rash consists of vesicles, weals, and papules which may become excoriated and secondarily infected.

Diagnosis
Diagnosis is clinical and may (if necessary) be confirmed by identification of mites or ova in scrapings from burrows or vesicles.

Treatment
Treatment is with lindane (1% gamma benzene hydrochloride) or malathion 0.5% in infants. These scabicides are applied on 2 consecutive days, and all close contacts should be treated with lotion covering the body from the neck downwards. In infants, the scalp and face should be included. Laundering of clothes and bedding is important.

It can take several weeks for the pruritus to subside after successful treatment as hypersensitivity persists. This can be managed with oral antihistamines and topical steroids.

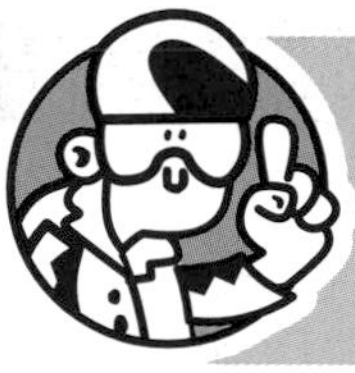

Itchy rash in the family—is it scabies?

Head lice (pediculosis capitis)
Pediculosis humanus capitis is a blood-sucking arthropod that infests the scalps of up to 10% of school children in some urban areas. Transmission is by head-to-head contact. The head louse prefers clean hair and does not discriminate between social groups.

Clinical features and diagnosis
The louse egg (nit) is attached to the base of the scalp hair and is visible as a small, white, grain-like particle. Eggs hatch after a week and the louse lives for 2–3 months. Many infestations are asymptomatic, but the most common manifestation is severe itching of the scalp often accompanied by enlarged cervical lymph nodes. The presence of nits is diagnostic.

Treatment
Treatment is with 0.5% malathion lotion which should be left on for 12 hours. The hair is then washed with ordinary shampoo and the dead nits removed with a metal fine-toothed comb. All the family should be treated. Clothing and bedding is disinfected by machine washing (cycles over 50°C inactivate lice and nits).

OTHER CHILDHOOD SKIN DISEASES

Pityriasis rosea
This common, acute, benign, and self-limiting condition is thought to be of viral origin. It begins with a 'herald patch', an oval or round, scaly, erythematous macule on the trunk, neck, or proximal part of limbs. This is followed within 1–3 days by a shower of smaller dull pink macules on the trunk in a so-called 'Christmas tree' pattern following the lines of the ribs. Spontaneous resolution occurs within 6–8 weeks.

No treatment is required.

Acne vulgaris
This is a chronic inflammatory disorder of the sebaceous glands and probably reflects an abnormal response to circulating androgens. It is an almost universal problem of adolescence, peaking in severity at age 16–18 years.

Clinical features
A variety of lesions occur on the face and upper trunk. Characteristically, comedones occur: plugs of keratin and sebum within the dilated orifice of a hair follicle. These may be open (blackheads) or closed (whiteheads). These progress to papules and pustules (bacterial superinfection) and in severe cases to cystic and nodular lesions, which may cause scarring.

Treatment
Treatment options include:

- Topical treatment with keratolytic agents, e.g. benzoyl peroxide.
- Ultraviolet light therapy: exposure to natural sunlight should be encouraged.
- Oral antibiotics: low-dose therapy with minocycline, oxytetracycline, or erythromycin is useful for moderate to severe pustular acne. Antibiotics are given for at least 3 months.
- Vitamin A analogue, 13-*cis*-retinoic acid: for severe acne that has not responded to conventional treatment.

Urticaria (hives)
Urticaria is a transient, itchy, erythematous rash characterized by the presence of raised weals (hives). It is induced by mast cell degranulation, in which histamine and other vasoactive mediators are released

causing vasodilatation and an increase in capillary permeability.

In childhood, most cases are acute and no cause is identified, although precipitating factors should be sought in the history.

Clinical features

It may be accompanied by oedema of the lips and eyes (angioedema). Involvement of the lips and tongue is an emergency because there is a risk of respiratory obstruction. Chronic urticaria may occur and usually clears spontaneously in about 6 months.

Management

Acute urticaria usually resolves spontaneously within a few hours. If itchy, it can be treated with an antihistamine, e.g. chlorpheniramine maleate. Precipitating factors should be avoided.

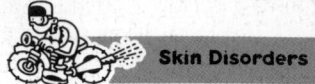

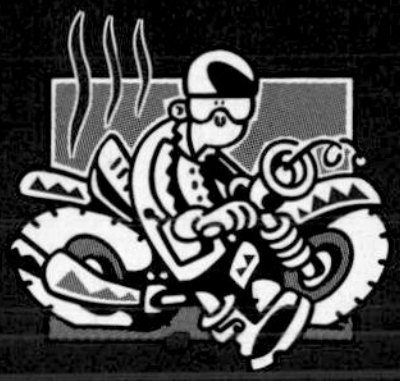

15. Cardiovascular Disorders

In developed countries, congenital heart disease (CHD) accounts for the majority of cardiovascular problems in infants and children. Worldwide, rheumatic fever remains the most important acquired form of heart disease. Ischaemic heart disease is rare in contrast to its incidence in adults, although it may occur in Kawasaki disease. Arrhythmias are very rare, with the exception of supraventricular tachycardias (SVTs). Important infections, affecting the cardiovascular system (CVS) are infective endocarditis and viral myocarditis.

CONGENITAL HEART DISEASE

This comprises the most common group of structural malformations affecting 6–8 out of 1000 live born infants. A number of important causative factors are recognized (Fig. 15.1), but in the majority, the cause is unknown.

CHD presents or may be diagnosed in a limited number of ways. These include:

- Antenatal diagnosis by ultrasound.
- Heart murmur.
- Cyanosis.
- Shock—low cardiac output.
- Cardiac failure (see Chapter 2).

Although there are over 100 different cardiac malformations, a small number account for the majority of cases (Fig. 15.2). These are conveniently classified into:

- Acyanotic forms.
- Cyanotic forms.

Initial evaluation should include a chest X-ray (CXR) and electrocardiogram (ECG), although these investigations do not usually provide a lesion diagnosis. Diagnosis is usually achieved by a combination of echocardiography including Doppler ultrasound.

Common investigations are shown in Fig. 15.3.

Acyanotic congenital heart disease

These are represented by lesions that allow blood to shunt from the left to the right sides of the circulation, or which obstruct flow due to the narrowing of a valve or vessel.

Causes of congenital heart disease

Genetic chromosomal disorders
- Down syndrome, e.g. atrioventricular septal defect
- Turner syndrome, e.g. aortic stenosis, coarctation of aorta
- chromosome 22 deletions
- Williams syndrome, e.g. supravalvular aortic stenosis

Teratogens
- congenital rubella, e.g. PDA, pulmonary stenosis
- alcohol, e.g. ASD, VSD

Fig. 15.1 Causes of congenital heart disease.

Common forms of congenital heart disease

Type	Name	Abbreviation	% of CHD
acyanotic	ventricular septal defect	VSD	32
	patent ductus arteriosus	PDA	12
	pulmonary stenosis	PS	8
	atrial septal defect	ASD	6
	coarctation of the aorta	COA	6
	aortic stenosis	AS	5
cyanotic	tetralogy of Fallot	—	6
	transposition of the great arteries	TGA	5

Fig. 15.2 Common forms of CHD.

Investigations in congenital heart disease	
Investigation	**Demonstrates**
CXR	cardiac shadow—may be enlarged or abnormal lung fields—pulmonary vascular markings may be: increased (plethora): signifiant L to R shunt, e.g. VSD decreased (oligaemia): reduced pulmonary blood flow, e.g. pulmonary stenosis
ECG	rate and rhythm of heart mean QRS axis hypertrophy of either ventricle
echocardiogram	precise anatomical abnormality
cardiac catheter	physiological/haemodynamic status rather than anatomy

Fig. 15.3 Investigations in CHD.

Left to right shunts (L to R)

Atrial septal defect (ASD)

There are two types of ASD:

- The most common ASD (6:10 000 live births) is a foramen secundum defect, high in the atrial septum. It is more common in girls (F:M = 2:1) and accounts for 6% of all cases of CHD.
- Much less common is the ostium primum type which occurs lower in the atrial septum (often associated with mitral regurgitation), and is a common defect in Down syndrome.

Secundum defects are usually asymptomatic in childhood. The L to R shunt develops very slowly and pulmonary hypertension is extremely uncommon.

Clinical features

The clinical features include:

- Abnormal right ventricular impulse.
- Widely split and fixed second sound (S2).
- Tricuspid flow murmur—rumbling mid-diastolic murmur at the left sternal edge.
- Pulmonary flow murmur—soft, ejection systolic murmur in the pulmonary area.

There is *no* murmur generated by the low velocity flow across the ASD. A significant L to R shunt generates flow murmurs at the tricuspid and pulmonary valves.

Diagnosis

The CXR shows pulmonary plethora and the ECG shows right ventricular hypertrophy with incomplete right bundle branch block.

Management

Treatment is surgical. Elective closure, which is low risk, should be carried out after about 7 years of age.

Ventricular septal defect (VSD)

Most are single, but multiple defects do occur and other heart defects coexist in about one third of children.

The natural history and prognosis depends on the:

- Size and position of the defect.
- Development of changes due to blood shunting from left to right through the defect. This includes narrowing of the right ventricular outflow tract and progressive pulmonary hypertension, both of which reduce the size of the shunt.

The clinical features, treatment, and outcome are best considered separately for the different sizes of defect.

Small VSD (maladie de Roger)

The child is asymptomatic and the murmur is often first noted on routine examination. The only abnormality is a pansystolic murmur (sometimes with a palpable thrill) at the lower left sternal border.

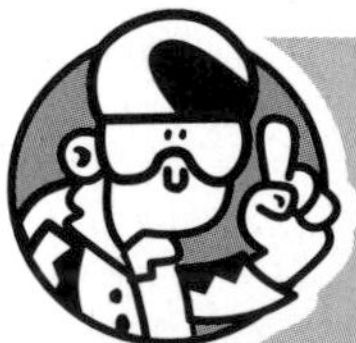

A ventricular septal defect is the most common variety of congenital heart disease. It accounts for one-third of all cases.

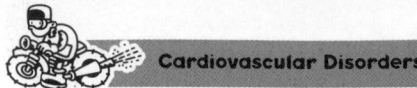

Antibiotic prophylaxis against bacterial endocarditis is necessary for dental extractions, but no other treatment is required. Spontaneous closure may occur.

Medium VSD

These usually present with symptoms during infancy including slow weight gain, difficulty with feeding and recurrent chest infections. In time, symptoms may actually disappear due to relative or actual closure of the defect.

On examination, there may be:

- An increased cardiac impulse.
- Palpable thrill.
- Harsh pansystolic murmur, loudest in the third and fourth left intercostal spaces.

If the pulmonary blood flow is high, a mid-diastolic murmur occurs due to blood flow across the normal mitral valve.

A CXR will show moderate cardiac enlargement, a prominent pulmonary artery, and increased vascularity of the lungs. Echocardiography will show the position of the defect. The shunt is measured by Doppler studies.

Heart failure, if present, should be treated with diuretics. In many of the children, spontaneous improvement occurs and surgical correction can be avoided. However, if there is still evidence of a significant shunt at 4 years closure, should be considered before the child starts school.

Large VSD

Heart failure develops early on, especially if a chest infection occurs. The cardiac signs are similar, but it is worth noting that the systolic murmur may be soft in a very large defect.

Initial medical treatment of the heart failure is required and surgical closure under cardiopulmonary bypass is usually necessary. In young infants with multiple defects, banding of the pulmonary artery allows a temporary respite until the child is big enough for definitive correction.

An example of a VSD is shown in Fig. 15.4.

Patent ductus arteriosus (PDA)

In this condition, the ductus arteriosus remains patent instead of closing soon after birth. It is most commonly seen in preterm infants during the neonatal period (PDA seen in newborn Intensive Care Units is caused by hypoxia and prematurity, and is a distinct entity from congenital PDA in term infants—see Chapter 27.)

Clinical features

A shunt develops between the aorta and pulmonary artery. The clinical features include:

- 'Bounding' pulses—wide pulse pressure.
- Murmur—initially 'systolic'. As pulmonary vascular resistance falls a continuous run-off from the aorta to the pulmonary artery occurs with a continuous 'machinery' murmur.

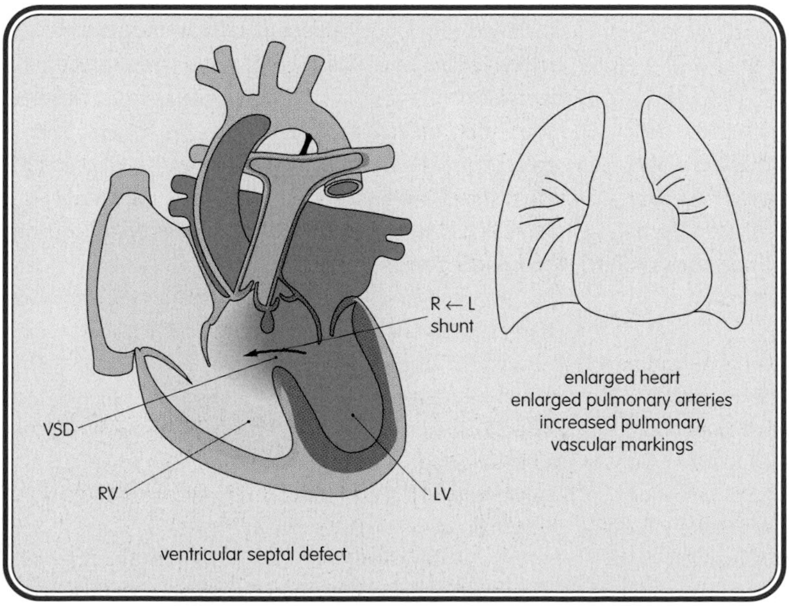

Fig. 15.4 Ventricular septal defect and chest X-ray changes.

A small duct may be asymptomatic. If the duct is large a significant L to R shunt develops as pulmonary vascular resistance falls and cardiac failure occurs.

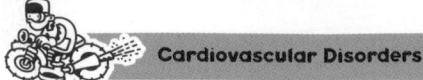

Diagnosis

CXR and ECG changes with a large symptomatic PDA are similar to those seen in a patient with a large VSD. The CXR shows cardiomegaly and increased pulmonary vascular markings.

A PDA can be directly visualized by two-dimensional echocardiography and the ductal shunt can be confirmed by Doppler ultrasound.

Management

Surgical closure is recommended. (In symptomatic preterm infants, medical treatment is an option.)

> **The risk of developing pulmonary vascular disease or infective endocarditis is higher in PDA than VSD and surgical closure is recommended for all PDAs. This can be achieved by division, ligation, or transvenous umbrella occlusion.**

Obstructive lesions

Coarctation of the aorta (COA)

This accounts for about 6% of CHDs and has a male preponderance (M:F=2:1). There is a narrowing of the aorta which may be preductal or postductal. The site and severity of the coarctation determines the clinical features, which range from a severely ill newborn to an asymptomatic child, or adult, with hypertension.

Preductal coarctation—symptomatic infants

In 40% of cases, there is an associated defect such as VSD or TGA. The systemic circulation is duct-dependent and supported predominantly by the right ventricle. Signs of heart failure and renal failure with general circulatory failure may develop in the first 2–6 weeks of life.

Surgical correction is indicated, subclavian flap aortoplasty being the most common procedure.

> **The key to clinical diagnosis of coarctation of the aorta is weak or absent femoral pulses.**

Postductal coarctation (asymptomatic children)

Although usually asymptomatic, there may be leg pains or headache. On examination, there is hypertension in the arm and weak or absent femoral pulses. There may be an ejection click (due to an associated bicuspid aortic valve) and a systolic ejection murmur audible in the left interscapular area.

Surgical correction is required. Options include:

- Balloon dilatation.
- Resection of the coarcted segment with end-to-end anastamosis.

Aortic stenosis (AS)

This accounts for 5% of all CHDs and has a male preponderance (M:F=4:1).

Symptoms and signs depend on the severity of the stenosis:

- Children with mild or moderate stenoses present with an asymptomatic murmur.
- Severe stenosis may present with heart failure in the infant, or with chest pain on exertion and syncope in older children.

Sustained, strenuous exercise should be avoided in children with moderate to severe AS. Surgical treatment depends on the severity and site of the stenosis. Options include balloon or surgical valvotomy. Aortic valve replacement is often required for neonates and children with a significant stenosis requiring early treatment.

Pulmonary stenosis (PS)

This accounts for about 8% of CHD and may be valvular (90%), subvalvular (infundibular), or supravalvular. Infundibular PS occurs in association with a large VSD as part of the tetralogy of Fallot.

Most cases are mild and asymptomatic. The clinical features include:

- Widely split S2, with soft pulmonary component (P2).
- Systolic ejection click (valvular PS).
- A systolic ejection murmur maximal at the upper left sternal border, radiating to the back.

Treatment options include transvenous balloon dilatation or pulmonary valvotomy.

Cyanotic congenital heart disease

There are two principal pathophysiological mechanisms for cyanosis in congenital heart disease:

- Decreased pulmonary blood flow with shunting of deoxygenated blood from the right side of the circulation to the left (systemic circulation), e.g. tetralogy of Fallot.
- Increased pulmonary blood flow with abnormal mixing of systemic and pulmonary venous return, e.g. transposition of great arteries (TGA).

Tetralogy of Fallot

This represents 6–10% of all CHDs and is the most common cause of cyanotic CHDs presenting beyond infancy. The four cardinal anatomical features are shown in Fig. 15.5.

The four cardinal anatomical features of the tetralogy of Fallot

- a large VSD
- right ventricular outflow tract (RVOT) obstruction:
  - infundibular stenosis (50%)
  - pulmonary valve stenosis (10%)
  - combination of above (30%)
- aorta over-riding the ventricular septum
- right ventricular hypertrophy

Fig. 15.5 The four cardinal anatomical features of tetralogy of Fallot.

Clinical features

Most patients present with cyanosis in the first 1–2 months of life. Hypoxic (hypercyanotic) spells are a characteristic feature, as is squatting on exercise which develops in late infancy.

Clinical signs include:

- Cyanosis with or without clubbing.
- Loud and single S2.
- Loud ejection systolic murmur maximal at the third, left intercostal space.

Diagnosis

The ECG shows right axis deviation and right ventricular hypertrophy. The CXR shows a characteristic 'boot-shaped' heart caused by right ventricular hypertrophy and a concavity on the left heart border where the main pulmonary artery and RV outflow tract normally create a convexity (Fig. 15.6). Pulmonary vascular markings are diminished.

Management

Prolonged hypercyanotic spells require treatment with:

- Morphine—relieves pain and abolishes hyperpnoea.
- Sodium bicarbonate (IV) to correct acidosis.
- Propranolol to cause peripheral vasoconstriction and relieve infundibular spasm. Oral propranolol may prevent hypoxic spells.

Definitive treatment is surgical. Palliative procedures may be required in infants with severe cyanosis or uncontrollable hypoxic spells. Pulmonary blood flow is

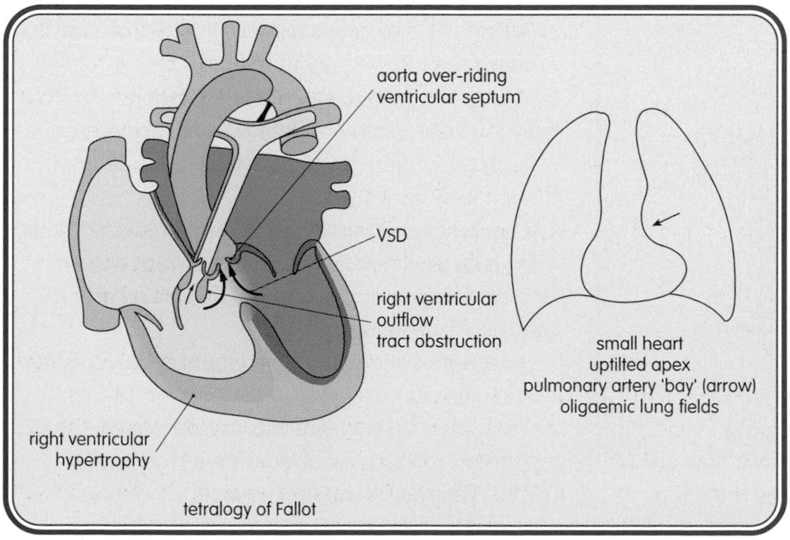

Fig. 15.6 Tetralogy of Fallot and CXR changes.

increased by creating a shunt between the subclavian artery and the pulmonary artery. Corrective total repair can now be carried out from 4–6 months of age. This involves patch closure of the VSD and widening of the right ventricular outflow tract.

Transposition of the great arteries

This accounts for about 5% of CHDs and is more common in males (M:F=3:1). In complete or D-transposition:

- The aorta arises anteriorly from the right ventricle.
- The pulmonary artery arises posteriorly from the left ventricle (Fig. 15.7).

Clearly, if completely separate, two such parallel circulations would be incompatible with life, but defects allowing mixing of the two circulations coexist. These include ASD, VSD, or PDA.

Clinical features

Most present with severe cyanosis often within the first day or two of life. Spontaneous closure of the ductus arteriosus reduces mixing of the systemic and pulmonary circulations. Arterial hypoxaemia is often profound (PaO_2 1–3 kPa) and unresponsive to O_2 inhalation.

The second sound is single and loud. If the ventricular septum is intact, no heart murmur is audible. The systolic murmur of a VSD or PDA may be present.

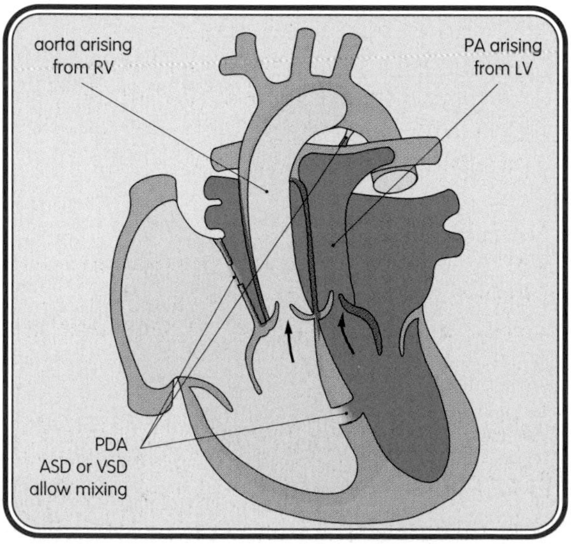

Fig. 15.7 Transposition of the great arteries.

Management

The immediate aim is to improve mixing of saturated and unsaturated blood. In the sick, cyanosed newborn, an infusion of PGE_1 is started to reopen the ductus arteriosus. Emergency cardiac catheterization and therapeutic balloon atrial septostomy (Rashkind procedure) is a life-saving palliative procedure. Definitive repair is usually achieved with an arterial switch procedure, which can be performed at a few weeks of age. The pulmonary artery and aorta are transected and switched over.

RHEUMATIC FEVER

Acute rheumatic fever is a sequela of group A β-haemolytic streptococcal infection, usually a tonsillopharyngitis. It is caused by an abnormal immune response which occurs in less than 1% of patients with streptococcal infection. Although the disease has largely been eradicated in developed countries with improved sanitation and the use of antibiotics for tonsillitis, it remains the most common cause of cardiac valvular disease worldwide. It mainly affects children aged between 5 and 15 years.

Clinical features

Polyarthritis, fever, and malaise develop 2–6 weeks after the pharyngeal infection. The arthritis is 'flitting', lasting less than a week in individual joints and commonly affects the large joints such as the knees and ankles.

There is a pancarditis in 50% of patients:

- Pericarditis may cause a friction rub and pericardial effusion.
- Myocarditis may cause heart failure.
- Endocarditis commonly affects the left-sided valves leading to murmurs, e.g. of mitral incompetence.

Erythema marginatum, pink macules on the trunk and limbs, is an uncommon painless, early manifestation. Hard subcutaneous nodules occur on the extensor surfaces in a minority of cases.

Sydenham's chorea is a late manifestation occurring 2–6 months after streptococcal infection in 10% of patients. There is emotional lability followed by involuntary, random, jerky movements lasting 2–3 months. Recovery is usually complete.

Diagnosis

The diagnosis is clinical and is based on a modified version of the Duckett Jones criteria (Fig. 15.8).

Diagnosis requires evidence of a preceding streptococcal infection together with two major criteria or one major and two minor criteria. The former is usually done serologically by finding an increase in antibodies to various streptococcal antigens, e.g. antistreptolysin 0 titre. Throat swab is often negative at the time of presentation.

Laboratory investigations in a suspected case include:

- ESR, C-reactive protein (CRP)—elevated.
- Antistreptolysin 0 titre—may be elevated.
- Throat swab—usually negative at time of presentation.
- ECG—prolonged P–R interval.
- Echocardiography—may show evidence of carditis.

Management

The acute episode is treated by:

- Bed rest.
- High-dose aspirin to suppress fever and arthritis.
- Steroids for severe carditis.
- Diuretics and ACE inhibitors for heart failure.
- Antibiotics if there is evidence of persisting streptococcal infection.

Recurrent attacks should be prevented by prophylactic penicillin (given either orally or as monthly intramuscular injections of benzathine penicillin). Lifelong prophylaxis has been advocated.

10 Duckett-Jones criteria for diagnosis of rheumatic fever

Major criteria
carditis
arthritis
chorea
erythema marginatum
subcutaneous nodules
Minor criteria
fever
arthralgia
prolonged PR interval on ECG
history of rheumatic fever
elevated acute-phase reactants: ESR, CRP, leucocytosis

Fig.15.8 Duckett Jones criteria for diagnosis of rheumatic fever.

Complications

Rheumatic valvular disease is the most common form of long-term damage, its severity increasing with the number of acute episodes. There is scarring and fibrosis of valve tissue, most commonly affecting the mitral valve.

CARDIAC INFECTIONS

These are uncommon and include:

- Infective endocarditis.
- Myocarditis.

Infective endocarditis

This inflammatory disorder, predominantly affecting the cardiac valves, is caused by infection with any of several types of organism including bacteria, fungi, and rickettsiae.

Clinical features

The early features are non-specific with fever, malaise, and weakness. The classical signs develop when vegetations form and throw off emboli.

Diagnosis

The following investigations may be of value in confirming the diagnosis:

- Blood cultures—at least three should be obtained in the first 24 hours of hospitalization. The causative organism, most commonly *Streptococcus viridans* (α-haemolytic streptococcus), is identified in 90% of cases.
- Cross-sectional echocardiography—this may confirm the diagnosis by the identification of vegetations, but can not exclude it.
- Acute-phase reactants—elevated.

Management

Treatment comprises 4–6 weeks of intravenous antibiotics, e.g. high-dose ampicillin with an aminoglycoside. Surgical removal of infected prosthetic material may be required.

All children with congenital heart disease are at risk of bacterial endocarditis.

Antibiotic prophylaxis against infective endocarditis is essential for dental or surgical treatment in all children with congenital heart disease.

Myocarditis

Myocarditis in infants and children is uncommon. It is usually viral. Most cases are caused by enteroviruses, e.g. Coxsackie B virus, echovirus.

Treatment is supportive. Most children recover, but some develop a chronic dilated cardiomyopathy as a sequela.

CARDIAC ARRHYTHMIAS

The most common symptomatic arrhythmia in the paediatric age group is supraventricular tachycardia (SVT). Sinus arrhythmia is common in normal children. The heart rate slows on inspiration and increases during expiration.

Supraventricular tachycardia

This is usually caused by a 're-entry' mechanism—the atrium is prematurely activated by an accessory pathway. It may present at any age including the fetus and newborn. The heart rate is usually between 200 and 300 beats per minute.

Clinical features

In utero it may cause hydrops fetalis and intrauterine death. In babies, if the tachycardia persists for more than 12–24 hours, cardiac failure and a low cardiac output state develop. Children may complain of fluttering in their chest, suggesting palpitations.

Diagnosis

The ECG usually shows a narrow complex tachycardia with P waves discernible after the QRS complex. In sinus rhythm, the Wolff–Parkinson–White syndrome may be evident if there is an accessory bundle allowing premature activation of the ventricles. The PR interval is short and there is a wide QRS with slurred upstroke (delta wave).

Management

An acute episode can be terminated and sinus rhythm restored by:

- Vagal stimulation—applying ice-cold compress to the face.
- Intravenous adenosine—safe and effective.
- Electrical cardioversion with a DC shock—the last resort if all the above fail in a sick infant.

The prognosis is good in the majority of cases. Ninety per cent of children will have no further episodes after infancy (over 1 year old). Radiofrequency ablation of the bypass tract has been used for those with persistent, frequently recurring paroxysms.

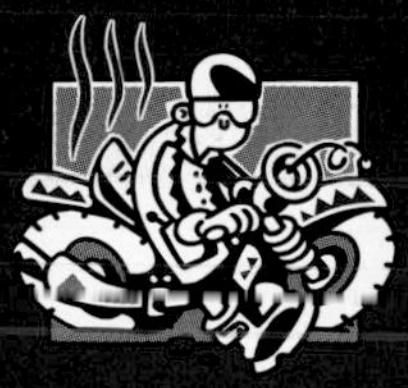

16. Disorders of the Respiratory System

Respiratory tract infections represent the most common infections of childhood and range from trivial to life-threatening illnesses. Ninety per cent of these are caused by viruses. They are classified into upper respiratory tract infections (URTIs) and lower respiratory tract infections (LRTIs). The other common and important diseases of this system are asthma and cystic fibrosis.

UPPER RESPIRATORY TRACT INFECTIONS

The upper respiratory tract comprises the ears, nose, throat, tonsils, pharynx, and sinuses, together with the extrathoracic airways.

The common cold (acute nasopharyngitis)

This is a viral infection (e.g. rhinovirus, coronavirus) causing a clear or mucopurulent nasal discharge (coryza) and nasal blockage. Symptomatic treatment (e.g. paracetamol) is all that is required for this self-limiting illness. Feeding difficulties may be experienced by young infants who are obligate nose-breathers.

Sore throat (pharyngitis and tonsillitis)

These are commonly viral (including EBV) but also may be caused by group A β-haemolytic streptococci. Children present with a sore throat, fever, and constitutional upset. It is very difficult to distinguish viral and bacterial infection clinically. However, a purulent exudate, lymphadenopathy, and severe pain suggest a bacterial cause.

Treatment

It is reasonable to give oral penicillin treatment for severe pharyngitis and tonsillitis, especially if a throat swab has been performed and confirms streptococcal infection.

Complications

These include:

- Retropharyngeal abscess.
- Peritonsillar abscess (quinsy).
- Post-streptococcal glomerulonephritis or rheumatic fever.

Tonsillectomy is now less commonly performed. Indications include recurrent tonsillitis, quinsy, or obstructive sleep apnoea.

Acute otitis media

This may be viral or bacterial (pneumococcus, *Haemophilus influenzae*, group B streptococci, *Moraxella catarrhalis*). It is very common in preschool children, who present with fever, vomiting, and distress. It is important to examine the eardrums in any ill and febrile toddler, as only the older child will localize the pain to the ear.

Clinical features

Examination reveals a red eardrum with loss of the light reflex. The drum may bulge and perforation may occur with a purulent discharge.

Management

Treat with amoxycillin and paracetamol.

Recurrent infections may be associated with otitis media with effusion. Mastoiditis and meningitis are now uncommon complications of acute otitis media.

Otitis media with effusion (OME, secretory otitis media, glue ear)

In young children who are prone to recurrent upper respiratory tract infections, it is common that the middle ear fluid persists (an effusion) causing a conductive hearing loss and an increased susceptibility to reinfection. An effusion may also occur without a history of acute infections and is probably due to poor Eustachian tube ventilation due to enlarged adenoids or allergy. The effusion and resulting hearing impairment is often transient, but if it is persistent it may be an indication for surgical drainage of the middle ear with grommet insertion. The grommet is a hollow plastic tube that ventilates the middle ear and only remains effective while patent. Ultimately it is extruded from the tympanic membrane. Decongestants and antibiotics are widely used but have unproven value. A low power hearing aid may be required.

Croup

Croup, or viral laryngotracheobronchitis, is most commonly caused by parainfluenza virus. This has a peak incidence in winter in the second year of life.

Clinical features

Symptoms of upper respiratory tract infection (coryza, fever) are usually present for a day or two before the onset of a characteristic barking ('sea lion') cough and stridor (which is caused by subglottic inflammation and oedema). Symptoms typically start, and are worse, at night.

Management

Most children are mildly affected and improve spontaneously within 24 hours. Management at home is supportive with paracetamol, fluids, and a warm humidified environment (although it remains unclear whether humidified air does improve outcome or hasten recovery).

About 1 in 10 children require hospitalization because of:

- More severe illness.
- Young age (under 12 months).
- Signs of dehydration and fatigue.

There is evidence that a single dose of nebulized steroid (e.g. budesonide 2 mg) has a beneficial effect in severe croup.

Nebulized adrenaline provides transient improvement by constricting local blood vessels and reducing swelling and oedema. It should only be given under close supervision in hospital where it may provide rapid, if transient, relief of airway obstruction, allowing time for transfer to the intensive therapy unit (ITU) and intubation in a child with severe airways obstruction.

Diphtheria

This potentially fatal and highly infectious disease is caused by a toxin produced by the *Corynebacterium diphtheriae*. In the UK, this scourge of childhood has been eliminated by an effective immunization programme, but it remains endemic in some countries and imported cases occur.

Acute epiglottitis

Acute bacterial epiglottitis is an uncommon life-threatening emergency caused by infection with *Haemophilus influenzae* type b. It has become rare since the introduction of Hib immunization. It is most common in children aged 1–6 years.

Clinical features

The onset is rapid over a few hours with the development of an intensely painful throat. The characteristic picture is of an ill, toxic, febrile child who is unable to speak or swallow, with a muffled voice and soft inspiratory stridor. The child tends to sit upright with an open mouth to maximize the airway and may drool saliva.

Management

It is vital to distinguish this illness from viral croup because the management is different:

- Minutes count if death is to be avoided.
- Urgent hospital admission should be arranged.
- No attempt should be made to lie the child down, to examine the throat with a spatula, or to take blood as these manoeuvres can precipitate total airway obstruction and death.

Examination under anaesthetic should be arranged without delay (preferably in the presence of a senior anaesthetist, paediatrician, and ENT surgeon) to allow confirmation of the diagnosis, followed by intubation. Once the airway is secured, blood should be taken for culture and intravenous antibiotics started using a third-generation cephalosporin, e.g. cefuroxime. Intubation is not usually required for longer than 24 hours.

Do not examine the throat if epiglottitis is suspected as complete airway obstruction may be provoked.

LOWER RESPIRATORY TRACT INFECTIONS

A minority of infections involve the lower respiratory tract, but these are more likely to be serious and are more common in infants. Causative agents include viruses and bacteria. They vary with the child's age and the site of infection. Infection may occur by direct spread from airway epithelium or via the bloodstream.

A number of well-defined clinical syndromes (determined by the predominant anatomical site of inflammation) are recognized (e.g. bronchiolitis and pneumonia) and often provide a clue to the likely pathogen. The term 'chest infection' should be avoided. The hallmarks of a lower respiratory tract infection are apparent on inspection (Fig. 16.1).

Pneumonia

Pneumonia is characterized by inflammation of the lung parenchyma with consolidation of alveoli. It may be caused by a wide range of pathogens with different organisms affecting different age groups (Fig. 16.2).

Clinical features

Usually, following an URTI the patient develops worsening fever, cough, and breathlessness. Tachypnoea is a key sign. The classical signs of consolidation (dullness to percussion, decreased breath sounds, and bronchial breathing) may be present, but they are difficult to detect in infants. Crackles may be present. In bacterial pneumonia, pleural inflammation causing chest (or abdominal pain) and an effusion more commonly develops.

Diagnosis

A chest X-ray (CXR) is required to confirm the diagnosis and blood cultures. A full blood count and nasopharyngeal aspirate for viral isolation should be carried out in hospitalized children.

It is often difficult to distinguish between viral and bacterial infections. Young children and babies are not good providers of sputum, and definitive diagnosis of bacterial infection remains difficult. However, the following all suggest bacterial pneumonia:

- Polymorph. leucocytosis.
- Lobar consolidation (Fig. 16.3).
- Pleural effusion.

Mycoplasma infection can be diagnosed by serology or by demonstration of cold agglutinins.

Management

Antibiotics are usually given if a diagnosis of pneumonia is made, and the choice is dictated by the child's age and the severity of illness:

- In severe illness requiring IV therapy, cefuroxime provides satisfactory cover.
- If *mycoplasma* is suspected, erythromycin should be given.

Rarely, pneumonia may be complicated by empyema. Recurrent or persistent pneumonia should raise the possibility of an inhaled foreign object (Fig. 16.4), cystic fibrosis, or TB.

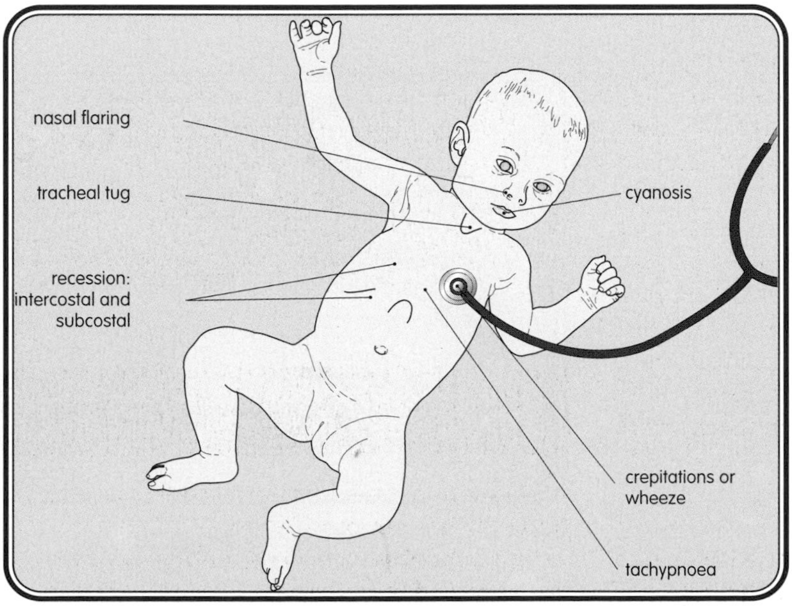

Fig. 16.1 Signs of lower respiratory tract infection in the infant.

Pathogens causing pneumonia in infants and children	
Age	**Pathogens**
neonates (<1 month)	group B streptococci *E. coli* *Chlamydia trachomatis*
infants	respiratory viruses, e.g. RSV, adenovirus *Streptococcus pneumoniae* *Haemophilus influenzae* *Bordetella pertussis*
children	*Streptococcus pneumoniae* *Haemophilus influenzae* group A streptococci *Mycoplasma pneumonia*

Fig. 16.2 Pathogens causing pneumonia in infants and children.

Bronchiolitis

This common, serious infection is caused by the respiratory syncytial virus (RSV). Annual winter epidemics occur in babies aged 1–9 months. An inflammatory response occurs predominantly in the bronchioles, hence the name.

Clinical features

Coryzal symptoms are followed by a cough with increasing breathlessness and associated difficulty in breathing. Small infants may develop apnoeic episodes. Ex-preterm infants with chronic lung disease and infants with congenital heart disease are at particular risk of being severely affected.

Examination reveals:

- Tachypnoea.
- Subcostal and intercostal recession.
- Chest hyperinflation.
- Bilateral fine crackles.
- High-pitched rhonchi on auscultation.

Whooping cough is most dangerous to very young infants.
Vaccination is given early to confer protection on this vulnerable group.

In severe disease, there may be cyanosis and circulatory failure with pallor and tachycardia.

Diagnosis

The CXR usually shows hyperinflation of the lungs and transcutaneous oxygen monitoring may reveal desaturation. A nasopharyngeal aspirate is examined by the fluorescent antibody test for RSV.

Management

Management is supportive (Fig. 16.5). Breathing (apnoea monitor), heart rate, and oxygen saturation

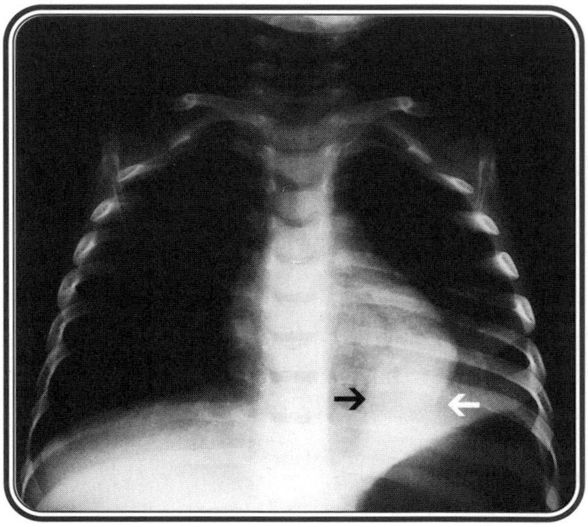

Fig. 16.3 CXR of lobar pneumonia. Consolidation is seen in the lower left lobe obscuring the left hemidiaphragm.

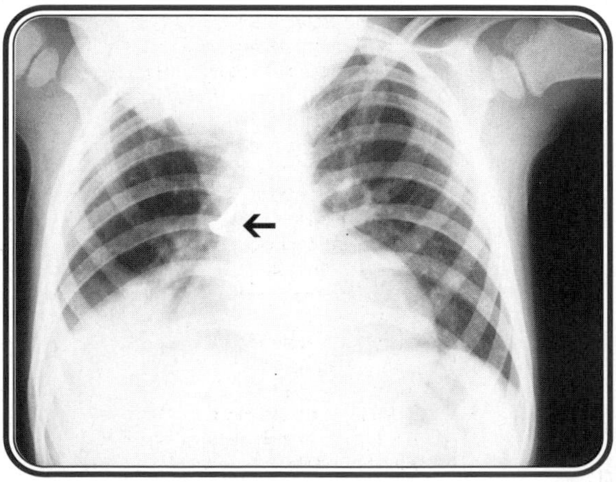

Fig. 16.4 CXR of an inhaled foreign object. Nail seen in the right intermediate bronchus with distal collapse of right middle and lower lobes.

Bronchiolitis is a common and severe infection in infants in the winter months.

(pulse oximeter) are monitored. Oxygen is the mainstay of treatment and is given via nasal cannulae or a head-box. Some infants may be well enough to continue oral feeds, but most require fluids to be given either by nasogastric tube or intravenously. A minority of hospitalized infants require assisted ventilation (only 1–2%). Secondary bacterial infection may occur, in which case antibiotic therapy is appropriate.

Sequela

Although most infants make a full recovery within 2 weeks, some have recurrent episodes of cough and wheeze over the subsequent few years, which may represent a sequela to the infection.

Whooping cough (pertussis)

Whooping cough or pertussis is a highly contagious clinical syndrome caused by a number of pathogens, most commonly *Bordetella pertussis*. It is endemic with epidemics occurring every 4 years. An effective vaccine exists and is a component of the routine triple vaccine containing diphtheria, tetanus, and pertussis (DTP).

Whooping cough is spread by droplet infection with an incubation period of 7–10 days. A case is infectious from 7 days after exposure to 3 weeks after the onset of the paroxysmal cough.

Clinical features

The clinical course can be divided into catarrhal, paroxysmal, and convalescent stages.

During a paroxysm of coughing (often worse at night) the child may go blue and vomit. The inspiratory whoop may be absent in infants. Nosebleeds and subconjunctival haemorrhage may occur after vigorous coughing. Symptoms can persist for 3 months (the '100 day' cough).

Complications

Complications, including pneumonia, convulsions, apnoea, bronchiectasis, and death, are more common in infants under 6 months of age.

Diagnosis

A marked lymphocytosis ($>15.0 \times 10^9$/L) is characteristic and the organism can be cultured from a nasal swab early in the disease.

Treatment

Erythromycin given early in the disease eradicates the organism and reduces infectivity, but does not shorten the duration of the disease.

Management of bronchiolitis	
Mild	feeding well respiratory rate <40/min minimal intercostal recession manage at home—regular review
Moderate	difficulty feeding moderate tachypnoea—rate >40/min marked intercostal recession moderate hypoxia in air—saturation >85% admit to hospital O_2 via nasal cannulae or head box fluids intravenously
Severe	not feeding tachypnoea—rate >60/min recurrent apnoea severe recession hypoxia in air—saturation <85% admit to ICU or high-dependency area high inspired O_2 intubation and assistive ventilation for respiratory failure or recurrent severe apnoea

Fig. 16.5 Management of bronchiolitis.

ASTHMA

Asthma is a chronic condition characterized by airway hyper-responsiveness due to inflammation. The characteristic clinical feature is recurrent episodes of airways narrowing associated with cough and wheeze.

Incidence

Asthma has increased in prevalence to become the most common chronic respiratory disorder of childhood. In the UK, one in five children will have had symptoms of asthma by the age of 10 years. During childhood, it is twice as common in boys as girls.

Aetiology

Asthma is a multifactorial disorder caused by a

combination of genetic predisposition and environmental factors. In most children, asthma is one manifestation of atopy; an inherited disorder characterized by:

- Raised serum IgE levels.
- Eosinophilia.
- Eczema.
- Allergic rhinitis and conjunctivitis (hay fever).
- Asthma.

Environmental factors, which increase the risk of developing asthma, include:

- Smoking—parental smoking and maternal smoking in pregnancy.
- Exposure to allergens during infancy.
- Viral infection during infancy.

Pathophysiology

The pathophysiology of airway narrowing in asthma includes chronic inflammation of the bronchial mucosa associated with mucosal oedema, secretions, and the constriction of airway smooth muscle (Fig. 16.6).

Diagnosis

Asthma is a clinical diagnosis. It is suggested by a history of recurrent episodes of cough, wheeze, and breathlessness. A diagnosis of asthma in infants (under 1 year) may be particularly difficult as their small airways predispose to wheeze during viral lower respiratory tract infections even in the absence of true bronchial hyper-reactivity. In the preschool child, a nocturnal cough may be the only symptom.

History

Enquiry should be made concerning a family history of asthma, trigger factors, and those features that allow the clinical evaluation of severity.

Seasonal exacerbations and remissions may be superimposed on this overall pattern. In addition, some children have little or no problems on a day-to-day basis but are prone to severe exercise-induced asthma or infrequent, sudden life-threatening attacks. Symptoms of mild, moderate, and severe asthma are shown in Fig. 16.7.

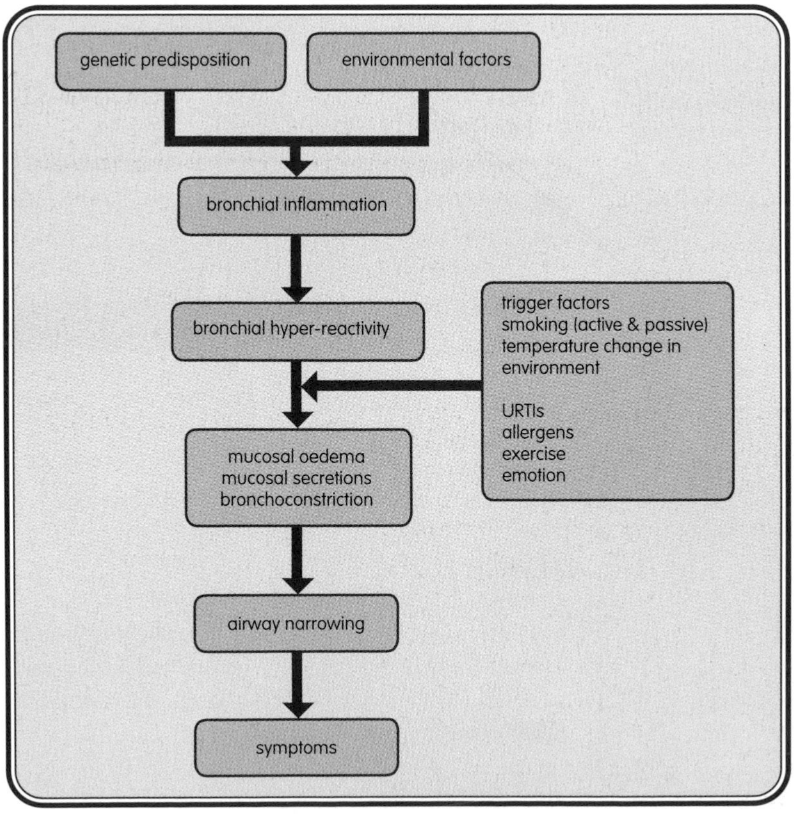

Fig. 16.6 Factors in the pathogenesis of asthma.

Examination

Auscultation of the chest is usually normal between attacks. Chronic, severe asthma is associated with thoracic deformity:

- Hyperexpansion.
- Pigeon chest (pectus carinatum).
- Harrison sulcus.

Investigations

A plain CXR may be useful at initial presentation. In children over the age of 5 years, the peak expiratory flow rate (PEFR) should be monitored and compared to the normal for height.

Asthma: mild, moderate, or severe	
Mild	infrequent symptoms sleep undisturbed occasional day off school no limitation of physical activity medication on 'as needed' basis
Moderate	unwell more often than well nocturnal symptoms common school absences exercise problematic regular medication—modest dosage
Severe	symptomatic most days sleep disturbed most nights prolonged school absences unable to exercise normally frequent hospital admissions regular medication—high dosage

Fig. 16.7 Asthma: mild, moderate, or severe.

Differential diagnosis

The differential diagnosis includes several important acute and chronic conditions. It must be remembered that 'all that wheezes is not asthma'. Alternative diagnoses are listed in Fig. 16.8. The diagnosis is more difficult in infants.

Management

Maintenance therapy and the treatment of an acute severe attack are considered separately.

Maintenance therapy

Children with asthma usually respond well to treatment and almost all should be able to lead full, normal lives. The main aspects of management are:

- Education of the child, family, and other carers (e.g. schoolteachers).
- Avoidance of provoking factors (e.g. allergens, smoke).
- Medication.

Education

A good understanding of the nature of asthma and its treatment is vital. Excellent written material is available from the National Asthma Campaign. The aims of education are to:

- Optimize compliance.
- Ensure proper use of inhaler devices.
- Work towards self-management commensurate with child's age and understanding.
- Ensure recognition of worsening asthma and safe response to acute attack.

Allergen avoidance

Allergy tests such as skin-prick testing or the measurement of specific IgE may be appropriate in

Differential diagnosis of asthma		
	Infants	**Children**
acute attack	acute bronchiolitis pneumonia cardiac failure	foreign body aspiration pneumonia acute laryngotracheobronchitis (croup)
recurrent wheeze	chronic lung disease of prematurity postbronchiolitic wheeze reflux with aspiration cystic fibrosis cardiac failure	foreign body aspiration primary ciliary dyskinesia cystic fibrosis

Fig. 16.8 Differential diagnosis of asthma.

some older children. Simple avoidance measures for the following allergens are worth trying:

- House dust mite: foam filling for pillows and duvets, lino floor, blinds in bedrooms, frequent vacuum cleaning, and damp dusting.
- Grass pollen: during the pollen season avoid walking in parks or fields and keep bedroom windows closed.
- Animal dander: remove cats from the home (never allow a cat to sleep on the bed).

There is little evidence that asthma is triggered by an allergic reaction to foods. Parental smoking should be discouraged.

Medication

The drugs used in the management of asthma in children can be classified into 'preventers' and 'relievers'.

A stepwise approach has been devised (British Guidelines for Asthma Management) and is summarized in Fig. 16.9. Patients should start treatment at the step most appropriate to the initial severity. Once control is achieved, treatment can be stepped down. A rescue course of oral prednisolone may be needed at any step (under 1 year old: 1–2 mg/kg/day; 1–5 years 20 mg/day; maximum dose 40 mg/day). In children with marked seasonal variation in asthma severity, the treatment should be varied according to the season.

Inhalation therapy is central to most asthma treatment. The basic systems available are considered in Figs. 16.10 and 16.11.

The mode of action, indications for use, and side effects of the most commonly used bronchodilator drugs are outlined in Fig. 16.12.

Stepwise management of chronic asthma in children	
Step 1	occasional use of relief bronchodilators
Step 2	regular inhaled preventer therapy: cromoglycate or low-dose inhaled steroids PLUS inhaled short-acting β_2 agonists as required
Step 3	increased dosage of inhaled steroids PLUS inhaled short-acting β_2 agonists as required
Step 4	regular high-dose inhaled steroids PLUS regular long-acting or nebulized β_2 agonists or oral slow-release xanthines
Step 5	as Step 4 with alternate-day, low-dose oral prednisolone instead of inhaled steroids
Stepping down	review treatment every few months and if symptoms are minimal, reduce treatment

Fig. 16.9 Stepwise management of chronic asthma in children.

Administration of medication by inhalation		
	Advantages	**Disadvantages**
metered dose inhaler with spacer	coordination not required usable at all ages	bulky
dry powder inhaler (DPI)	coordination unimportant small and portable easy to operate	requires rapid inspiration unsuitable for children <5 years
nebulizer	coordination unimportant usable at all ages effective in severe attack	expensive, noisy, cumbersome treatment takes a long time, >5 min frightens some infants

Fig. 16.10 Administration of medication by inhalation.

Steroid therapy in asthma

Glucocorticoids are key drugs in the management of asthma, both in prophylaxis and the treatment of acute attacks. They are the only drugs that have been shown to reduce inflammation in asthmatic airways. They may be given:

- By inhalation.
- Orally.
- Intravenously.

Inhaled steroids

Inhaled steroids are now the 'preventers' of choice in the management of childhood asthma. However, some paediatricians still prefer to use sodium cromoglycate as first line prophylaxis and then move on to the inhaled steroids if control is not achieved.

Features of inhaled steroids are:

- They inhibit synthesis of inflammatory mediators (cytokines, leukotrienes, and prostaglandins).

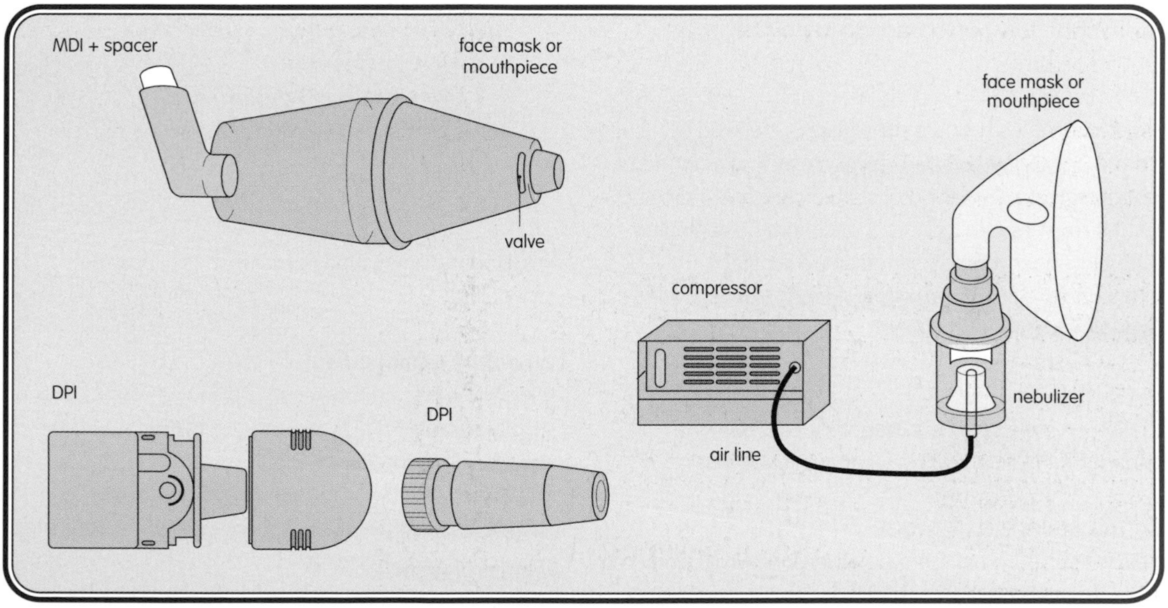

Fig. 16.11 Inhaler devices.

Asthma drug therapy: mode of action, indications, and side effects of bronchodilators			
Relievers (bronchodilators)	**Mode of action**	**Use**	**Side effects**
short-acting β_2 agonists, e.g. salbutamol, terbutaline	smooth muscle relaxation	relief of bronchospasm	tachycardia hypokalaemia restlessness
long-acting β_2 agonists, e.g. salmeterol	smooth muscle relaxation	nocturnal asthma exercise-induced asthma trial alternative to high-dose inhaled steroids	
theophylline	phosphodiesterase inhibition	oral theophylline for nocturnal asthma IV aminophylline in acute severe asthma	restlessness diuresis cardiac arrhythmias
anticholinergics, e.g. ipratropium bromide	inhibit cholinergic bronchoconstriction; add on to β_2 agonists in acute attack	first-line bronchodilator in infants	dry mouth urinary retention

Fig. 16.12 Asthma drug therapy: mode of action, indications, and side effects of bronchodilators.

- They are effective in nearly all children.
- They reduce airway hyper-responsiveness.
- They reduce both the symptoms and frequency of attacks.
- They prevent irreversible airway narrowing.

Local side effects such as oral thrush or dysphonia are uncommon. At high doses, systemic side effects may occur due to absorption of steroid from the gut. Ninety per cent of the dose is deposited in the mouth and pharynx, but this can be reduced by the use of a spacer (with MDIs) and mouth washing (with DPIs).

Oral steroids

Prednisolone as a single daily dose is the drug of choice. Short courses (5–7 days) are indicated for acute exacerbations. Regular oral steroids are only indicated for the most severe asthma that cannot be controlled with high-dose inhaled steroids and regular bronchodilators. Alternate day dosage is preferred to reduce systemic side effects.

Intravenous steroids

Hydrocortisone given intravenously is used in the management of an acute severe asthma attack.

Acute severe asthma

This is considered in more detail in Chapter 28. Features of acute severe asthma include:

- Respiratory rate over 50 breaths/min.
- Pulse over 140 beats/min.
- Use of accessory muscles.
- Too breathless to talk.

Life-threatening features include:

- Cyanosis.
- Silent chest (insufficient airflow to generate wheeze).
- Exhaustion, poor respiratory effort.

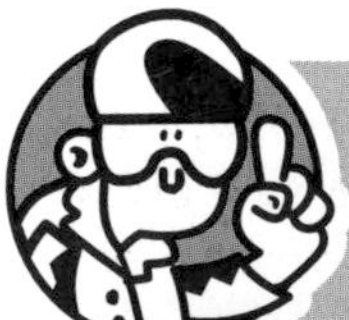

There is a colour code for asthma drug inhaler devices:

- **'Preventers' are brown, e.g. inhaled steroid.**
- **'Relievers' are blue, e.g. inhaled salbutamol.**

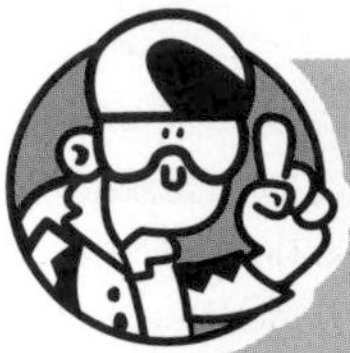

Which inhaler device for which patient?

- **Nebulizers: these can be used at any age.**
- **Metered dose inhaler (MDI): only suitable for competent older children (breath-activated MDIs are available and do not require such a high level of coordination).**
- **MDI and spacer: useful in infants, young children.**
- **Dry powder inhaler (DPI): children from age 5 years.**

- Agitation, diminished consciousness (indicate hypoxia).

Immediate management

- High-flow O_2 via facemask.
- Salbutamol (2.5–5.0 mg) or terbutaline (5.0–10.0 mg) via an oxygen -driven nebulizer.
- Prednisolone (1–2 mg/kg bodyweight) orally.
- Pulse oximetry—O_2 saturation <92% in air indicates need for hospitalization.

If life-threatening features (or poor response):

- Intravenous aminophylline 5 mg/kg over 20 minutes followed by maintenance infusion at 1 mg/kg/h (omit the loading dose if the child is on oral theophylline).
- Intravenous hydrocortisone 100 mg 6-hourly.
- Add ipratropium bromide to nebulized β_2-agonist.

CYSTIC FIBROSIS

Incidence and aetiology

Cystic fibrosis (CF) is the most common serious genetic disease in white people with a carrier rate of 1:25 and incidence of 1:2500 live births. It is an autosomal recessive disease arising from mutations in a gene on chromosome 7 which encodes an ABC (ATP-binding casette) transporter, the cystic fibrosis transmembrane regulator (CFTR protein). The most common mutation is a three base-pair deletion that removes the phenylalanine at position 508 (ΔF508). This is found in

70% of disease chromosomes, but several hundred different mutations have now been identified.

The mutations in the CFTR cause defective chloride ion transport across epithelial cells and increased viscosity of secretions, especially in the respiratory tract and exocrine pancreas. This predisposes to recurrent chest infections and pancreatic insufficiency. In addition, abnormal transport in sweat gland epithelium results in high concentrations of sodium and chloride in sweat, which form the basis of the most useful diagnostic test, the sweat test.

Clinical features

Cystic fibrosis should be considered in any child with recurrent chest infection and failure to thrive. Viscid mucus in the small airways predisposes to infection with *Staphylococcus aureus, Haemophilus influenzae,* and *Pseudomonas* species. Repeated infection leads to bronchial wall damage with bronchiectasis and abscess formation.

There is a cough productive of purulent sputum and on examination there may be:

- Hyperinflation.
- Crepitations.
- Rhonchi.

An example of typical chest X-ray changes is shown in Fig. 16.13.

In most children, deficiency of pancreatic enzymes (protease, amylase, and lipase) leads to malabsorption, steatorrhoea, and failure to thrive. Stools are pale, greasy, and offensive. About 10% of CF infants present with 'meconium ileus' in the neonatal period in which inspissated meconium causes internal obstruction.

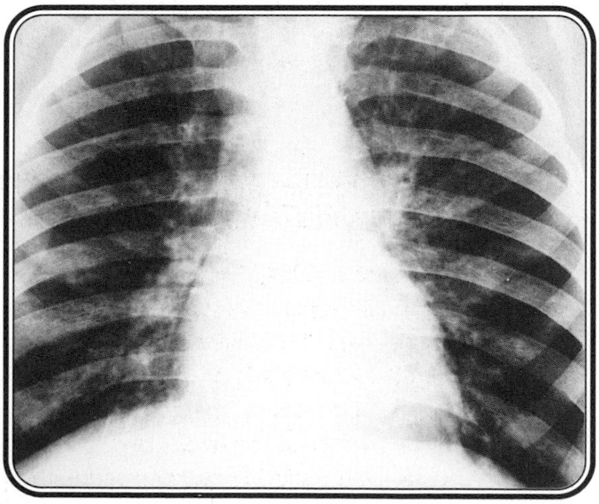

Fig.16.13 Typical CXR of a child with cystic firbrosis, showing bilateral severe lung pathology: hyperinflated lungs with bronchial wall thickening.

Diagnosis

Diagnosis is made using the 'sweat test'. Failure of the normal reabsorption of sodium and chloride by the sweat duct epithelium leads to abnormally salty sweat: chloride concentrations of 80–125 mmol/L are found in contrast to the normal value of less than 15 mmol/L.

DNA analysis is also available for the more common mutations.

Management

Cystic fibrosis is a multisystem disease and management requires a multidisciplinary approach, which is most effectively delivered by a specialist centre. The main aims are to:

- Prevent progression of lung disease.
- Promote adequate nutrition and growth.

A team approach is required involving paediatricians, physiotherapists, dieticians, nurses, the primary care team, and last, but not least, the child's parents.

Respiratory management

Physiotherapy (chest percussion, breathing exercises and postural drainage) is the mainstay of respiratory management. Many centres recommend continuous prophylactic antibiotics, which may be taken orally or inhaled using a nebulizer. Acute exacerbations require vigorous treatment with intravenous antibiotics directed against the common bacterial pathogens (*Haemophilus influenzae, Staphylococcus aureus, and Pseudomonas aeruginosa*), and guided by recent sputum culture results if available.

Many children have reversible small airways obstruction and benefit from inhaled bronchodilators.

Nutritional management

The combined threats of malabsorption due to pancreatic insufficiency, poor appetite, and increased metabolism due to chronic infection, and increased respiratory work render nutritional management of vital importance in CF. The following supplements may be given:

- A high-calorie diet with vitamin supplements, especially of fat soluble vitamins A, D, E, and K.
- Pancreatic enzyme supplementation using enteric-

coated microspheres in gelatin-coated capsules (e.g. Creon) which contain amylase, lipase and protease. This usually has a marked effect on steatorrhoea and allows 'catch-up' growth.

Genetic screening

Isolation of the CF gene and identification of the common mutations has made it technically possible to screen the population in order to identify carriers, and to offer counselling and prenatal diagnosis to couples at risk of having a child with CF. However, a variety of logistical, ethical, technical, and psychological problems need to be solved before any national programme can be introduced. For example, exclusion of the common mutation is easy but the hundreds of rare mutations remain difficult to screen for.

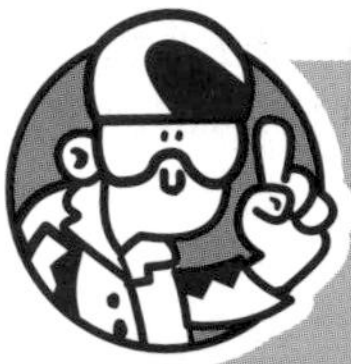

The CFTR protein:

- **Acts as a cAMP-dependent chloride channel in the apical membranes of epithelial cells.**
- **Is composed of 1480 amino acid residues.**
- **Contains functional domains including membrane-spanning regions, ATP-binding domains, and a regulatory domain.**
- **Is an ATP-binding cassette (ABC) transporter.**

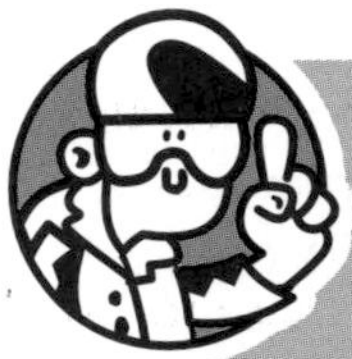

Mutations in the CFTR gene:

- **The ΔF508 mutation is found on 70% of CF chromosomes.**
- **A three base-pair deletion causes the loss of the phenylalanine (F) at residue number 508.**
- **700 mutations have now been reported in the CFTR gene, but few of these occur at a worldwide frequency of more than 1%.**

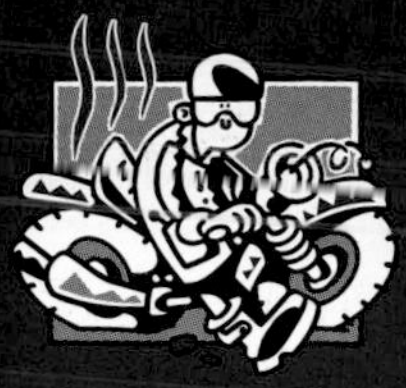

17. Disorders of the Gastrointestinal System

Both medical and surgical disorders of the gastrointestinal tract are common in paediatric practice. At least 5 million young children die each year from diarrhoeal diseases.

The range of pathological processes affecting the gastrointestinal tract is broad. It includes:

- Congenital abnormalities.
- Infection.
- Immune-mediated allergy or inflammation.

INFANTILE COLIC

This is a common syndrome characterized by recurrent inconsolable crying or screaming accompanied by drawing up of the legs during the first few months of life. It may occur several times a day, particularly in the evening.

Diagnosis

The differential diagnosis of inconsolable screaming includes some important conditions (see HInts & Tips). Occasionally 'colic' may be due to cow's milk protein intolerance or gastro-oesophageal reflux.

Treatment and prognosis

The condition is benign with a good prognosis, although it may provoke non-accidental injury in infants at risk. Sympathetic counselling is important. In severe or persistent cases, a trial of a cow's milk-free diet followed by a trial of anti-reflux treatment may be indicated.

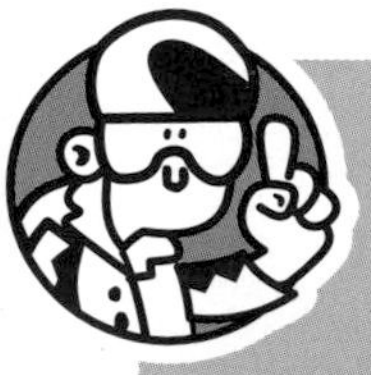

Inconsolable crying in an infant, consider:

- **Colic.**
- **Otitis media.**
- **Incarcerated hernia.**
- **Urinary tract infection.**
- **Anal fissure.**
- **Intussusception.**

GASTRO-OESOPHAGEAL REFLUX

The involuntary passage of gastric contents into the oesophagus is a common problem especially in babies during the first year of life. Functional immaturity of the lower oesophageal sphincter, liquid milk rather than solid feeds, and a supine posture are all contributory factors.

Clinical features

Symptoms are usually mild (regurgitation/posseting) and no treatment is required. In a minority, symptoms are severe and complications such as failure to thrive, oesophagitis, or recurrent aspiration pneumonia may occur.

Infants at risk of severe gastro-oesophageal reflux include the following:

- Preterm infants—especially those with chronic lung disease (bronchopulmonary dysplasia).
- Infants with cerebral palsy.
- Infants with congenital oesophageal anomalies, e.g. after repair of a tracheo-oesophageal fistula.

The main symptom is recurrent regurgitation or vomiting. About 10% of infants with symptomatic reflux develop complications. Oesophagitis may be manifested by:

- Irritability.
- Features of pain after feeding.
- Blood in the vomit.
- Iron-deficiency anaemia.

Reflux can cause recurrent aspiration pneumonia, cough, bronchospasm (with wheezing), and exacerbation of chronic lung diseases such as cystic fibrosis or bronchopulmonary dysplasia.

Diagnosis

Most reflux can be diagnosed clinically, but several techniques are available for confirming the diagnosis and assessing the severity:

- 24-hour ambulatory oesophageal pH monitoring—this is a popular way of diagnosing and quantifying acid reflux.

- Barium studies—may be required to exclude underlying anatomical abnormalities.
- Endoscopy—this is indicated in patients with suspected oesophagitis.

In the majority of mildly affected infants, reassurance and the early introduction of solids at 3 months are all that is required. Nursing the baby in an upright position after feeds may help. More troublesome reflux may respond to an alginate and antacid combination (e.g. Gaviscon Infant) or thickening the feed with inert carob-based agents.

In more severe reflux, the following drugs may be used:

- Prokinetic drugs such as cisapride—these speed gastric emptying and increase lower oesophageal sphincter pressure.
- Drugs to reduce gastric acid secretion—used especially if there is evidence of oesophagitis. H_2 antagonists, e.g. ranitidine, are the first choice.

Surgery is required for very severe cases with complications. The most commonly used procedure is Nissen fundoplication in which the fundus of the stomach is wrapped around the lower oesophagus.

GASTROENTERITIS

Gastroenteritis is an infection of the gastrointestinal tract, usually viral, which presents with a combination of diarrhoea and vomiting (D & V).

Incidence and aetiology

In developed countries, it is usually mild and self-limiting (affecting 1 in 10 children under the age of 2 years) but in the developing world approximately 5 million children, under 5 years old die from gastroenteritis each year.

Rotavirus is the most common pathogen in the UK. Gastroenteritis may also be caused by:

- Bacteria, including *Shigellae, Salmonellae, Campylobacter*, and *Escherichia. coli.*
- Three parasites: *Entamoeba histolytica, Giardia lamblia,* and *Cryptosporidium.*

Clinical features

Viral infection may cause a prodromal illness followed by vomiting and diarrhoea:

- The vomiting may precede diarrhoea and is not usually bile or bloodstained.
- Abdominal pain and blood or mucus in the stool suggests an invasive bacterial pathogen.
- The severity of diarrhoea may be underestimated if it pools in the large bowel or very watery stool is mistaken for urine in the nappy.

On examination, the most important physical signs relate to the presence and severity of dehydration (Fig. 17.1). The high surface area to bodyweight ratio in babies and infants renders them susceptible to rapid derangement of fluid and electrolyte balance.

Diagnosis

The differential diagnosis includes at least two important surgical conditions:

- In young infants, especially boys (aged 2–12 weeks), vomiting may be due to pyloric stenosis. Stool output is reduced and visible peristalsis with a palpable pyloric mass may be evident.
- In older infants and toddlers (aged 1–2 years), intussusception presents with vomiting. Paroxysmal abdominal pain and the eventual passage of 'redcurrant jelly' stools should raise suspicion of this condition, which is *lethal* if overlooked.

Investigations should include:

- Measurement of the plasma urea and electrolytes.
- Stool culture.
- Stool microscopy.

Dehydration may be further classified according to whether the plasma sodium concentration is normal, low (hyponatraemia), or high (hypernatraemia). This has a bearing on the fluids used for rehydration (see below).

Management

Rehydration

The key to management is rehydration with correction of the fluid and electrolyte imbalance. The strategy depends on the severity of dehydration.

Mild dehydration

Oral rehydration solutions (ORS), e.g. Dioralyte, Rehidrat are used. These contain dextrose to stimulate sodium and water reabsorption across the bowel wall, and various salts.

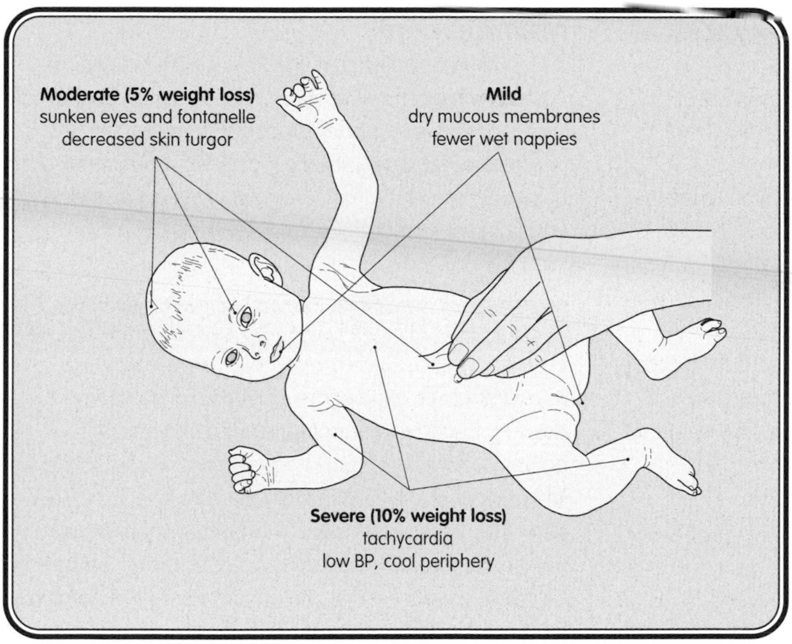

Fig. 17.1 Clinical features of dehydration.

Moderate to severe dehydration

If there are signs of circulatory failure, immediate resuscitation is achieved by intravenous administration of 10–20 mL/kg of 0.9% NaCl (normal saline) or 'plasma' (human albumin 5%).

Further rehydration can usually be achieved satisfactorily with 4% dextrose/0.18% NaCl with KCl added at a concentration of 20–40 mmol/L.

The volume required in 24 hours is calculated from estimated deficit + maintenance + ongoing losses:

1. Deficit = % dehydration x bodyweight in kg (1 kg = 1000 mL).

2. Maintenance—allow:

100 mL/kg/24 h for 0–10 kg bodyweight

50 mL/kg/24 h for 10–20 kg bodyweight

20 mL/kg/24 h for >20 kg bodyweight

3. Ongoing losses:

Estimate volume of vomit and diarrhoea.

How to calculate the volume required is shown in this example:

Child weighing 10 kg with estimated 10% dehydration

- Deficit = 10% of 10 kg = 1 kg=1000 mL.
- Maintenance in 24 h = 100 mL/kg = 1000 mlL.
- Total required in 24 h = 2000 mL.

Give IV 0.9% NaCl 20 mL/kg over 30 min = 200 mL.

Give 1800 mL 4% Dex/0.18% NaCl over 24 hours, i.e. IV infusion at 75 mL/h.

Medication

There is no role for antiemetic or antidiarrhoeal medication in gastroenteritis. Antibiotics are rarely indicated except for specific bacterial infections, such as invasive salmonellosis or severe *Campylobacter* infection, and amoebiasis or giardiasis.

PYLORIC STENOSIS

Pyloric stenosis is due to hypertrophy of the smooth muscle of the pylorus and is an important cause of vomiting in babies.

Incidence

Pyloric stenosis is five times more common in boys and is familial with multifactorial inheritance.

Clinical features

It presents with persistent, projectile non-bilious vomiting between 2 and 6 weeks of age (it does not occur in the newborn or beyond 3 months of age). The infant remains hungry and eager to feed after vomiting. Weight loss, constipation, mild jaundice, and dehydration develop after a few days (Fig. 17.2).

Diagnosis

Diagnosis is clinical and made by palpation of the hypertrophied pylorus during a test feed. Peristaltic waves may be visible.

Ultrasound of the abdomen may be helpful in demonstrating the hypertrophied pylorus.

In addition, a characteristic electrolyte disturbance develops with a hypochloraemic metabolic alkalosis (serum HCO_3^- elevated to 25–35 mEq/L). This is due to the loss of acidic gastric contents.

Incidence of pyloric stenosis is 1–5 per 1000 live births:

- **More common in boys.**
- **Causes a metabolic alkalosis.**
- **Surgical treatment by Ramstedt's procedure.**

Management

The definitive treatment is the Ramstedt's procedure, in which the hypertrophied pyloric musculature is divided. This is not an emergency procedure and it is of vital importance to correct the dehydration and biochemical abnormality with IV fluid therapy before anaesthesia and surgery is undertaken.

INTUSSUSCEPTION

Intussusception is a condition in which one segment of bowel telescopes into an adjacent distal part of the bowel. It most commonly begins just proximal to the ileocaecal valve (ileum invaginates into caecum). The peak age is between 6 and 9 months, when the lead point is believed to be Peyer's patches that have been enlarged by a preceding viral infection. An anatomical lead point, such as a Meckel's diverticulum or polyp, is more likely to be present in an older child.

Clinical features

The classical presenting 'triad' is:

- Colicky abdominal pain.
- Vomiting.
- An abdominal mass.

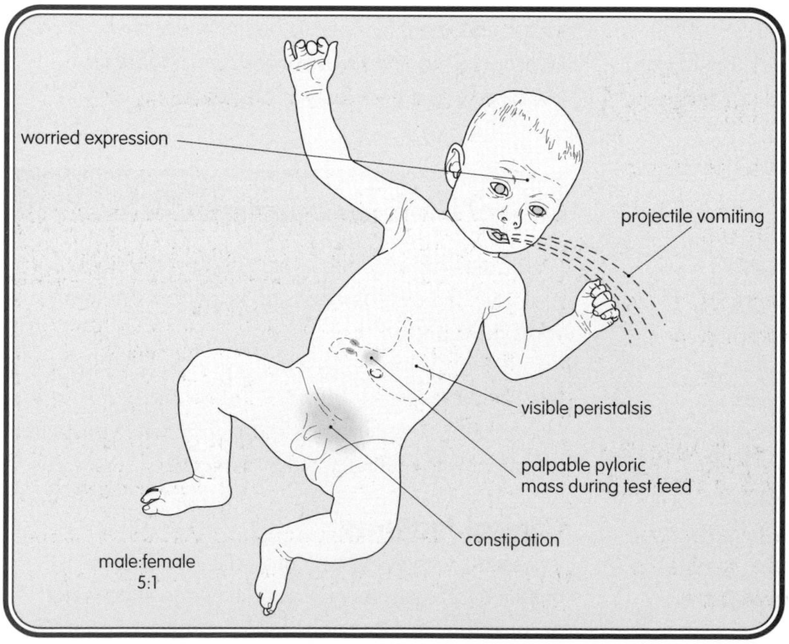

Fig. 17.2 Clinical features of pyloric stenosis.

The typical history is of episodes of screaming during which the infant draws up his legs and becomes pale. Vomiting occurs and the vomit may be bile-stained. As the blood supply to the bowel becomes progressively compromised, the characteristic 'redcurrant jelly' stool may be passed.

Examination may reveal a 'sausage-shaped' mass formed by the intussusceptum which is usually palpable in the right upper quadrant.

Rectal examination (PR) is an essential part of the assessment. The tell-tale bloodstained mucus may only be revealed on PR. Signs of intestinal obstruction and shock develop over 24–48 hours.

Plain X-ray of the abdomen is often normal, but may on occasion show small bowel obstruction, paucity of gas in the right iliac fossa, or the soft tissue outline of the intussusception itself.

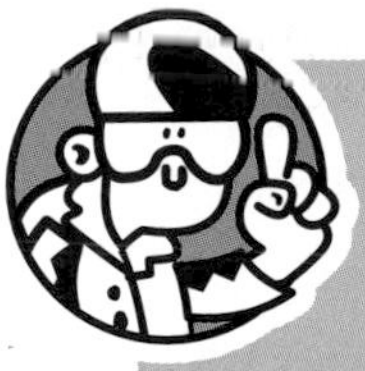

Suspect intussusception if there is:

- **An infant aged 6–9 months.**
- **Paroxysmal colicky abdominal pain.**
- **Vomiting.**
- **'Redcurrant jelly' stool.**
- **'Sausage-shaped' mass in right upper quadrant.**

Management

Intussusception is a life-threatening condition which it is easy for the unwary to misdiagnose as gastroenteritis. If suspected, an immediate diagnostic enema using air or contrast material (barium or gastrograffin) should be carried out.

In most cases, hydrostatic reduction is possible. If this is unsuccessful, operative reduction is necessary.

Enema and attempts at hydrostatic reduction are contraindicated if the history is long (24–48 hours) or if there are signs of intestinal obstruction, peritonitis, or shock.

MECKEL'S DIVERTICULUM

This remnant of the fetal vitello intestinal duct occurs in 2% of the population. It is usually 5 cm long and found 60 cm proximal to the ileocaecal valve. It contains ectopic gastric mucosa.

The majority are asymptomatic, but the most typical presentation is painless, severe rectal bleeding due to peptic ulceration. Treatment is surgical.

ACUTE APPENDICITIS

This important cause of acute abdominal pain occurs when the appendix becomes obstructed (usually by a faecolith) or inflamed by lymphatic hyperplasia. It occurs at any age, although it is rare in infants when the lumen of the appendix is wider and well drained.

Clinical features

The classic symptoms are a central abdominal pain that moves to the right iliac fossa (RIF) over a period of hours. The pain is of increasing severity and aggravated by movement (as the peritoneum is exquisitely pain sensitive).

Anorexia is usual and often associated with nausea and vomiting. Constipation may be a feature.

Clinical signs include:

- Mild fever.
- Tachycardia.
- Dehydration.
- RIF tenderness.
- Guarding in a toxic child.

The differential diagnosis is shown in Fig. 17.3.

The differential diagnosis of acute abdominal pain	
Surgical	**Medical**
appendicitis intussusception volvulus Meckel's diverticulum strangulated hernia ovarian torsion	mesenteric adenitis gastroenteritis constipation UTI lower lobe pneumonia diabetic ketoacidosis Henoch–Schönlein purpura sickle cell crisis

Fig. 17.3 The differential diagnosis of acute abdominal pain.

Diagnosis

The diagnosis is usually made clinically. If there is diagnostic uncertainty, useful investigations include:

- Urine: microscopy and culture.
- Full blood count.
- Chest X-ray.
- Abdominal ultrasound.

Management

A short period of observation can be undertaken before appendicectomy when there is uncertainty, although progression to peritonitis can occur within a few hours in young children.

Other complications include septicaemia, appendix abscess, and appendix mass. An abscess requires surgical drainage.

Conservative management is given for an appendix mass with elective appendectomy carried out 6 weeks later.

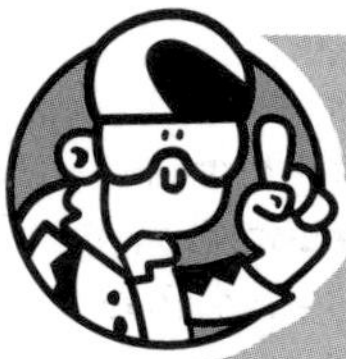

Atypical presentations with poorly localised pain are common in young children (<5 years) or when the inflamed appendix is retrocaecal or pelvic.

MESENTERIC ADENITIS

This non-specific inflammation of mesenteric lymph nodes is thought to provoke a peritoneal reaction causing acute abdominal pain that mimics appendicitis.

Clinical features

It occurs commonly in children and is often associated with other systemic symptoms and signs including fever, headache, pharyngitis, and cervical lymphadenopathy. It is likely to be viral in origin.

Diagnosis and management

Observation in hospital is often required due to the difficult diagnosis. Management is conservative, as the symptoms are self-limiting, although persisting right iliac fossa tenderness warrants surgical exploration to identify appendicitis.

COELIAC DISEASE

Incidence and aetiology

Coeliac disease arises from malabsorption caused by gluten-mediated immunological damage to the mucosa of the proximal small intestine with subsequent atrophy of the villi and loss of the absorptive surface. The incidence varies between 1 in 250 and 1 in 4000 live births, and appears to be increasing in some areas of the world.

There is a familial predisposition with 10% of first degree relatives affected.

Clinical features

A few children present with failure to thrive following weaning when gluten-containing foods are introduced to the diet. Malabsorption of fat (steatorrhoea) occurs first, with bulky, light-coloured, offensive stools.

On examination, there is:

- Poor weight gain.
- Abdominal distension.
- Buttock wasting.

The majority of cases present with more subtle problems such as:

- Diarrhoea.
- Transient poor weight gain.
- Irritability.
- Growth failure.
- Anaemia due to iron or folate deficiency.

Diagnosis

Diagnosis requires the demonstration of a flat mucosa on jejunal biopsy followed by clinical improvement on dietary gluten withdrawal. Specific IgA antigliadin or antiendomysial antibodies are a useful screening test. Empirical withdrawal of gluten from the diet should *not* be used as a diagnostic test.

Management

A diet free of gluten-containing products should be adhered to for life. Dietary supervision is required—a special sign indicates foods that are gluten-free.

Coeliac disease is associated with a variety of autoimmune disorders, including thyroid disease and pernicious anaemia, and the risk of small bowel malignancy (especially lymphoma) is increased 20-fold. A strict gluten-free diet may protect against this risk of malignancy.

FOOD INTOLERANCE

Adverse reactions to specific foods or food ingredients are not uncommon and may be transitory or permanent. The majority are immune-mediated reactions, usually to proteins, and are properly referred to as food allergies. However, non-immune-mediated intolerance also occurs, e.g. lactose intolerance due to intestinal disaccharidase deficiency.

Transient dietary protein intolerances

These are more common in infants with a strong family history of atopy or IgA deficiency. They are most commonly manifested by protracted diarrhoea with or without vomiting and failure to thrive. However, allergy to specific proteins may also play a role in eczema and migraine and, occasionally, may cause acute anaphylaxis.

Intolerance to the following foods has been described:

- Cow's milk.
- Soya.
- Wheat.
- Fish, egg, chicken, and rice.
- Nuts.

Diagnosis

Diagnosis is made when the symptoms are relieved by removal of specific foods or food constituents, and recur on reintroduction. Laboratory tests such as IgE levels or skin-prick testing are rarely helpful.

Management

Cow's milk protein intolerance, if severe, may cause a protein-losing enteropathy and blood loss. It is best managed with a casein hydrolysate-based formula as up to 30% of infants will also be, or will become, intolerant to soya. Most patients grow out of their intolerance by the age of 2 years which is therefore an appropriate time to conduct a dietary challenge.

Lactose intolerance

Lactose is the predominant disaccharide in milk and requires the intestinal brush-border enzyme lactase for its digestion. Lactase deficiency is most commonly encountered as a secondary and transient phenomenon after gastroenteritis. Congenital lactase deficiency is rare, and hereditary late-onset lactose intolerance is predominantly seen in Afro-Carribean and oriental people.

Clinical features

Accumulation of intestinal sugar results in watery diarrhoea and bacterial production of organic acids, which lowers stool pH and causes excoriation of the perianal region.

Diagnosis

Lactose is a reducing sugar and may therefore be detected in the stool by the Clinitest method.

Treatment

Treatment is with a diet free of products containing lactose and milk.

INFLAMMATORY BOWEL DISEASE

Up to one-quarter of cases of inflammatory bowel disease have their onset during childhood or adolescence.

Crohn's disease

Crohn's disease, or regional enteritis, is a transmural and focal inflammatory process that may affect any portion of the gastrointestinal tract from the mouth to the anus. The distal ileum or the colon are most frequently involved. Its cause is unknown, although there is a clear genetic predisposition. Affected intestine is thickened and non-caseating epithelioid cell granulomata are found on histology.

Ulcerative colitis

Ulcerative colitis is a chronic, recurrent inflammatory disease involving the mucous membrane of the colon. The disease process is restricted to the mucosa and begins in the rectum, extending proximally.

Clinical features of inflammatory bowel disease

It presents with:

- Cramping lower abdominal pain.
- Bloody diarrhoea.
- Weight loss.

Extra intestinal features may be present including arthritis, spondylitis, and erythema nodosum.

HIRSCHSPRUNG'S DISEASE (CONGENITAL AGANGLIONIC MEGACOLON)

This is a rare genetic disorder of bowel innervation. There is an absence of ganglion cells in the myenteric and submucosal plexuses for a variable segment of bowel extending from the anus to the colon. The aganglionic segment is narrow and contracted. It ends proximally in a normally innervated and dilated colon. It is more common in males.

Clinical features

Infants with the disease usually present in the neonatal period with:

- Delayed passage of meconium.
- Subsequent intestinal obstruction with bilious vomiting and abdominal distension.

Enterocolitis is a severe, life-threatening complication.

Older children present with:

- Chronic, severe constipation present from birth.
- Abdominal distension.
- An absence of faeces in the narrow rectum.

Diagnosis and management

Diagnosis is made by demonstrating the absence of ganglion cells on a suction biopsy of the rectum. Surgical resection of the involved colon is required. An initial colostomy is usually followed by a definitive pull-through procedure to anastomose normally innervated bowel to the anus.

BILE DUCT OBSTRUCTION

Obstruction of bile flow due to biliary atresia or a choledochal cyst are rare, but treatable, causes of persistent neonatal jaundice. Early recognition and diagnosis of these liver diseases is important.

Biliary atresia

This is a rare disorder of unknown aetiology in which there is either destruction or absence of the extrahepatic biliary tree. It represents a rare but important cause of persistent neonatal jaundice (Fig. 17.4).

Clinical features

The jaundice persists from the second day after birth and is distinguished by being due to a predominantly conjugated hyperbilirubinaemia accompanied by dark urine and pale stools.

As the disease progresses there is failure to thrive due to:

- Malabsorption.
- Enlargement of the liver and spleen.

A bleeding tendency may develop due to Vitamin K deficiency.

Diagnosis

Abdominal ultrasound, liver biopsy, and intra-operative cholangiography may be required to clarify the diagnosis.

Treatment

Treatment consists of the Kasai procedure (hepatoportoenterostomy) which needs to be carried out ideally before the age of 6 weeks.

Liver disease presenting in the newborn period: causes of conjugated hyperbilirubinaemia	
bile duct obstruction	biliary atresia choledochal cyst
neonatal hepatitis	congenital infection inborn errors: α_1 antitrypsin deficiency galactosaemia

Fig. 17.4 Liver disease presenting in the newborn period: causes of conjugated hyperbilirubinaemia.

18. Renal and Genitourinary Disorders

Structural abnormalities of the kidney and urinary tract are common, and many are now identified on antenatal ultrasound screening. The most common disease encountered in this system is urinary tract infection, which has special significance because of its potential to damage the growing kidneys.

URINARY TRACT ANOMALIES

Congenital abnormalities of the kidneys and urinary tract can be identified in about 1 in 400 fetuses. They may be detected on antenatal ultrasound screening or present with a variety of symptoms and signs in infancy or later childhood (see Hints & Tips).

Congenital anomalies of the urinary tract include:

- Renal anomalies.
- Obstructive lesions of the urinary tract.
- Vesicoureteric reflux.

Presentation of urinary tract anomalies:

- **Urinary tract infection.**
- **Recurrent abdominal pain.**
- **Palpable mass.**
- **Haematuria.**
- **Failure to thrive.**

Renal anomalies

Absence of both kidneys (renal agenesis) results in Potter syndrome in which oligohydramnios (caused by lack of fetal urine) is associated with lung hypoplasia and postural deformities (see Hints & Tips).

Other anomalies include:

- Abnormalities of ascent and rotation.
- Duplex kidney (Fig. 18.1).
- Horseshoe kidney (Fig. 18.1).
- Cystic disease of the kidney.
- Renal dysplasia.

Ectopia of the kidney is common and pain arising from an ectopic kidney may be misleading on account of its site.

Duplex systems are commonly associated with other abnormalities such as renal dysplasia and vesicoureteric reflux. The upper pole ureter may be ectopic (draining into the urethra or vagina) and the lower pole ureter often refluxes.

There are many conditions associated with cystic kidneys including:

- Autosomal recessive infantile polycystic kidney disease.
- Autosomal dominant adult-type polycystic kidney disease.
- Tuberous sclerosis.

Obstructive lesions of the urinary tract

The site of obstruction may be at the pelviureteric (PU) junction, the vesicoureteric (VU) junction, the bladder, or the urethra (Fig. 18.2).

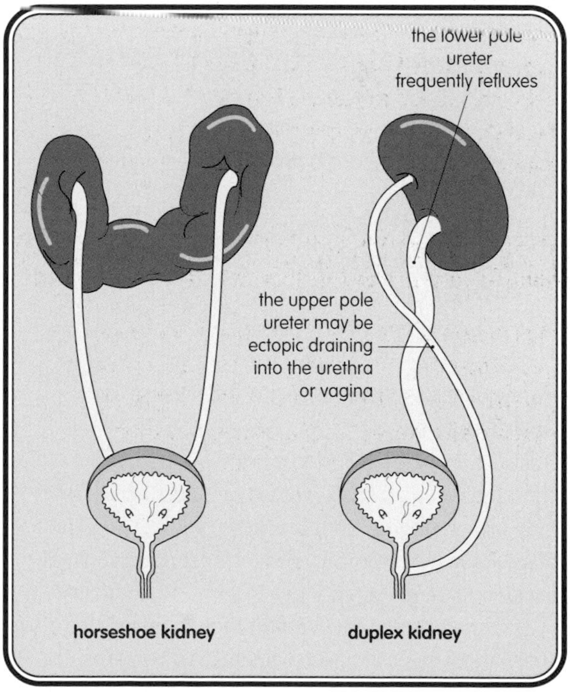

Fig. 18.1 Urinary tract anomalies.

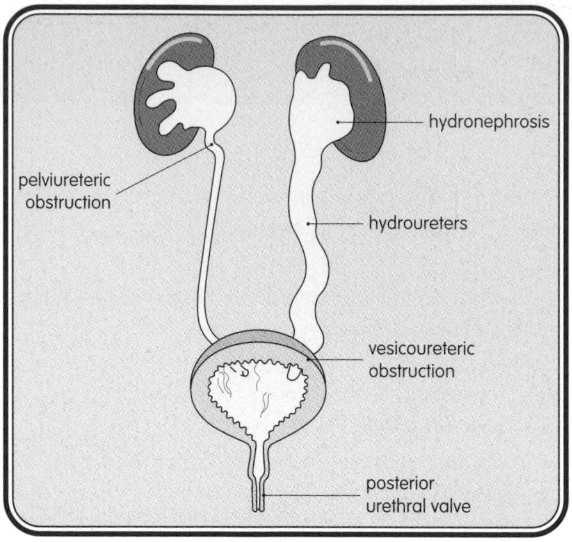

Fig. 18.2 Sites of urinary tract obstruction and dilatation.

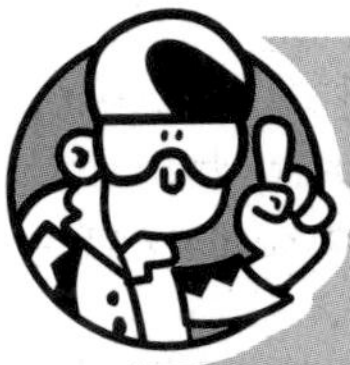

Features of Potter syndrome:
- **Renal agenesis.**
- **Oligohydramnios.**
- **Lung hypoplasia.**
- **Characteristic facies.**
- **Postural deformities, e.g. talipes.**

If undetected before birth, the patient may present with:
- A urinary tract infection.
- Abdominal or loin pain.
- Haematuria.
- A palpable bladder or kidney.

Pelviureteric obstruction (congenital hydronephrosis)

Obstruction may be due to a narrow lumen or compression by a fibrous band or blood vessel, and may vary in degree from partial to almost complete obstruction (with gross hydronephrosis and minimal remaining renal tissue).

Mild degrees of obstruction may resolve spontaneously, but severe obstruction requires surgical treatment with conservation of renal tissue wherever possible.

Vesicoureteric obstruction

Obstruction may be due to stenosis, kinking, or dilatation of the lower part of the ureter (ureterocele) and may be unilateral or bilateral. There is a combination of hydroureter and hydronephrosis.

Posterior urethral valves

These are abnormal folds of the urethral mucous membrane, which occur in males in the region of the verumontanum. They impede the flow of urine with back-pressure on the bladder, ureters, and kidneys.

The degree of obstruction varies from the very severe (with death *in utero* from renal failure or after birth from Potter syndrome), to the less severe (which presents usually with urinary tract infection, poor urinary stream, and renal insufficiency in a male).

Vesicoureteric reflux

Primary vesicoureteric reflux (VUR) is caused by a developmental anomaly of the vesicoureteric junction. The ureters enter directly into the bladder, rather than at an angle and the segment of ureter within the bladder wall is abnormally short. Urine refluxes up the ureter during voiding, predisposing to infection and exposing the kidneys to bacteria and high pressure. There is a spectrum of severity which is graded I–V (Fig. 18.3).

Clinical features

VUR is often associated with other genitourinary anomalies and may be secondary to bladder pathology, e.g. neuropathic bladder.

The important consequences of VUR include:
- Predisposition to urinary tract infection.
- Urinary tract infection and pyelonephritis.
- Reflux nephropathy. This is destruction of renal tissue with scarring due to infection and back-pressure. If severe, it may result in high blood pressure and chronic renal failure.

Diagnosis

VUR is diagnosed by a micturating cystourethrogram (MCUG). In the older child, it can also be diagnosed by dynamic nuclear medicine scanning using MAG3 or DTPA (indirect cystography).

Management

The management depends on severity. Mild VUR resolves spontaneously (10% each year), but

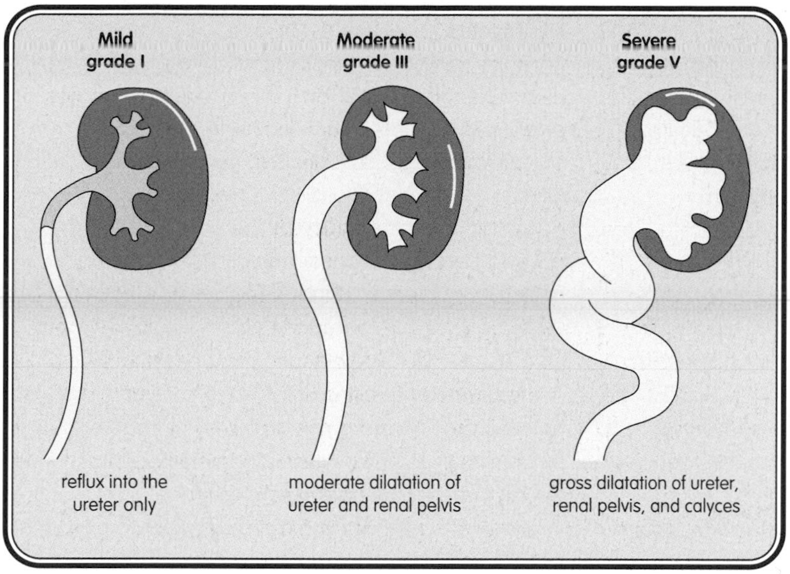

Fig. 18.3 Grades of vesicoureteric reflux.

prophylactic antibiotics (e.g. trimethoprim) are given to prevent infection. Severe grades of VUR may benefit from surgical reimplantation of the ureters.

GENITALIA

Inguinoscrotal disorders

Inguinoscrotal disorders include:

- Undescended testis.
- Inguinal hernia and hydrocele.
- The acute scrotum.

Undescended testis

The testes develop intra-abdominally and migrate through the inguinal canal to the scrotum in the third trimester. The testes are therefore normally in the scrotum in term newborns, but are frequently undescended in preterm infants.

Clinical features and examination

A testis that has not reached the scrotum (undescended testis) may be:

- Incompletely descended: lying along normal pathway (the minority, 20%).
- Maldescended or ectopic: deviated from the normal path after emerging from the superficial inguinal ring (the majority, 80%).

An undescended testis must be distinguished from a 'retractile' testis that can be coaxed down into the scrotum. (Examination should be undertaken in a warm room with warm hands.)

The testes are examined during routine surveillance in the newborn, at 6 weeks and at 18 months. Referral to a surgeon should be made if either testis is impalpable or an ectopic testis is found at the 6 week check.

Further investigations may be helpful if one or both testes are impalpable in order to determine their existence and location. These may include:

- Ultrasound.
- Magnetic resonance imaging.
- Laparoscopy.
- Endocrine investigations.

The testes may be absent in cases of intersex.

Management

Treatment is by orchidopexy and this is best performed between the age of 1 and 2 years. Potential, but unproven, benefits include:

- A reduced risk of torsion.
- Psychological and cosmetic benefits.
- Reduced risk of malignancy.
- Improved fertility.

Orchidectomy is indicated for a unilateral intra-abdominal testis that is not amenable to orchidopexy.

Inguinal hernias and hydroceles

The testis descends into the scrotum taking with it a connecting fold of peritoneum (the processus vaginalis) which normally becomes obliterated at or around birth. Failure of the processus vaginalis to close results in an inguinal hernia or a hydrocoele (Fig 18.4).

Inguinal hernias

Inguinal hernias are more common in boys, premature babies, and infants, with a positive family history. A minority are bilateral. The parents notice an intermittent swelling in the groin or scrotum.

The main concern is the risk of strangulation which is higher in young infants. Referral for prompt surgery is indicated.

Danger signs in the initially irreducible hernia are:

- Hardness.
- Tenderness.
- Vomiting.

These suggest entrapment of bowel within the sac and compromise of its vascular supply (strangulation). Urgent referral is imperative.

Sedation, analgesia, and expert manipulation may allow reduction which is followed by surgical repair.

Hydroceles

If the connection with the processus vaginalis is small, a hydrocele forms rather than an inguinal hernia. The swelling is painless and being full of fluid it transilluminates. It is possible to get above the swelling, which cannot be reduced.

Spontaneous resolution by the age of 12 months is common and treatment during infancy is not required unless it is extremely large.

The acute scrotum

Acute pain and swelling of the scrotum is an emergency because of the possibility of testicular torsion. It occurs most frequently in the neonatal period and at puberty, but can occur at any age.

Inadequate fixation to the tunica vaginalis allows the testis to rotate and occlude its vascular supply. Doppler studies may assist in diagnosis.

Surgical exploration must not be delayed, as the testis may become non-viable. The defect is often bilateral, so the contralateral testis should also be fixed at surgery.

The differential diagnosis includes:

- Torsion of the testicular appendix (hydatid of Morgagni).
- Epididymo-orchitis.
- Idiopathic scrotal oedema.

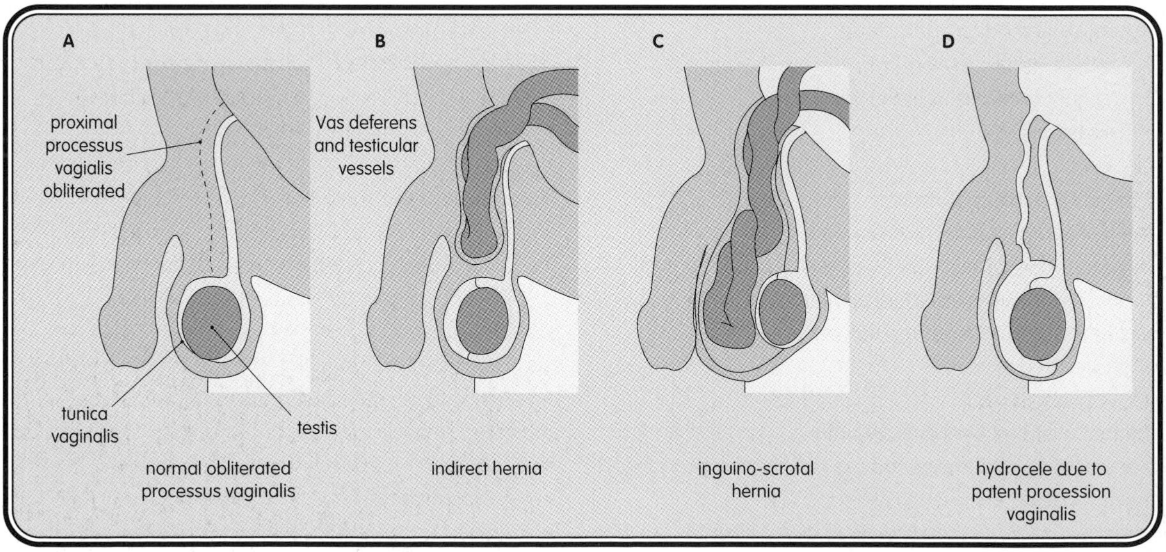

Fig 18.4 (A) The normal testis. Following normal testicular descent, the processus vaginalis, an evagination of the parietal peritoneum between the internal inguinal ring and testis, disappears leaving only the tunica vaginalis around the testis. Persistence of the processus vaginalis results in an inguinal hernia (B, C), or a hydrocele (D).

Penile abnormalities

Penile abnormalities include:

- Hypospadias.
- Phimosis.

Hypospadias

A spectrum of congenital abnormalities of the position of the urethral meatus occurs. Severe forms are associated with chordee, a ventral curvature of the penis.

Phimosis

This refers to adhesion of the foreskin to the glans penis after the age of 3 years. Mild degrees can be managed with periodic, gentle retraction. Paraphimosis is irreducible retraction of the foreskin beyond the coronal sulcus.

Circumcision

Non-retractility of the foreskin and preputial adhesions are normal in small boys, and forcible attempts to retract the foreskin are ill-advised as this may lead to scarring and phimosis.

Ballooning of the prepuce during urination is not uncommon and this usually resolves as the prepuce becomes more retractile.

Balanitis xerotica obliterans (lichen sclerosis) causes a thickened, scarred, white prepuce that is fixed to the glans. This, recurrent balanitis (infection of the glans), and sometimes recurrent urinary tract infection (UTI), are the only medical indications for circumcision. Most circumcisions are performed for religious reasons.

Complications of circumcision include:

- Haemorrhage.
- Infection.
- Damage to the glans.

The procedure should not be undertaken lightly.

An infant with hypospadias must not be circumcised as the foreskin is used at surgical correction.

Vulvovaginitis

Inflammation of the vulva and vaginal discharge is a not uncommon problem in young girls. Predisposing factors include poor hygiene, tight-fitting clothing, and threadworm infection. A vulval swab may detect a yeast or streptococcal infection which can be treated with the appropriate topical or oral therapy. Often, general measures are the most important. These include the avoidance of bubble bath, strong soaps and synthetic underwear. If these measures fail, examination under anaesthetic to exclude a vaginal foreign body may be indicated.

Rarely, vulvovaginitis may result from sexual abuse.

URINARY TRACT INFECTION

Infection of the urinary tract is common in children. About 3–5% of girls and 1–2% of boys will have a symptomatic UTI during childhood. Sex-specific infection rates vary with age.

In children, most infections are caused by *Escherichia coli* originating from the bowel flora. Other pathogens include *Proteus spp.* (especially in boys), *Klebsiella spp., Pseudomonas spp.*, and *Enterococcus spp.* The most common host factor predisposing to UTI is urinary stasis. Important causes of urinary stasis include:

- Vesicoureteric reflux (VUR).
- Obstructive uropathy, e.g. ureterocoele, urethral valves.
- Neuropathic bladder, e.g. spina bifida.
- Habitual infrequent voiding and constipation.

Clinical features

The clinical features vary markedly with age:

- In neonates and very young infants jaundice may occur and septicaemia may develop, rapidly leading to shock and hypotension.
- In infants, UTI may occur with or without fever and symptoms are non-specific: vomiting, diarrhoea, irritability, failure to thrive.
- Between 1 and 5 years of age, fever, malaise, abdominal discomfort, urinary frequency, and nocturnal enuresis are the presenting features. In this age group, dysuria may also be due to balanitis or vulvovaginitis.

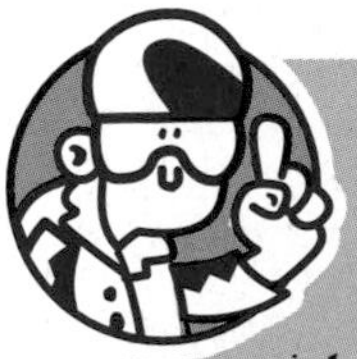

UTIs occur:

- **Predominantly in boys up to age 3 months.**
- **Equally in boys and girls from 3–12 months.**
- **Increasingly in girls rather than boys after age 1 year.**

- **UTI presents with non-specific features in infants.**
- **UTI must be suspected in any febrile infant with no obvious clinical source.**

- Over 5 years of age, the classical presenting features of cystitis (frequency, dysuria, fever, and enuresis) or pyelonephritis (fever and loin pain) occur. Asymptomatic bacteriuria is common in school-age girls.

Diagnosis

Confirmation of diagnosis requires culture of a pure growth of a single pathogen of at least 10^8 colony-forming units per litre of urine. However, obtaining an uncontaminated urine sample from infants and children is not always easy (Fig. 18.5). Specimens should be chilled without delay to 4°C (i.e. refrigerate) to prevent bacterial multiplication. The presence or absence of pyuria is an unreliable guide.

A positive nitrite stick test is a reliable test for coliform infection, but false negatives occur if the urine has been in the bladder for less than an hour or the organism does not convert nitrate (e.g. enterococci).

Treatment of the acute infection

Prompt treatment with antibiotics is indicated to reduce the risk of renal scarring. This should be initiated as soon as a urine sample has been taken for culture, using the 'best guess' antibiotic. Treatment can be modified when urine culture results are available and stopped if the culture is negative.

A urine sample should be cultured from:

- **Any infant with a fever and no obvious clinical source.**
- **Any child with recurrent or prolonged fever.**
- **Any child with unexplained abdominal pain.**
- **Any child with dysuria or frequency, enuresis or haematuria.**

Antibiotic choice:

- Oral trimethoprim is a suitable initial choice for uncomplicated UTI in an older child.
- Parenteral antibiotics, e.g. ampicillin plus gentamicin or cefuroxime, should be given to infants or any systemically unwell older child, and to children with signs of acute pyelonephritis or a known urinary tract abnormality.
- Prophylactic antibiotics should be given in low dose after treatment of the acute infection, until investigation of the urinary tract is complete.

Further investigation

All children require further imaging of their urinary tract after a first confirmed UTI. The aim of this is:

- To identify any predisposing underlying anatomical or functional abnormality of the urinary tract such as vesicoureteric reflux.
- To identify renal scars.

Although the outcome for the majority of infants and

Collecting a urine sample

Method	Indication
suprapubic aspiration	appropriate in a severely ill infant requiring urgent diagnosis. Success is enhanced by ultrasound guidance
'clean-catch' midstream specimen	possible in a male infant or continent child
'bag urine'	a plastic bag is attached and removed immediately urine is passed. Sample emptied into a sterile container through a snipped corner

Fig. 18.5 Collecting a urine sample.

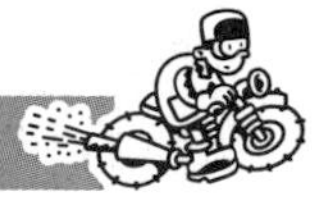

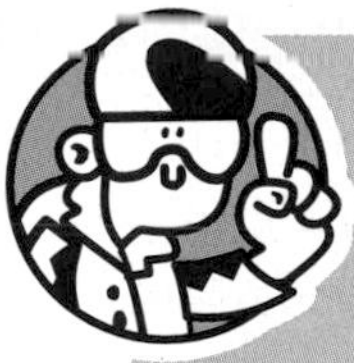

All children require further investigation after a first confirmed UTI to identify anatomical or functional abnormalities and renal scars.

children with UTI is benign, a small minority are at risk of renal damage, especially those with recurrent infection associated with vesicoureteric reflux.

The exact scheme depends on the age of the child. No single imaging investigation provides a full assessment.

An initial ultrasound of the kidneys and urinary tract is performed on all infants and young children. A renal ultrasound scan is valuable for:

- Demonstrating the presence of two kidneys.
- Identifying obstruction with urinary tract dilatation.

It is *not* reliable for detecting renal scars or vesicoureteric reflux.

Infants aged under 1 year

In addition to ultrasonography, recommendations include:

- Micturating cystourethrogram (MCUG), to identify vesicoureteric reflux.
- Static radioisotope scan (DMSA), to identify renal scars.

These investigations are deferred until 3 months after the acute infection to avoid detecting transient abnormalities. Prophylactic antibiotics should be given in the interim.

Children aged between 1 and 7 years

Ultrasonography and a radioisotope scan are recommended. MCUG can be reserved for:

- Children in whom the radioisotope scan shows an abnormality.
- Children with recurrent infection.
- Children with a family history of reflux or reflux nephropathy.

The risk of developing renal scarring becomes less with increasing age and is uncommon with infection in children over 5 years of age.

Simple advice should be given concerning measures, which can reduce recurrence risk, i.e.

- High fluid intake.
- Regular unhurried voiding.
- Good perineal hygiene.

If investigations reveal vesicoureteric reflux or renal scarring, prophylactic antibiotics are given at least until the child is 2–3 years old (i.e. past the period of greatest risk for renal scarring).

Children with recurrent UTI or scarring require regular follow-up with a repeat urine culture, BP monitoring, and further renal imaging to check for new scar formation and resolution of vesicoureteric reflux.

ACUTE NEPHRITIS

Acute nephritis is a clinical condition caused by inflammatory changes in the glomeruli. It is characterized by:

- Fluid retention (oedema, hypertension).
- Haematuria.
- Proteinuria.

The majority of cases are postinfectious and follow a streptococcal throat or skin infection with Group A β-haemolytic streptococci. Less common causes include:

- Henoch–Schönlein purpura.
- IgA nephropathy.
- Mesangiocapillary glomerulonephritis.

Clinical features

The presenting history may be of discoloured 'smoky' urine. Physical examination reveals signs of fluid overload such as oedema and raised blood pressure.

Diagnosis

The urine is positive for blood and protein, and microscopy may reveal red cells and casts. Renal function should be evaluated by measuring plasma urea, electrolytes, and creatinine.

An abdominal X-ray and ultrasound may be required to exclude other causes of haematuria.

The aetiology is pursued with a throat swab, antistreptolysin 0 titre, complement C3 levels, and ESR.

Management

Management centres around:

- Control of fluid and electrolyte balance by monitoring intake and output.
- Use of diuretics and antihypertensives as required.

The prognosis of poststreptococcal nephritis is good. However, rarely, a rapidly progressive glomerulonephritis with renal failure may occur, especially in nephritis from other causes. Diagnostic renal biopsy is indicated in these circumstances as immunosuppression may prevent irreversible renal failure if used early.

NEPHROTIC SYNDROME

The nephrotic syndrome is a clinical condition characterized by heavy proteinuria, oedema, and a low plasma albumin. Prolonged glomerular leakage of protein leads to hypoalbuminaemia that is associated with loss of fluid into the extracellular space, manifested as oedema. Reduction in circulating volume stimulates renal retention of salt and water.

In 90% of cases, childhood nephrotic syndrome is accounted for by an immune-mediated process associated with 'minimal change' histology and responsiveness to steroid therapy.

Clinical features

The usual presenting feature is oedema which manifests as:

- Puffiness around the eyes.
- Swelling of the feet and legs.
- In severe cases, gross scrotal oedema, ascites and pleural effusions.

Reduced urine output and 'frothiness' of the urine may have been noticed.

Diagnosis

Diagnosis is confirmed by documentation of proteinuria (+++ on dipstix testing) and hypoalbuminaemia, usually less than 25 g/L (normal range 35–40 g/L). Additional investigations should include biochemical renal function tests (urea, electrolytes, creatinine), urine microscopy, and Hep. B antigen.

The following features should prompt consideration of renal biopsy to identify rarer causes such as focal segmental glomerulosclerosis or membranoproliferative glomerulonephritis, which are usually steroid resistant:

- Age—below 1 year or over 10 years.
- Presence of macroscopic haematuria.
- Hypertension.
- Evidence of renal failure.

Management

If the clinical features are consistent with classical steroid-sensitive nephrotic syndrome, treatment is begun with oral steroids (prednisolone, 60 mg/m^2/day). Remission usually occurs within 10 days.

Several serious complications may occur including hypovolaemia (manifested by a high PCV, hypotension, and peripheral vasoconstriction) and thrombosis or infection (due to the hypercoagulable state and loss of immunoglobulins).

Penicillin prophylaxis is given in the acute phase to prevent pneumococcal infection.

Subsequent relapses may occur which, if frequent, may require the use of additional immunosuppressive agents such as cyclophosphamide.

HAEMOLYTIC URAEMIC SYNDROME

This uncommon syndrome is the most common cause of acute renal failure due to intrinsic renal disease in children under the age of 4 years. It is usually caused by a preceding infection, most often gastroenteritis due to a verotoxin-producing strain of *Escherichia coli*.

As the name suggests, there is a microangiopathic haemolytic anaemia associated with parenchymal renal disease characterized by haematuria, proteinuria, and acute renal failure.

Management is supportive and most children recover full renal function.

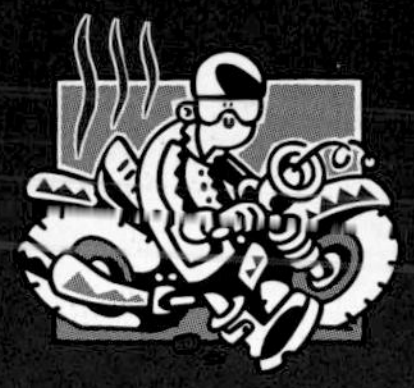

19. Neurological Disorders

The developing nervous system is susceptible to damage by a host of diverse pathological processes, inherited and acquired. Malformations, infections, trauma, genetic diseases, and tumours all affect the nervous system. Several important conditions affecting the nervous system are considered elsewhere:

- Neonatal hypoxia–ischaemia (see Chapter 27).
- Head injury (see Chapter 28).
- Coma (see Chapter 28).
- Brain tumours (see Chapter 22).
- Neural tube defects (see Chapter 9).

MALFORMATIONS OF THE CENTRAL NERVOUS SYSTEM (CNS)

If severe, these cause fetalloss or early death. They encompass such important conditions as:

- Hydrocephalus.
- Craniosynostosis.
- Neural tube defects.

Hydrocephalus

Hydrocephalus is enlargement of the cerebral ventricles due to excessive accumulation of cerebrospinal fluid (CSF). This condition is the most frequent cause of an enlarged and rapidly expanding head in newborn infants.

The causes include a variety of acquired pathological mechanisms as well as malformations (Fig. 19.1). Hydrocephalus is classified according to whether or not the ventricles communicate with the subarachnoid space:

- In non-communicating hydrocephalus, the obstruction is intraventricular.
- In communicating hydrocephalus, it is extraventricular.

Clinical features

The presenting clinical features vary with age. Dilated ventricles can be detected on antenatal ultrasound.

In infants:

- The head circumference is disproportionately large and its rate of growth is excessive.
- The anterior fontanelle's pressure is increased, sutures become separated, and scalp veins are prominent. If untreated, the eyes deviate downward (setting-sun sign).

In older children, the clinical features are those of raised intracranial pressure:

- Headache.
- Vomiting.
- Lethargy.
- Irritability.
- Papilloedema.

Diagnosis

Diagnosis is confirmed by imaging. If the anterior fontanelle is still open, ultrasound can be used to assess ventricular dilatation. A computed tomography scan (CT) or magnetic resonance imaging (MRI) will establish the diagnosis, evaluate the cause, and is useful for monitoring treatment and detecting complications.

Treatment

The mainstay of treatment is insertion of a ventriculoperitoneal shunt. Complications of shunts include obstruction and infection.

Craniosynostosis

This is premature fusion of the cranial sutures. Most affected infants present soon after birth with an abnormal skull, the shape of which depends on which

Causes of hydrocephalus

Non-communicating (intraventricular obstruction)
congenital malformation:
- aqueduct stenosis
- Dandy–Walker syndrome

intraventricular haemorrhage
ventriculitis
brain tumour

Communicating (extraventricular obstruction)
subarachnoid haemorrhage
tuberculous meningitis
Arnold–Chiari malformation

Fig. 19.1 Causes of hydrocephalus.

sutures have fused. The sagittal suture is most commonly involved, causing a long, narrow skull.

Generalized craniosynostosis is a cause of microcephaly.

Neural tube defects

These were the most common congenital defects of the CNS and are considered in detail in Chapter 9. In the UK, the birth prevalence has fallen because of antenatal screening. There has also been a natural decline, of which, the cause is uncertain.

A range of lesions occur:

- Spina bifida occulta: the vertebral arch fails to fuse. There may be associated tethering of the cord.
- Meningocele: meninges herniate through a vertebral defect.
- Myelomeningocele: meninges and spinal cord herniate: the most severe form of spinal dysrhaphism.
- Encephalocoele: extrusion of the brain and meninges through a midline skull defect.
- Anencephaly: cranium and brain fail to develop (detected on antenatal ultrasound and termination of pregnancy is usually performed).

INFECTIONS OF THE CNS

Meningitis

A range of bacteria and viruses (Fig. 19.2) may cause acute meningitis. Rare causes include TB, fungal infections, and malignant infiltration. The serious and potentially lethal nature of bacterial meningitis renders it most important. Although more common, viral meningitis is a relatively benign and self-limiting disease.

Acute meningitis: common pathogens

Bacterial
Neisseria meningitidis
Streptococcus pneumoniae
Haemophilus influenzae type B
During the neonatal period:
- Group B streptococci
- *E. coli*
- *Listeria monocytogenes*

Viral
mumps
enteroviruses
Epstein–Barr virus

Fig. 19.2 Meningitis: common pathogens.

Early signs of meningitis in infants are non-specific. Immediate treatment with parenteral penicillin is indicated for suspected meningococcal septicaemia.

Bacterial meningitis

The peak age of incidence is younger than 5 years old, and 80% of all cases occur in children under 16 years. Meningococcal meningitis accounts for over half of all cases and in the UK, Group B is the most common variety. Pneumococcal meningitis is less common and tends to affect the children under 2 and older adults. It has a high fatality rate (10%) and a high risk of neurological sequelae (30%). Since the introduction of Hib vaccination in the UK in 1992, meningitis due to *H. influenzae* type B has become rare.

The pathogens are carried in the nasal passages and invade the meninges via the bloodstream. In the early stages, symptoms and signs are non-specific, making diagnosis difficult, especially in infants.

Clinical features

There may be irritability, poor feeding, vomiting, fever, and drowsiness. More specific signs develop later, including:

- A bulging fontanelle in babies.
- Neck stiffness and photophobia in the older child.
- A convulsion.

Meningococcal infection may present with a characteristic non-blanching purpuric rash.

Diagnosis

Lumbar puncture (LP) and examination of the CSF is diagnostic. A high index of suspicion (and low threshold for performing an LP) is necessary in young children in whom signs and symptoms of meningitis are non-specific.

If there are focal neurological signs or clinical signs of raised intracranial pressure (coma, papilloedema), treatment can be initiated without performing a LP as there is a risk of coning.

Rapid diagnostic tests are available (Chapter 12). Blood cultures should also be taken.

Treatment

Broad-spectrum intravenous antibiotic treatment is initiated using a third-generation cephalosporin, e.g. cefotaxime. A febrile child with a purpuric rash (i.e. suspected meningococcal sepsis) should be treated *immediately* with benzylpenicillin (IM or IV) and transferred urgently to hospital. Meningococcal septicaemia can kill within hours and early antibiotic treatment significantly reduces fatality rates. In infants under 3 months, ampicillin may be added empirically to cover *Listeria monocytogenes*.

There is evidence that a component of the tissue damage in meningitis is caused by the host's inflammatory response. Attempts have been made to suppress this with steroids: dexamethasone has been shown to reduce the incidence of some neurological sequelae in non-neonatal meningitis caused by *H. influenzae* and *S. pneumoniae*.

Complications

Acute complications of meningitis include:

- Inappropriate ADH secretion (fluids should be restricted).
- Subdural effusion.
- Cerebral oedema.
- Convulsions.

Neurological sequelae include sensorineural deafness: all children should have their hearing tested following meningitis. Rifampicin is given to the patient, and to all household contacts, following infection with meningococcus or *H. influenzae* type B in order to eradicate nasopharyngeal carriage.

Encephalitis

In encephalitis there is inflammation of the brain substance. Acute encephalitis is usually viral. The most common causes in the UK are:

- Herpes simplex virus 1 and 2.
- Enteroviruses.
- Varicella.

The common viral exanthems (measles, rubella, mumps, and varicella) can all cause encephalitis by direct viral invasion of the brain or can be complicated by an immune-mediated postinfectious encephalomyelitis (see below).

Clinical features

The clinical features include early non-specific symptoms and signs such as fever, headache, and vomiting, followed by the abrupt development of an encephalopathic illness characterized by altered consciousness, seizures, and raised intracranial pressure.

Diagnosis and management

Early recognition of herpes simplex encephalitis is important as specific treatment with acyclovir improves prognosis if given early.

Diagnosis is difficult acutely, but EEG and MRI may show evidence of the characteristic temporal lobe abnormalities.

Supportive management for severe encephalitis may require:

- Admission to an Intensive Care Unit for intracranial pressure monitoring.
- Treatment of cerebral oedema with mannitol and dexamethasone.

Postinfectious syndromes

These may affect the brain or peripheral nervous system.

- Postinfectious encephalomyelitis: delayed brain swelling caused by an immune-mediated inflammatory reaction to viral infection. It may follow any of the common viral exanthems.
- Varicella zoster typically causes an acute cerebellitis.

Acute postinfectious polyneuropathy (Guillain–Barré syndrome)

This demyelinating polyneuropathy follows 2–3 weeks after a viral infection with, for example, cytomegalovirus or Epstein–Barr virus, or infection with *Mycoplasma pneumoniae* or *Campylobacter jejuni*.

Clinical features

It usually begins with fleeting sensory symptoms in the toes and fingers and progresses to a symmetrical, ascending paralysis with loss of tendon reflexes. Autonomic involvement may occur and respiratory depression may be life-threatening. The disease may progress over several weeks. The CSF protein is characteristically markedly raised.

Management
Supportive care including assisted ventilation may be required. Respiratory function must be closely monitored. Specific therapy includes immunoglobulin infusion and plasma exchange. There may be residual neurological problems.

CEREBRAL PALSY

Cerebral palsy (CP) is defined as a disorder of motor function due to a non-progressive (static) lesion of the developing brain. It is useful to remember that:

- Although the lesion is non-progressive, the clinical manifestations evolve as the nervous system develops.
- Children with cerebral palsy often have problems in addition to disorders of movement and posture, reflecting more widespread damage to the brain.

The cause is unknown in many patients, but identified risk factors can be categorized into antenatal, intrapartum, and postnatal (Fig. 19.3).

Clinical features

There may be a history of risk factors and motor delay. Cerebral palsy may present with:

- Delayed motor milestones.
- Abnormal tone and posturing in infancy.
- Feeding difficulties due to lack of oromotor coordination.
- Speech and language delay.

Causes of cerebral palsy

Antenatal (80%)
cerebral dysgenesis
congenital infections:
- rubella
- CMV
- toxoplasmosis

Intrapartum (10%)
birth asphyxia

Postnatal (10%)
preterm birth:
- hypoxic–ischaemic encephalopathy
- intraventricular haemorrhage

hyperbilirubinaemia
hypoglycaemia
head injury
intracranial infection:
- meningitis
- encephalitis

Fig. 19.3 Causes of cerebral palsy.

Diagnosis

The diagnosis is made on clinical examination which may show abnormalities of:

- Tone—e.g. hypertonia or hypotonia.
- Power—e.g. hemiparesis.
- Reflexes—e.g. brisk tendon reflexes or abnormal absence (or persistence) of primitive reflexes.
- Abnormal movements—e.g. athetosis or chorea.
- Abnormal posture or gait.

Classification

Cerebral palsy is classified according to the anatomical distribution of the lesion and the main functional abnormalities (Fig. 19.4).

Spastic cerebral palsy
Damage to the pyramidal pathways causes increased limb tone (spasticity) with brisk deep-tendon reflexes, and extensor plantar responses. Hypotonia may precede spasticity. The distribution of affected limbs allows further classification:

- Hemiparesis: arm may be affected more than leg or vice versa.
- Diplegia: all four limbs are affected, but legs more than arms. This is the characteristic CP of the preterm infant.
- Quadriplegia: all four limbs are affected, but arms worse than legs. Often there is truncal involvement, with seizures, and intellectual impairment. This is the most severe form and is the characteristic CP of severe birth asphyxia.

Ataxic cerebral palsy
Caused by damage to the cerebellum or its pathways. Features include early hypotonia with poor balance, uncoordinated movements, and delayed motor development.

Dyskinetic cerebral palsy
Caused by damage to the basal ganglia or extrapyramidal pathways (e.g. in kernicterus). The clinical presentation is often with hypotonia and delayed motor development. Abnormal involuntary movements may appear later which include chorea (abrupt, jerky movements), athetosis (slow writhing

Classification of cerebral palsy

Spastic (70%)
hemiplegic
diplegic
quadriplegic
Dyskinetic (10%)
athetoid
dystonic
Ataxic (10%)
hypotonic
Mixed (10%)

Fig. 19.4 Classification of cerebral palsy.

continuous movements), or dystonia (sustained abnormal postures).

Management of CP

Management requires a multidisciplinary approach. Accurate diagnosis and prognosis must be given to the parents. Prognosis in early infancy can be uncertain. A programme of physiotherapy may be indicated and orthopaedic intervention is often beneficial (braces, surgery, special shoes). Attention must be paid to associated problems such as sensory deficits, learning difficulties, and epilepsy.

EPILEPSY

Epilepsy is common, affecting 5 out of 1000 school-age children.

It is useful to distinguish between an 'epileptic seizure', which is a transient event, and epilepsy, which is a disease or syndrome:

- An epileptic seizure is a transient episode of abnormal and excessive neuronal activity in the brain that is apparent either to the subject or an observer.
- Epilepsy is a chronic disorder of the brain characterized by recurrent, unprovoked epileptic seizures.

Several important features of these definitions require emphasis.

With epileptic seizures:

- The abnormal neuronal activity during an epileptic seizure may be manifested as a motor, sensory, autonomic, cognitive, or psychic disturbance. The neurophysiological basis is inferred on clinical grounds.
- A convulsion is a subtype of seizure in which motor activity occurs.
- An electrophysiological disturbance unaccompanied by any clinical change is *not* classified as an epileptic seizure.
- There are many paroxysmal disturbances ('funny turns') that mimic epileptic seizures (see Chapter 5).

In epilepsy, a diagnosis is made in a patient *in whom epileptic seizures recur spontaneously*.

However, it is important to recognize that an 'epileptic seizure' can be provoked in individuals who do *not* have epilepsy (examples of provoking insults include fever, hypoglycaemia, trauma, and hypoxia).

Classification and terminology

The International League Against Epilepsy has devised a useful classification system for epileptic seizures and for epilepsies and epilepsy syndromes. In any patient, an attempt should be made:

- To identify the types of seizure occurring.
- To diagnose the epilepsy or epilepsy syndrome present.

Terms such as grand mal and petit mal are outdated and should be avoided.

Classification of epileptic seizures

The initial division is into (Fig. 19.5):

- Generalized seizures—in which the first clinical change indicates initial involvement of both cerebral hemispheres.
- Partial seizures—in which there is initial activation of part of one cerebral hemisphere.

Partial seizures are further classified into:

- Simple, in which consciousness is retained.
- Complex, in which consciousness is impaired or lost.

A partial seizure may become secondarily generalized.

Classification of epilepsies and epilepsy syndromes

The initial division is according to the seizure type into (Fig. 19.6):

- Generalized epilepsies and syndromes.
- Localization-related epilepsies and syndromes.

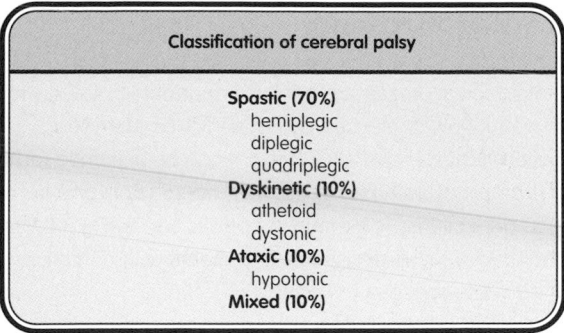

Classification of epileptic seizures

Generalized
- absence seizures
- myoclonic seizures
- clonic seizures
- tonic seizures
- tonic–clonic seizures
- atonic seizures

Partial

simple (consciousness not impaired)
- with motor symptoms (Jacksonian)
- with somatosensory or special sensory symptoms
- with autonomic symptoms
- with psychic symptoms

complex (with impairment of consciousness)
- beginning as simple partial seizure
- with only impairment of consciousness
- with automatisms

partial seizure with secondary generalization

Fig. 19.5 Classification of epileptic seizures.

An additional category is provided for those in which it is undetermined whether seizures are focal or generalized, either because the seizure type is uncertain or because both focal and generalized seizures occur.

Further subdivision is according to aetiology into
- Idiopathic (or primary)—in which there is no apparent cause except perhaps for genetic predisposition.
- Symptomatic—in which the cause is known or suspected.

Causes of epilepsy

Epilepsy can result from a very diverse group of pathological processes, but it is important to realize that in about 75% of children no cause will be identified, even after extensive evaluation. It can be assumed that the aetiology in these cases of so-called idiopathic or primary epilepsy is genetic. A specific cause (Fig. 19.7) is more likely to be identifiable in patients with partial or intractable epilepsy.

Diagnosis

A careful and complete history is the mainstay of diagnosis. A detailed description is required of the events before, during, and after a suspected seizure (a video recording is a potentially useful adjunct). The first aim is to distinguish true epileptic seizures from the many paroxysmal disturbances (see Chapter 5) that may mimic them:
- Breath-holding attacks.
- Reflex anoxic seizures.
- Vasovagal syncope (simple faints).
- Cardiac dysrhythmias.

Enquiry should be made concerning possible predisposing events (head injury, intracranial infection) and any family history of epilepsy.

Physical examination in a child with uncomplicated epilepsy is frequently normal. Careful attention should

Classification of epilepsy

Generalized epilepsies and epilepsy syndromes

idiopathic generalized epilepsy (IGE), defined syndromes include:
- benign familial neonatal convulsions
- childhood absence epilepsy (CAE)
- juvenile absence epilepsy (JAE)
- juvenile myoclonic epilepsy (JME)

symptomatic generalized epilepsy, defined syndromes include:
- infantile spasms (West syndrome)
- Lennox–Gastaut syndrome
- cerebral malformations
- progressive myoclonic epilepsies including:
  - inborn errors of metabolism
  - neurodegenerative diseases

Localization-related epilepsies and epilepsy syndromes

idiopathic partial epilepsy, defined syndromes include:
- benign childhood epilepsy with centrotemporal spikes (benign rolandic epilepsy)

symptomatic partial epilepsy, defined syndromes include:
- epilepsy caused by focal lesions of the brain associated with:
  - cortical dysgenesis
  - CNS infection
  - head injury
  - AV malformations
  - brain tumours

Fig. 19.6 Classification of epilepsy.

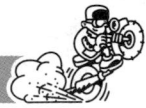

be paid to the skin to identify the stigmata of neurocutaneous syndromes and to the fundi as retinal changes may provide a clue to aetiology.

Investigations

EEG

This may be useful as an aid to diagnosis, in identifying a particular epilepsy syndrome or in identifying an underlying anatomical lesion or neurodegenerative disorder. However, it must be born in mind that a single interictal EEG will be normal in up to 50% of children with epilepsy, and non-specific or even so-called 'epileptiform' abnormalities may be found in normal asymptomatic children. A routine interictal EEG does not therefore prove or disprove a diagnosis of epilepsy. Additional information may be obtained from ambulatory EEG monitoring, telemetry with simultaneous video recording, or recordings during sleep or after sleep deprivation.

Neuroimaging

Not all children with epilepsy require a brain scan. Indications for neuroimaging include:

- Partial seizures.
- Intractable, difficult to control seizures.
- A focal neurological deficit.
- Evidence of a neurocutaneous syndrome or of neurodegeneration.

CT is more readily available and quicker to perform. However, MRI has greater sensitivity in the detection of small lesions, e.g. in temporal lobe or subtle cortical dysgeneses.

Causes of 'symptomatic' epilepsy

cortical dysgenesis
cerebral malformations
genetic diseases:
- neurocutaneous syndromes
- Down syndrome
- fragile X syndrome
- neurodegenerative disorders
- inborn errors of metabolism

cerebral tumours
cerebral damage due to:
- head trauma
- birth asphyxia, hypoxia–ischaemia
- intracranial infection (meningitis, encephalitis)

Fig. 19.7 Causes of 'symptomatic' epilepsy.

Other investigations

Additional specific investigations, which may be appropriate if there is clinical suspicion of an underlying neurometabolic disorder, include:

- Plasma and urine amino acids.
- Biopsy of skin or muscle.
- Measurement of white blood cell enzymes.
- DNA analysis.

Some important epilepsy syndromes

Infantile spasms (West syndrome)

This is a sinister but happily uncommon variety of epilepsy with peak onset between 4 and 6 months of age. Myoclonic seizures occur, often as 'salaam attacks'—violent flexor spasms of head, trunk, and limbs followed by extension of the arms. They are often multiple and may be misdiagnosed as colic. The EEG shows hypsarrhythmia, a chaotic pattern of large amplitude slow waves with spikes and sharp waves. Seventy per cent of the patients have the symptomatic form, and important causes include tuberous sclerosis and perinatal hypoxic–ischaemic encephalopathy. The prognosis is poor but may be improved by early treatment. Until recently, treatment with ACTH was the approved approach, but the anti-epilepsy drug vigabatrin has been shown to have a good clinical effect.

Childhood absence epilepsy

This relatively common variety of epilepsy has a peak onset at 6–7 years (range 4–12 years). The absence seizures comprise transient unawareness (blank spells). They typically last for 5–15 seconds but may be very frequent with up to several hundred daily. Episodes may be induced by hyperventilation. The ictal EEG is characteristic with generalized, bilaterally synchronous three per second spike–wave discharges (Fig. 19.8). The prognosis is good with spontaneous remission in adolescence in the majority of children. Sodium valproate is the drug of first choice, although medication is not required for infrequent absences.

Management of epilepsy

Effective management of a child with epilepsy involves far more than the prescription of anti-epilepsy drugs (AEDs). Both the child and parents need to be educated about the condition, the prognosis, and the nature of the particular epilepsy or epilepsy syndrome.

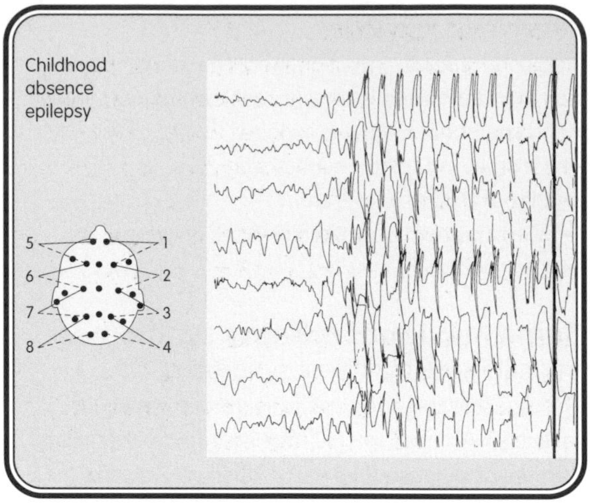

Fig. 19.8 EEG in a typical absence seizure. There is 3/sec spike and wave discharge which is bilaterally synchronous.

Children with epilepsy should be encouraged to participate in and enjoy a full social life. Certain activities do, however, require special precautions:

- Swimming: a competent adult swimmer should be present to provide supervision.
- Domestic bathing: patients should be supervised in the bath.
- Cycling: a helmet must be worn and traffic avoided.
- Climbing: climbing trees and rocks is best avoided.

It is important to consider the psychological and educational implications. Overprotection by the parents should be sympathetically discouraged. Behavioural and emotional difficulties may occur in the teenage years with loss of self-esteem, anxiety, or depression. The diagnosis should be discussed with school staff. Learning difficulties may be present in a proportion of children with epilepsy, but only a minority require special schooling.

- **Epilepsy affects 5 per 1000 school-age children.**
- **Up to 75% of childhood epilepsy will have no identifiable cause.**
- **Children with partial seizures require brain imaging.**

Use of anti-epilepsy drugs (AEDs)

Not all children with epilepsy require drug treatment. Many clinicians would not start treatment after a single brief generalized tonic–clonic seizure or for infrequent myoclonic or absence seizures.

Commonly used AEDs include:

- Sodium valproate.
- Carbamazepine.
- Phenobarbitone.

The currently recommended first line treatment is :

- Sodium valproate for generalized epilepsy
- Carbamazepine for partial epilepsy.

Monotherapy will achieve total seizure control in 70% of children. Blood level monitoring is rarely required. A number of newer AEDs are now available, including lamotrigine and vigabatrin. The latter is particularly effective in treating infantile spasms.

FEBRILE SEIZURES

A febrile seizure is a seizure associated with fever in a child between 6 months and 6 years of age in the absence of intracranial infection or an identifiable neurological disorder.

Febrile seizures are the most common cause of seizures in childhood and occur in about 3% of children. There may be a familial predisposition. The seizures usually occur when body temperature rises rapidly. They are typically brief (1–2 minutes), generalized, tonic–clonic seizures.

The underlying infection causing the fever may be a viral illness or a bacterial infection such as otitis media, tonsillitis, pneumonia or urinary tract infection.

Clinical features

Meningitis may present with seizures and fever, so it is very important to exclude this diagnosis. This often requires a lumbar puncture in young children (under 18 months) presenting with a first febrile seizure in whom specific signs of meningitis may be absent.

Management

Management includes:

- Identification and treatment of underlying infection. This may be apparent on clinical examination but additional investigations to consider include CXR,

FBC, blood culture, urine microscopy and culture, and lumbar puncture.
- Keeping the patient cool with regular antipyretics and tepid sponging.
- Termination of a prolonged convulsion (i.e. for longer than 5–10 minutes) with rectal diazepam.
- Parental education (Fig. 19.9).

NEUROCUTANEOUS SYNDROMES

Neurofibromatosis type 1 (von Recklinghausen disease)

This is an autosomal dominant disorder affecting about 1 in 4000 live births. About 50% of cases result from new mutations and have no family history.

The important clinical features include:
- *Café-au-lait* patches on the skin.
- Axillary freckles.
- Neurofibromas, which may be palpable on peripheral nerves.

Neurofibromatosis type 2 (NF2)

Also known as central neurofibromatosis, NF2 is a distinct disease due to mutations in a different gene on chromosome 22. It is much rarer (affecting 1 in 40 000 people) and characterized by bilateral acoustic neuromata.

Tuberous sclerosis

This is an autosomal dominant disorder affecting 1 in 7000 live births. Up to 75% of cases represent new mutations. It is genetically heterogeneous with one disease gene on chromosome 9 and a second gene on chromosome 16.

It is a multisystem disease affecting not only the skin and brain, but also the heart, kidneys, and lungs.

Sturge–Weber syndrome

This sporadic disorder is characterized by
- Unilateral facial naevus (port-wine stain) in the distribution of the trigeminal nerve.
- Leptomeningeal angiomatosis.

There are abnormal blood vessels over the surface of the brain which may be associated with seizures, hemiplegia, and learning difficulties.

A CT of the brain typically shows unilateral intracranial calcification with a double contour like a railway line and cortical atrophy.

NEURODEGENERATIVE DISORDERS

A large number of individually rare but important inherited diseases are associated with progressive neurodegeneration in childhood. Most are autosomal

Information for parents about febrile seizures	
Will it happen again?	about one third of children have recurrent febrile seizures recurrence is more likely if the first seizure occurs under the age of 18 months or if there is a family history
Can I prevent further episodes?	during febrile illnesses, the child should be kept cool with antipyretics, removal of clothing, and tepid sponging
What should I do if a convulsion occurs?	place child in recovery position parents of children at risk of frequent or prolonged seizures can be supplied with rectal diazepam to administer if a seizure lasts longer than 5 minutes
Is it epilepsy?	febrile seizures are not classified as epilepsy about 3% of children with febrile seizures go on to develop afebrile recurrent seizures, i.e. epilepsy, in later childhood risk factors for epilepsy include: • seizures that are focal, prolonged (>15 minutes) or recur in the same illness • first-degree relative with epilepsy • neurological abnormality

Fig. 19.9 Information for parents about febrile seizures.

recessively inherited and genetic and biochemical defects have been established at a molecular level in many cases.

Clinical features

The clinical hallmark is a progressive, worsening deficit. Features may include:

- Progressive dementia.
- Epilepsy.
- Visual loss.
- Ataxia.
- Alterations in tone and reflexes (depending on the precise pattern of nervous system involvement).

Parental consanguinity increases the risk of such disorders (Fig. 19.10).

Inherited neurodegenerative diseases—some examples
Lysosomal storage diseases
sphingolipidosis, e.g. Tay–Sachs disease
mucopolysaccharidosis, e.g. Hurler syndrome (MPS1)
Peroxisomal disorders
adrenoleucodystrophy
Trace metal metabolism
Wilson's disease
Menke's syndrome

Fig. 19.10 Inherited neurodegenerative diseases—some examples.

NEUROMUSCULAR DISORDERS

These are best considered according to their anatomical site (Fig. 19.11) in the lower motor pathway. Genetic, infective, inflammatory, and toxic factors may cause this group of diseases.

Clinical features

The hallmark of these disorders is weakness. They may present with:

- Floppiness (hypotonia).
- Delayed motor milestones.
- Weakness, fatiguability.
- Abnormal gait.

Clinical features on examination may include hypotonia, muscle weakness or wasting, abnormal gait, and reduced tendon reflexes.

Diagnosis

Special investigations useful in the diagnosis of neuromuscular diseases include:

- Muscle enzymes: serum creatine kinase is elevated in Duchenne and Becker dystrophies.
- Electrophysiology: nerve conduction studies and electromyography.
- Biopsy: muscle or nerve may be biopsied.
- DNA analysis: direct mutational analysis of disease genes in certain disorders.
- Imaging: ultrasound, CT, or MRI of muscle.
- Edrophonium test: for myasthenia gravis

Muscular dystrophies

This is a group of inherited disorders characterized by progressive degeneration of muscle. The most common and important is Duchenne muscular dystrophy.

Duchenne muscular dystrophy

This X-linked recessive disease affects 1 in 4000 male infants. About one third of cases are new mutations. The disease gene is very large (2 Mb) and encodes dystrophin, a sarcolemmal membrane protein.

Affected boys usually develop symptoms between 2 and 4 years of age. Independent walking may be delayed and affected children never run normally. Patients are wheelchair bound by 12 years of age and die from congestive heart failure or pneumonia by 25 years of age.

Clinical features

Associated clinical features include:

- Pseudohypertrophy of calf muscles.

Neuromuscular disorders
Anterior horn cell
spinal muscular atrophy
poliomyelitis
Peripheral nerve
hereditary neuropathy
Guillain–Barré syndrome
Bell's palsy
Neuromuscular junction
myasthenia gravis
Muscle
muscular dystrophies
myotonia
congenital myopathies

Fig. 19.11 Neuromuscular disorders.

- Positive Gower's sign (evident at 3–5 years). Hands are used to push up on the legs to achieve an upright posture, indicating weakness of the lower back and pelvic girdle muscles.
- Scoliosis.
- Cardiomyopathy.
- Mild learning difficulties.

Diagnosis

Investigations to confirm the diagnosis include:

- Serum creatine kinase level (10–20 times normal).
- Muscle biopsy.
- DNA analysis (identification of mutations in the dystrophin gene).

Management

Treatment is supportive. Walking can be prolonged by provision of orthoses and scoliosis can be helped by a truncal brace or moulded seat. Early diagnosis is important to allow identification of female carriers and genetic counselling.

Becker muscular dystrophy

This is a milder disease due to mutation in the same gene. The average age of onset is much later (in the second decade) with prolonged survival.

Loss of acquired skills is the hallmark of a neurodegenerative disorder. Most are genetic, but acquired forms do occur such as prion disease and subacute sclerosing panencephalitis.

20. Musculoskeletal Disorders

DISORDERS OF THE HIP AND KNEE

Developmental dysplasia of the hip

Developmental dysplasia of the hip (DDH) encompasses congenital dislocation of the hip (CDH).

DDH represents a spectrum of hip instability ranging from a dislocated hip to hips with various degrees of acetabular dysplasia (in which the femoral head is in position but the acetabulum is shallow). It was previously thought to be entirely congenital, but is now known to also occur after birth in previously normal hips.

There is a national screening programme for its detection because early diagnosis is so important. However, clinical examination is unreliable. True dislocations occur in about 2:1000 and abnormalities detected on screening amount to 6:1000.

Clinical features

Risk factors for DDH include:

- Female sex.
- Prematurity.
- Breech or caesarean delivery.
- Family history.
- Neuromuscular disorders.

Babies are screened at birth and at the 6-week check using the Barlow and Ortolani manoeuvres. With increasing age, joint laxity lessens and these tests are then unhelpful. Warning signs may be:

- Delayed walking.
- A limp.
- A waddling gait.

Asymmetrical skin creases are an unreliable guide.

Diagnosis

Typically on examination, there is limited abduction (a supine child should be able to abduct fully the flexed hip up until the age of 2 years).

Ultrasound scanning is diagnostic (Fig. 20.1). Hip X-rays are not useful until after 4–5 months of age when the femoral head has ossified (Fig. 20.2).

Management

This involves:

- Fixing the hip in abduction with a Pavlik or Von Rosen harness.
- Avoiding weight-bearing.

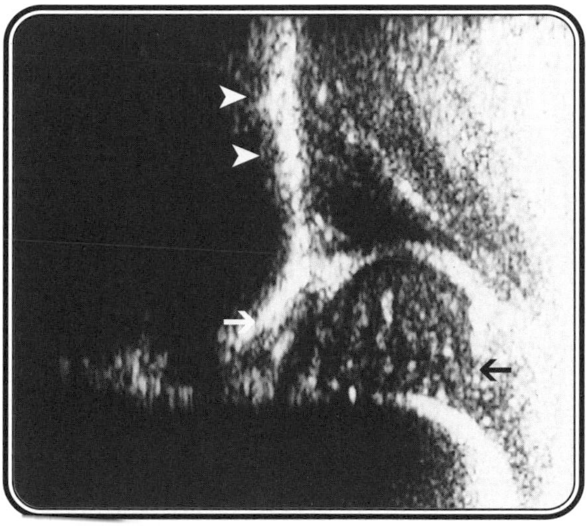

Fig. 20.1 Ultrasound scan of the hip. The femoral head (black arrow) is dislocated out of the acetabulum (white arrow). The white arrowheads demonstrate the ileum.

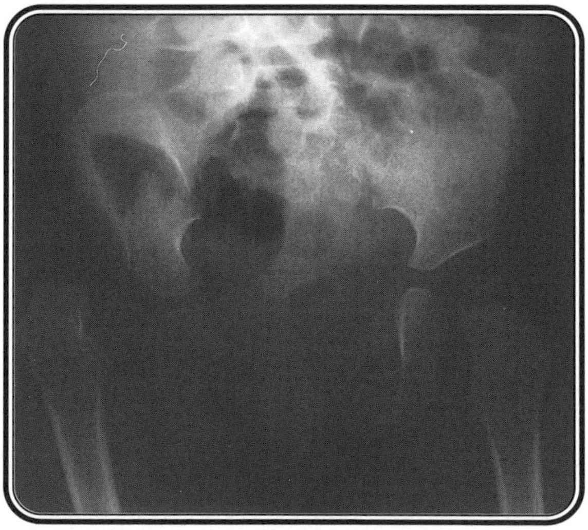

Fig. 20.2 X-ray of congenital dislocation of the right hip in an older child.

For children in whom the diagnosis has been delayed, open reduction and derotation femoral osteotomy needs to be performed. In these cases, accelerated degenerative changes may necessitate total hip replacement in early adult life.

Perthes' disease

In this condition of unknown aetiology, there is a growth disturbance associated with temporary ischaemia of the upper femoral epiphysis. This leads to a cycle of avascular necrosis with flattening and fragmentation of the femoral head. Revascularization and reossification occurs with the resumption of growth (which may not be normal); the whole cycle takes 3–4 years. Risk factors include:

- A previous family history.
- Male sex: it is five times more common in boys.

The incidence is 1:2000.

Clinical features

There is an insidious onset of limp between the ages of 3–12 years (though the majority occur between 5 and 7 years). Pain, which may be intermittent, may be felt in the hip, thigh, or knee. Between 10–20% of cases are bilateral. Abduction and rotation is limited on examination.

Diagnosis

Hip X-rays are diagnostic (Fig. 20.3). Bone scans and MRI may be necessary.

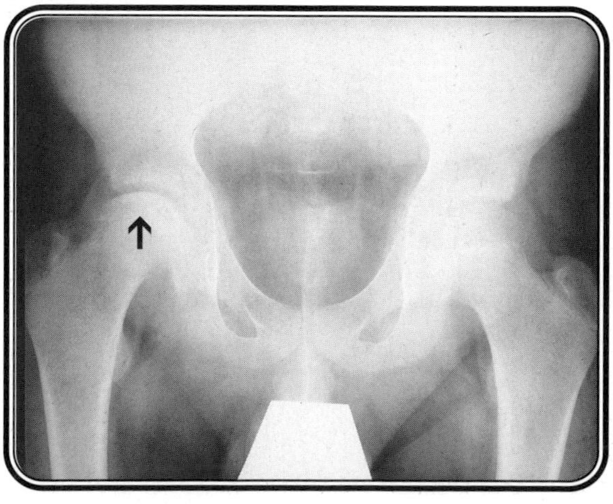

Fig. 20.3 Perthe's disease. Increased density in the right femoral head, which is reduced in height.

Management

In most children, the prognosis is good especially in those under 6 years of age or if less than half of the femoral head is involved. Treatment involves bed rest and traction. Early osteoarthritis is uncommon.

In older children, and those in whom more than half of the epiphysis is involved, permanent deformity of the femoral head occurs in over 40%, resulting in earlier degenerative arthritis. In severe disease, the hip needs to be fixed in abduction allowing the femoral head to be covered and moulded by the acetabulum as it grows. Plaster, callipers, or femoral or pelvic osteotomy may achieve fixation.

Transient synovitis (irritable hip)

This common self-limiting condition occurs in children between 2 and 12 years of age often following a viral infection.

Clinical features

Typical features are:

- Sudden onset of hip pain.
- Limp.
- Refusal to bear weight on the affected side.

There is no pain at rest. Examination reveals limited passive abduction and rotation in an otherwise well and afebrile child. The critical differential diagnosis is septic arthritis, in which the child is febrile and unwell with pain at rest.

Diagnosis

All investigations are essentially normal, but it is often necessary to perform them, as this is a diagnosis of exclusion. Investigations include:

- Acute-phase reactants (WBC, C-reative protein (CRP), and erythrocyte sedimentation rate (ESR).
- Blood cultures.
- Hip X-ray.

An ultrasound scan may show a small effusion.

Management

Treatment is supportive (bed rest and paracetamol) as the condition spontaneously resolves within 7 days.

Slipped upper femoral epiphysis (SUFE)

In this relatively uncommon condition of unknown aetiology, there is progressive posterior and inferior

Irritable hip is a diagnosis of exclusion. Septic arthritis must always be considered.

slippage of the femoral head on the femoral neck.
SUFE:

- Is most common in boys (obese White or tall thin Black).
- Typically presents between 10 and 15 years of age, during the adolescent growth spurt.
- Presents with limp.

Thirty per cent have a family history and one quarter are bilateral although not necessarily synchronous.

DISORDERS OF THE SPINE AND NECK

Back pain

Back pain is uncommon before adolescence. In infants and young children, it is usually associated with significant pathology such as connective tissue disorders. Referral is warranted.

In adolescence back pain may be caused by:

- Muscle spasm or soft tissue pain: this is usually a sports-related injury.
- Scheuermann's disease: this is osteochondritis (idiopathic avascular necrosis of an ossification centre) of the lower thoracic vertebrae causing localized pain, tenderness, and kyphosis.
- Spondylolysis and spondylolisthesis: there is a defect in the pars interarticularis of usually L4 or L5 (spondylolysis). If there is anterior shift of the vertebral body (graded according to severity), there is lower back pain exacerbated by bending backwards (spondylolisthesis).
- Vertebral osteomyelitis or discitis: this presents with severe pain on weight-bearing and walking associated with local tenderness.
- Tumours: these may be benign or malignant and may cause cord or root compression.
- Idiopathic: this is a diagnosis of exclusion, but pain may be exacerbated by stress and poor posture.

Scoliosis

This is lateral curvature of the spine and affects 4% of children. It is classified according to cause:

- Vertebral abnormalities, e.g. hemivertebra, osteogenesis imperfecta.
- Neuromuscular, e.g. polio, cerebral palsy.
- Miscellaneous, e.g. idiopathic (most common), Marfan syndrome.

Idiopathic scoliosis

As well as lateral curvature, there is rotation of the thoracic region which can be demonstrated as the child bends forwards and a rib hump is noted (Fig. 20.4). More than 85% cases occur in adolescence. It is most commont in girls and often there is a family history. Pain is not a typical feature.

The scoliosis is monitored clinically, radiologically, and chronologically.

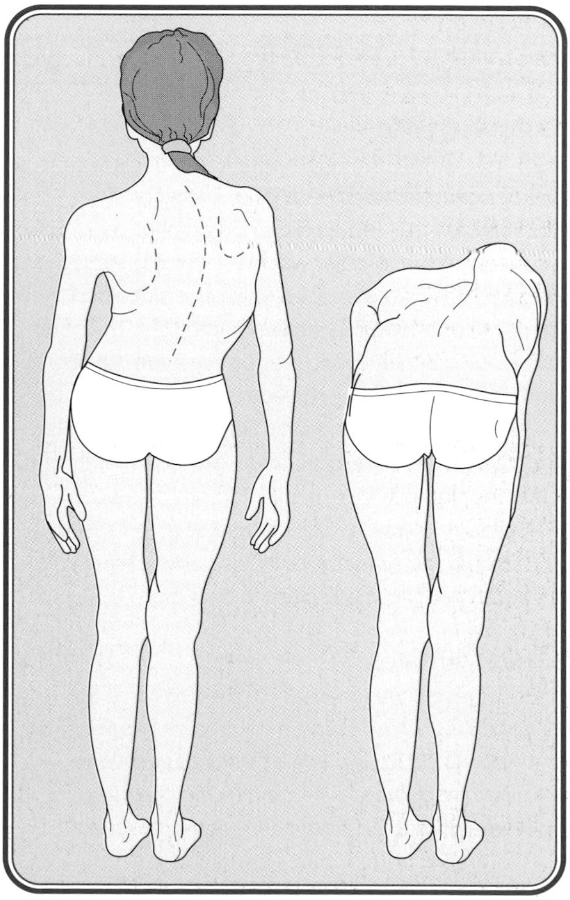

Fig. 20.4 Idiopathic adolescent scoliosis showing vertebral rotation (rib hump) when bending forward.

- Mild curves are not treated.
- Moderate curves are braced (23 hours a day until growing has stopped).
- Severe curves (>40°) require surgery that fuses the spine and therefore terminates further growth. Untreated severe curves may lead to later degenerative changes, pain, and unwanted cosmetic appearance.

Torticollis

Acute torticollis (wry neck) is a relatively common and self-limiting condition in young children often associated with an upper respiratory tract infection.

The most common cause of torticollis in infants is a sternomastoid tumour. A mobile non-tender nodule within the sternomastoid muscle is noticed in the first few weeks of life. The cause is unknown. It usually resolves by 1 year and may benefit from passive stretching by a physiotherapist.

BONE AND JOINT INFECTIONS

Osteomyelitis

Early recognition and aggressive treatment is essential for a favourable outcome in bone infections. The infection is usually haematogenous in origin or may be secondary to an infected wound. It typically starts in the metaphysis where there is relative stasis of blood. Two thirds of cases occur in the femur and tibia. The peak incidence is bimodal: occurring in the neonatal period and in older children (9–11 years).

In all age groups, the most common pathogen is *Staphylococcus aureus,* although group B streptococci and *Haemophilus influenzae* infections also occur.

Children with sickle-cell disease have increased susceptibility to salmonella osteomyelitis. *Escherichia Coli* is an important pathogen in neonates.

Clinical features

Infants present with fever and refusal to move the affected limb. Older children will localize the pain and are also systemically unwell. Examination reveals exquisite tenderness over the affected bone usually with warmth and erythema. Pain limits movement.

Diagnosis

The acute-phase reactants (WBC, CRP, and ESR) are usually significantly elevated.

Blood cultures are positive in more than half of the cases, therefore, aspiration of the bone is necessary to identify the organism and its sensitivity. Bone scans are more sensitive in the early phase of the illness (24–48 hours) compared with X-rays which tend to be normal in the first 10 days. Periosteal elevation or radiolucent necrotic areas can usually be demonstrated between 2 and 3 weeks.

Treatment

Early treatment with intravenous antibiotics is imperative until there is clinical improvement and normalizing of the acute-phase reactants. Several weeks of oral antibiotics follow. Failure to respond to medical treatment is an indication for surgical drainage (rarely necessary).

Complications include:

- Chronic osteomyelitis.
- Septic arthritis.
- Growth disturbance and limb deformity (occurs if the infection affects the epiphyseal plate).

Septic arthritis

Purulent infection of a joint space is more common than osteomyelitis and can lead to bone destruction and considerable disability. The incidence is highest in children younger than 2 years of age and is usually haematogenous in origin. Other causes include:

- Osteomyelitis.
- Infected skin lesions.
- Puncture wounds.

In infants, the hip is the most common site (the knee is the most common site in older children). *Stapylococcus aureus* is the most common pathogen in all age groups. More recently, *Kingella kingae* (Gram-negative rod) has emerged as an important cause of septic arthritis.

Clinical features

The typical presentation is a painful joint with:

- Fever.
- Irritability.
- Refusal to bear weight.

Infants often hold the limb rigid (pseudoparalysis) and cry if it is moved. There is tenderness and a variable degree of warmth and swelling on examination.

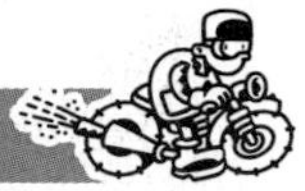

Investigation

The acute-phase reactants are usually elevated. Aspiration of the joint space may reveal organisms and the presence of white cells. The aspirate can then be cultured.

Ultrasound may identify effusions, but X-rays are often initially normal or show a non-specific, widened joint space.

Management

Early and prolonged intravenous antibiotics are necessary; these may be converted to oral therapy according to the clinical response. Surgical drainage is indicated only if the infection is overwhelming, resistant, or advanced.

Complications include destruction of the articular cartilage and bone.

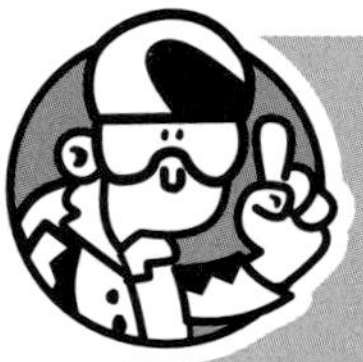

Bacterial bone and joint infections: *Staphylococcus. aureus* is the most common pathogen in all age groups.

RHEUMATIC DISORDERS

These include:

- Juvenile chronic arthritis (JCA).
- Dermatomyositis.
- Systemic lupus erythematosus.

Juvenile chronic arthritis

JCA is a group of disorders in which there is chronic arthritis lasting more than 3 months (6 weeks in the USA) and presenting before 16 years of age.

Features of the different subtypes are shown in Fig. 20.5.

Systemic (Still's disease)

This often presents with an acute illness characterized by:

- High fever.
- A salmon-pink rash.
- Lymphadenopathy.
- Organomegaly together with aches and pains in the joints and muscles (arthralgia and myalgia).

There is often no arthritis at presentation.

Classification of juvenile chronic arthritis

Feature	Systemic (Still's disease)	Polyarticular	Pauciarticular
joint number	variable	>5	<4
joints involved	any, often peripheral	knees, ankles, elbows, wrists	large, e.g. knees and ankles
pattern	symmetrical	symmetrical	asymmetrical
sex ratio (F:M)	1:1	3:1	5:1
total cases	10–20%	40–50%	40–50%
median age of onset	4 years	all ages	3 years
systemic involvement	predominant and self-limited	mild to moderate	absent
rheumatoid factor	negative	positive in 10%	negative
antinuclear antibodies	10%	50%	80%
course	arthritis is chronic and destructive in 50%	arthritis may be unremitting	uveitis is major cause of morbidity

Fig. 20.5 Classification of juvenile chronic arthritis.

Polyarticular

This is more common in girls. Symmetrical involvement of the limb joints is the usual pattern, but the cervical spine and temporomandibular joint may be affected.

Rheumatoid factor:

- Positive subtype: this occurs in older girls and resembles adult rheumatoid arthritis. It may progress to severe debilitating arthritis.
- Negative: this polyarticular JCA has a milder course.

Pauciarticular

Early onset is the most common subtype and typically occurs in young girls with asymmetric arthritis involving knees, ankle, and elbows. Antinuclear antibodies are nearly always present and one third will develop chronic iridocyclitis (inflammation of the iris and ciliary body, which comprise the anterior uveal tract—anterior uveitis).

The late-onset subtype affects older boys and usually presents with arthritis in a large joint.

Diagnosis

Useful tests for the evaluation of JCA include:

- FBC: anaemia occurs in systemic disease.
- Acute-phase reactants: elevated.
- Rheumatoid factor: negative in the majority.
- Antinuclear antibodies.
- X-rays: soft tissue swelling in early stages. Bony erosion and loss of joint space later.

Management

A multidisciplinary team approach is required. This will encompass:

- Physiotherapy: to optimize joint mobility, to prevent deformity, and to increase muscle strength.
- Medication: pain control and suppression of inflammation are provided by: non-steroidal anti-inflammatory agents (NSAIDs), e.g. ibuprofen or aspirin. Systemic steroids may be indicated for severe systemic disease or severe uveitis.

GENETIC SKELETAL DYSPLASIAS

Achondroplasia

This is a disorder of endochondral ossification. Inheritance is autosomal dominant with about half of all cases due to new mutations. Children with achondroplasia have:

- Short stature due to marked shortening of limbs.
- A large head with frontal bossing and depression of the nasal bridge.
- Short broad hands.
- Kyphoscoliosis and lumbar lordosis.

Osteogenesis imperfecta (brittle bone disease)

Osteogenesis imperfecta is a heterogeneous group of disorders:

- Caused by mutations in collagen genes.
- Characterized by fragile bones and frequent fractures.

There are two forms:

- Type 1 (the most common form) is an autosomal dominant disorder. Affected children have recurrent fractures, blue sclerae, and conductive hearing loss.
- Type II is a severe, lethal form with multiple fractures present before birth. Many affected infants are stillborn. Inheritance is usually autosomal recessive.

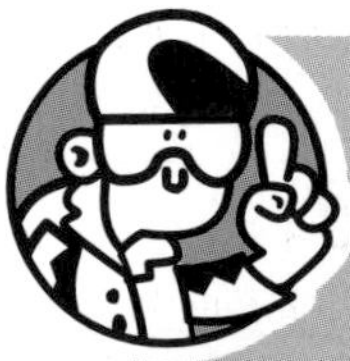

Ophthalmological screening with a slit lamp to detect anterior uveitis is especially important in children with pauciarticular JCA.

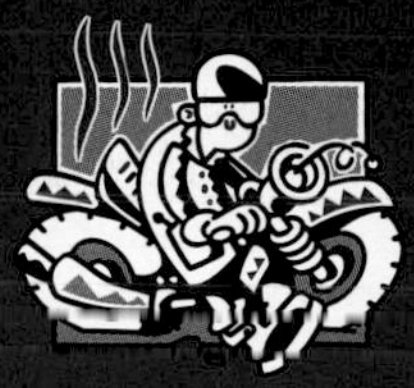

21. Haematological Disorders

These encompass defects in the cellular elements of the blood or in those soluble elements involved in haemostasis. Neoplastic diseases of the white cells or lymphatic system are considered separately (see Chapter 22). The most common problem encountered is iron deficiency anaemia.

Normal developmental variations are important in the interpretation of changes in the blood in infancy and childhood.

HAEMATOPOIESIS

Early prenatal haematopoiesis occurs in the liver, spleen, and lymph nodes. It commences in the bone marrow at about the fourth or fifth month of gestation. At birth, haematopoietic activity is present in most of the bones, especially long bones.

Cells in the peripheral blood have a relatively short life span (see Hints & Tips). Continuous replenishment in massive amounts from the bone marrow is required to maintain adequate blood counts.

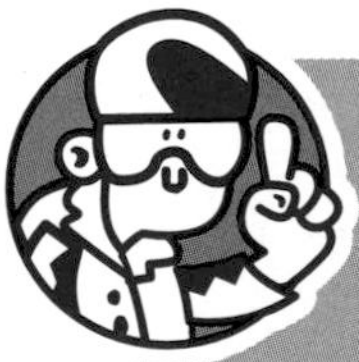

Life span of peripheral blood cells:
- **Red cells: 120 days.**
- **Platelets: 10 days.**
- **Neutrophils: 6–7 hours.**

Normal developmental changes in haemoglobin

The haemoglobin concentration and haematocrit are relatively high in the term newborn infant because of the low oxygen tension prevailing *in utero*. The wide range encountered, 14–20 g/dl, is accounted for by:
- Variation in how rapidly the umbilical cord is clamped.
- The infant's position after delivery.

If cord clamping is delayed and the baby is held lower than its placenta, haemoglobin and blood volume are both increased by a placental transfusion.

These values subsequently decline, reaching a nadir at:
- About 7 weeks in preterm infants.
- 2–3 months for term infants.

The lower limit of normal for this 'physiological' anaemia is 9.0 g/dl. During this period, there is erythroid hypoplasia of the marrow and a change from fetal to adult haemoglobin.

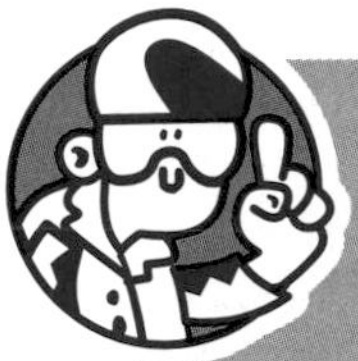

Developmental changes in haemoglobin concentration:
- **Haemoglobin concentration is high at birth, 14–20 g/dl.**
- **It falls to a nadir of 9–13 g/dl at 2–3 months in term infants.**
- **HbF values decline postnatally to 2% of total at 9–12 months.**

ANAEMIA

Anaemia is a decrease of the haemoglobin concentration in the blood to below normal. Dietary iron deficiency is the most common cause but there are many others. In clinical practice, anaemia can be classified initially according to the red cell:
- Colour intensity (normochromic/hypochromic).
- Size (microcytic/normocytic/macrocytic).

Important causes based on this classification are shown in Fig. 21.1.

Iron deficiency anaemia (IDA)

This is the most common cause of anaemia in childhood. It usually results from inadequate dietary intake rather than loss of iron through haemorrhage.

Classification and causes of anaemia

Microcytic, hypochromic anaemia
- defects of haem synthesis
  - iron deficiency
  - chronic inflammation
- defects of globin synthesis
  - thalassaemia

Normocytic, normochromic anaemia
- haemolytic anaemias
  - intrinsic red cell defects
    - membrane defects: spherocytosis
    - haemoglobinopathies: sickle cell disease
    - enzymopathies: G6PD deficiency
  - extrinsic disorders
    - immune-mediated: Rh incompatibility
    - microangiopathy
    - hypersplenism
- haemorrhage (acute or chronic)
  - hookworm infestation
  - Meckel's diverticulum
  - menstruation
- hypoproduction disorders
  - red cell aplasia, e.g. renal disease
  - pancytopenia, e.g. marrow aplasia, leukaemia

Macrocytic anaemia
- bone marrow megaloblastic
  - vitamin B_{12} deficiency
  - folic acid deficiency
- bone marrow not megaloblastic
  - hypothyroidism
  - Fanconi anaemia

Fig. 21.1 Classification and causes of anaemia.

Iron requirements

The fetus absorbs iron from the mother across the placenta.

- Term infants have adequate reserves for the first 4 months of life.
- Preterm infants have limited iron stores and because of their higher rate of growth, they outstrip their reserves by 8 weeks of age.

Both breast milk and unmodified cow's milk are low in iron concentration (0.05–0.10 mg/100 mL). However, 50% of the iron is absorbed from breast milk, in comparison to just 10% from cow's milk. Most formula milks are fortified with iron and contain 10 times the concentration in breast milk (1.0 mg/100 mL). However, only 4% is absorbed.

Dietary sources of iron include red meat, fortified breakfast cereals, dark green vegetables, and bread. About 10–15% of dietary iron is absorbed. Absorption is

- Enhanced by ascorbic acid (vitamin C).
- Reduced by tannin in tea.

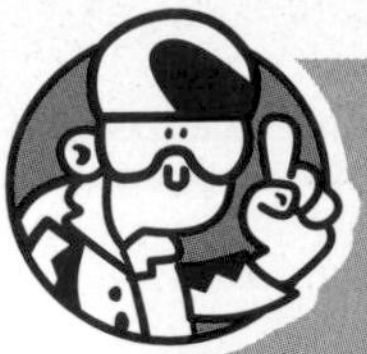

Concerning iron in milk:

- **Breast and unmodified cow's milk are low in iron.**
- **Iron is better absorbed from breast milk (50%) compared to cow's milk (10%).**
- **Formula milks are fortified with iron.**

Iron requirements increase during adolescence, especially for girls who lose iron through menstruation.

Causes of iron deficiency

Nutritional deficiency is common in certain at-risk groups (Fig. 21.2). Malabsorption may be complicated by iron deficiency. Blood loss is a less common cause but may occur with:

- Menstruation.
- Hookworm infestation.
- Repeated venesection in babies.
- Meckel's diverticulum.
- Recurrent epistaxis.

Clinical features

Mild iron deficiency is asymptomatic. As it becomes more severe there may be:

- Irritability.
- Lethargy.
- Fatigue.
- Anorexia.

On examination, the only signs may be pallor of the skin and mucous membranes. Severe anaemia may cause congestive cardiac failure. IDA in infancy and early childhood is associated with developmental delay and poor growth, which is reversible by long-term oral iron treatment.

Diagnosis

Diagnosis is confirmed by the blood count and film, supplemented by investigations of iron status. If dietary deficiency is likely, the latter can be omitted and diagnosis confirmed by a positive response to a therapeutic trial of iron.

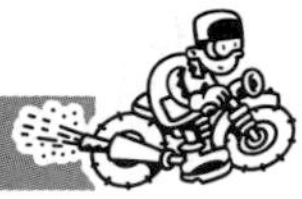

Dietary iron deficiency	
Infants	preterm infants require iron supplements from 6–8 weeks term infants will develop iron deficiency after 4 months if • mixed feeding is unduly delayed • unmodified cow's milk is introduced early
Children	poor diet associated with low socio-economic status or strict vegetarian diets

Fig. 21.2 Dietary iron deficiency.

Management

Primary prevention in infants can be achieved by:

- The avoidance of unmodified cow's milk.
- The use of iron-supplemented formulae.

Mild to moderate anaemia is treated with dietary counselling and oral iron using, for example, sodium iron edetate. Therapy should be continued for 3 months to allow replenishment of tissue iron stores.

Severe anaemia with cardiac decompensation may require transfusion. Investigation for occult gastrointestinal tract bleeding is indicated if there is a failure of response to treatment or recurrence despite an adequate intake.

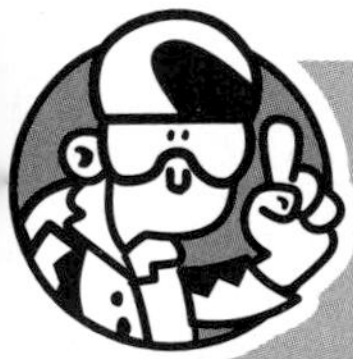

Children need to *absorb* 0.8 mg of elemental iron per day.
Reference nutrient *intakes* of iron are:

- **6 months: 4 mg/day.**
- **12 months: 8 mg/day.**
- **Adult male: 9 mg/day.**
- **Adult female: 15 mg/day.**

Thalassaemias

The thalassaemias are a group of hereditary anaemias caused by defects of globin chain synthesis. They are classified into:

- α-thalassaemia: reduced synthesis of α-globin chains.
- β-thalassaemia: reduced synthesis of β-globin chains.

Mutations in the globin genes lead to a reduction or absence of the corresponding globin chains. Excess unpaired globin chains produce insoluble tetramers that precipitate causing membrane damage and:

- Either cell death within the bone marrow (ineffective erythropoiesis).
- Or premature removal by the spleen (resulting in haemolytic anaemia).

β-thalassaemia

This occurs most frequently in people from the Mediterranean and Middle East. Over 150 million people carry β-thalassaemia mutations. There are two main types:

- Homozygous β-thalassaemia (β-thalassaemia major, Cooley's anaemia).
- Heterozygous β-thalassaemia (β-thalassaemia minor, ♣β-thalassaemia trait).

β-thalassaemia major

There is usually a complete absence of β-globin chain production (genotype β^o/β^o), although some mutations allow partial synthesis (genotype β^+/β^+). Haemoglobin A cannot be synthesized.

Clinical features

Affected infants usually present at 6 months with severe haemolytic anaemia, jaundice, failure to thrive, and hepatosplenomegaly. If untreated, bone marrow hyperplasia occurs with development of the classical facies.

- Maxillary hypertrophy.
- Skull bossing.

Diagnosis

Haemoglobin electrophoresis reveals a markedly reduced or absent HbA with increased HbF (30–90%) (see Chapter 12).

Treatment

The mainstay of treatment is regular blood transfusion, aiming to maintain the haemoglobin concentration above 10 g/dl. Unfortunately, chronic transfusion therapy is complicated by iron overload. Iron accumulates in parenchymal organs including the heart, liver, pancreas, gonads, and skin.

Chelation therapy with subcutaneous desferrioxamine, given regularly overnight, is used to promote iron removal, but negative iron balance is rarely achieved. Many patients succumb to congestive heart failure due to cardiomyopathy in their second or third decade.

Splenectomy is useful in selected patients and bone marrow transplantation can restore haematopoietic function. In the future, the developments of oral chelating agents and gene therapy hold promise.

β-thalassaemia minor (β-thalassaemia trait)

The only abnormality is a mild, hypochromic, microcytic anaemia. Most are asymptomatic.

β-thalassaemia trait may be misdiagnosed as iron deficiency anaemia. The important diagnostic feature is the raised HbA_2 and about 50% have a mild elevation of HbF (1–3%) on electrophoresis.

α-thalassaemia

This is caused by absence or reduced synthesis of α-globin genes. Most result from gene deletion. The manifestations and severity depend on the number of genes deleted (Fig. 21.3).

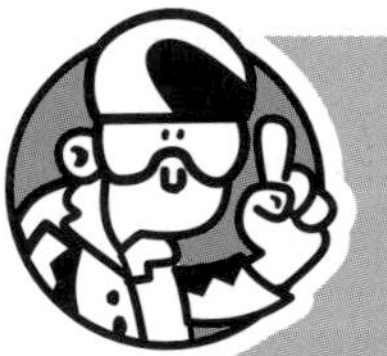

The only treatment for severe thalassaemias is regular and frequent blood transfusions. Genetic counselling is important in all haemoglobinopathies.

HAEMOLYTIC ANAEMIA

Haemolytic anaemia occurs when the life span of the red blood cell is shorter than the normal 120 days. Haemolytic anaemia may be caused by:

- Intrinsic red cell defects, e.g. spherocytosis, sickle-cell disease, glucose-6-phosphate dehydrogenase deficiency.
- Extrinsic defects, e.g. Rh incompatibility, microangiopathy, and hypersplenism.

It is characterized by:

- Anaemia.
- Reticulocytosis.
- Increased erythropoiesis in the bone marrow.
- Unconjugated hyperbilirubinaemia.

Hereditary spherocytosis

This is an autosomal dominant disorder caused by abnormalities in spectrin, a major supporting component of the red blood cell membrane. About 25% of cases are sporadic with no family history and are due to new mutations. As the name suggests the red cell shape is spherical and the life span is reduced by early destruction in the spleen.

Clinical features

The clinical features are highly variable and include:

- Mild anaemia: 9–11 g/dl.
- Jaundice: hyperbilirubinaemia.
- Splenomegaly: mild to moderate.

Clinical manifestations of α-thalassaemia variants

Variant	Number of genes deleted	Hb pattern	Clinical features
α-thalassaemia major	four	4F (Hb Bart)	hydrops foetalis/ death *in utero*
haemoglobin H disease	three	B4A (Hb H) (beyond early infancy)	severe anaemia, persists through life
α-thalassaemia minor	two	normal	mild anaemia
silent carrier	one	normal	no anaemia normal RBC indices

Fig. 21.3 Clinical manifestations of α-thalassaemia variants.

Complications include:

- Aplastic crises secondary to parvovirus B_{19} infection.
- Gall stones caused by increased bilirubin excretion.

Diagnosis

Spherocytes are seen on peripheral blood film. Diagnosis is confirmed by the osmotic fragility test (spherocytes already have maximum surface area to volume and rupture more easily than biconcave red cells in hypotonic solutions).

Management

Mild disease requires no treatment other than folic acid to meet the increased demands of the marrow.

Splenectomy is indicated for more severe disease, but should be deferred until school age because of the subsequent risk of overwhelming infection. The child should receive:

- Hib, meningococcal and pneumococcal vaccines before splenectomy.
- Prophylactic penicillin for life afterwards.

Sickle-cell disease

This chronic haemolytic anaemia occurs in patients homozygous for a mutation in the β-globin gene (which causes substitution of valine for glutamine in the sixth amino acid position of the β-globin chain). This causes a solubility problem in the deoxygenated state: HbS aggregates into long polymers that distort the red cells into a sickle shape.

The heterozygous state (sickle cell trait) confers resistance to falciparum malaria; this 'heterozygote advantage' explains the high incidence of the mutation in populations originating in malarious areas such as tropical Africa, the Mediterranean, the Middle East, and parts of India.

Sickled red cells have a reduced life span and are trapped in the microcirculation causing ischaemia.

Clinical features

The synthesis of HbF during the first few months affords protection until the age of 4–6 months. Progressive anaemia with jaundice and splenomegaly then develops, and the infant may present with an episode of dactylitis or overwhelming infection. The subsequent course of the disease is punctuated by crises of which 'vaso-occlusive' crises are by far the most common.

Vaso-occlusive crises

These episodes are often precipitated by infection, dehydration, chilling, or vascular stasis.

The clinical features depend on the tissue involved, but most commonly manifests as a 'painful' crisis, with pain in the long bones or spine. Cerebral or pulmonary infarction are less common but more serious. The latter may present as 'acute chest syndrome', which is characterized by:

- Fever.
- Crepitations.
- Chest pain.
- Pulmonary shadowing on chest X-ray arising from a combination of infarction and infection.

In infancy, patients with sickle-cell disease have a functional hyposplenism despite splenomegaly. Repeated vaso-occlusive episodes lead to infarction and fibrosis so that the spleen is no longer palpable from 5 years of age (so-called 'autosplenectomy'). These patients are, therefore, at risk of overwhelming infection with encapsulated organisms (*Haemophilus influenzae, Streptococcus pneumoniae*). There is an increased risk of osteomyelitis due to *Salmonella* and other organisms.

Long-term consequences of sickle-cell disease may include:

- Myocardial damage and heart failure.
- Aseptic necrosis of long bones.
- Leg ulcers.
- Gall stones.
- Renal papillary necrosis.

Management

Antenatal screening is available and this allows initiation of antibiotic prophylaxis early in life. Prophylactic penicillin should be taken to prevent pneumococcal infection. Daily folic acid supplements help to meet the demands of increased red cell breakdown. Pneumococcal and meningococcal vaccine should be given as well as the standard course of Hib vaccine.

The treatment of a vaso-occlusive crisis includes:

- Analgesia—opioids for severe pain.
- Oxygenation.
- Adequate hydration—IV fluids.

Exchange transfusion, designed to reduce the proportion of sickle cells, is indicated for brain or lung

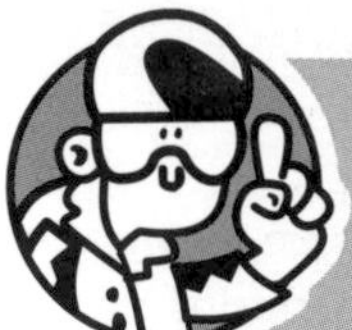

Sickle-cell disease:
- **HbS differs from HbA by the substitution of valine for glutamine at position 6 in the β-globin chain.**
- **HbS forms insoluble polymers in the deoxygenated state.**
- **The heterozygous state confers some protection against malaria.**

infarction and priapism. Transfusion with packed red cells may be required if a sudden fall in haemoglobin occurs during an aplastic sequestration or haemolytic crisis.

Sickle cell trait

The heterozygote with sickle cell trait (HbAS) is asymptomatic unless subjected to hypoxic stress (e.g. general anaesthesia). Sickle cells are not seen on peripheral smear and diagnosis requires a solubility test (e.g. sodium metabisulfate slide test) or Hb electrophoresis. The trait is worth detecting to allow genetic counselling and precautions to be taken against hypoxemia during flying and general anaesthesia.

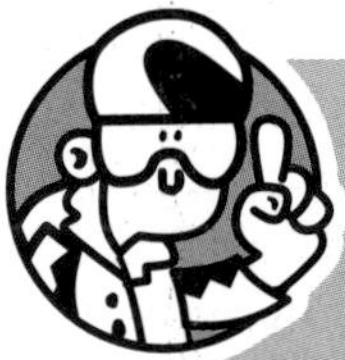

The spleen in sickle-cell disease:
- **In infancy, there is splenomegaly.**
- **Recurrent infarction and 'autosplenectomy' causes the spleen to regress and become impalpable after age 5 years.**
- **Splenic hypofunction renders patients susceptible to encapsulated organisms.**

Red cell enzyme deficiencies

These include glucose-6-phosphate dehydrogenase (G6PD) deficiency and the much rarer pyruvate kinase deficiency.

G6PD deficiency

This is an X-linked recessive disorder with variable clinical severity. Over 100 million people are affected worldwide particularly in the Mediterranean, Middle Eastern, Oriental, and Afro-Carribean populations. G6PD-deficient red cells do not generate enough glutathione to protect the cell from oxidant agents. Males are more severely affected, but females may manifest the phenotype.

Clinical features

G6PD deficiency may manifest with:
- Neonatal jaundice: worldwide it is the most common cause of neonatal jaundice requiring exchange transfusion
- Haemolytic episode: induced by infection, oxidant drugs, or fava beans. Intravascular haemolysis occurs with fever, malaise, and the passage of dark urine (haemoglobinuria).

BLEEDING DISORDERS

Normal haemostasis requires a complex interaction between three factors:
- Blood vessels.
- Platelets (thrombocytes).
- Coagulation factors.

A bleeding diathesis may result from a deficiency or disorder of any of these elements. Clinical presentation of a generalized bleeding diathesis may include:
- Petechiae or purpura.
- Prolonged bleeding after dental extraction, surgery, or trauma.
- Recurrent bleeding into muscles or joints.

Disorders of blood vessels

Injury to blood vessels provokes two responses that limit bleeding:
- Vasoconstriction.
- Activation of platelets and coagulation factors by subendothelial collagen.

Rare inherited disorders include Ehlers–Danlos syndrome associated with excessive capillary fragility and hereditary haemorrhagic telangiectasia.

Acquired disorders include vitamin C deficiency (scurvy) and Henoch–Schönlein purpura.

Henoch–Schönlein purpura (anaphylactoid purpura)

This is a multisystem vasculitis involving the small blood vessels. It commonly follows an upper respiratory tract infection or exposure to a drug or allergen, and is assumed to be immune-mediated.

It is more common in boys and mainly affects children aged between 2 and 8 years.

Clinical features

The condition affects skin, joints, gastrointestinal tract, and kidneys. Clinical features are described in Fig. 21.4.

Diagnosis and management

Diagnosis is clinical. Normal platelet count and coagulation studies exclude other causes of purpura.

Treatment is symptomatic and supportive. Steroids may be of benefit in severe gastrointestinal disease. The prognosis is excellent. Most children recover within 4–6 weeks, although, rarely, chronic renal disease may develop.

Disorders of platelets

These may be quantitative or qualitative, with the former (thrombocytopenia) being most common.

Thrombocytopenia

A decreased number of platelets (from the normal count of 150–450 x 10^9/L) is the most common cause of abnormal bleeding. Purpura usually occurs when the count is below 30 x 10^9/L. The cause may be decreased platelet production or reduced platelet survival (Fig. 21.5).

Idiopathic thrombocytopenic purpura (ITP)

This is the most common cause of thrombocytopenia in childhood and refers to an immune-mediated thrombocytopenia for which an exogenous cause is not apparent. The platelets are destroyed within the reticuloendothelial system, mainly in the spleen.

Clinical features

ITP mainly affects children between 2 and 10 years of age. Presentation is with purpura and superficial bleeding which may be accompanied by bleeding from mucosal surfaces, e.g. epistaxis. The spleen is palpable in a minority of cases.

Diagnosis

The differential diagnosis includes:

- Acute leukaemia.
- Non-accidental injury.
- Henoch–Schönlein purpura.

A full blood count reveals thrombocytopenia but no pancytopenia. Bone marrow aspiration to exclude marrow infiltration, or aplasia, is advocated by some. This should be done if there is doubt about the diagnosis or steroid therapy is contemplated (see below). An increase in megakaryocytes (platelet precursors) is characteristic.

Treatment

In most children, the disease is acute, benign, and self-limiting, and no therapy is required. The most important potential complication is intracranial haemorrhage—rare but serious. Several management options exist for more severe disease. Platelet infusions are rapidly destroyed and have no role except in life-threatening emergencies. Intravenous gamma globulin infusions

Clinical features of Henoch–Schönlein purpura	
skin	a purpuric rash typically affects the legs and buttocks
GI tract	colicky abdominal pain accompanied by gross or occult bleeding intussusception may occur
joints	pain and swelling of the large joints, e.g. knees and ankles
kidneys	glomerulonephritis manifested by microscopic haematuria rarely severe and progressive

Fig. 21.4 Clinical features of Henoch–Schönlein purpura.

Causes of thrombocytopenia
Decreased production bone marrow failure • aplastic anaemia • leukaemia Wiskott–Aldrich syndrome **Reduced survival** immune-mediated thrombocytopenia • idiopathic thrombocytopenic purpura (most common) • secondary to viral infection, drugs hypersplenism giant haemangioma disseminated intravascular coagulation

Fig. 21.5 Causes of thrombocytopenia.

cause a rise in the platelet count and may be indicated in severe disease.

A short course of oral steroids is an alternative. These act by reducing capillary fragility and inhibiting platelet destruction.

Thrombocytopenia in teenagers, especially girls, is more likely to become chronic and to reflect an underlying disorder such as systemic lupus erythematosus.

Coagulation disorders

Haemophilia A and B and von Willebrand disease account for the majority of inherited coagulation disorders.

Haemophilia A (factor VIII deficiency)

This is an X-linked recessive disorder due to reduced or absent factor VIII. The incidence is 1 in 5000–10 000 males. It is the result of a new mutation in one third of cases. The factor VIII molecule is a complex of two proteins:

- VIII:C—small molecular weight unit, antihaemophiliac factor.
- VIII:R—large molecular weight unit, von Willebrand factor.

Clinical features

Haemophilia A results from deficiency of VIII:C. Clinical severity varies greatly and depends on the factor VIII levels (Fig. 21.6). The characteristic clinical feature is spontaneous or traumatic bleeding which can be:

- Subcutaneous.
- Intramuscular.
- Intra-articular.

Mild haemophilia may remain undetected until excessive bleeding occurs, e.g. after dental extraction. Even severely affected boys often have few problems in the first year of life (unless circumcision is performed), but early bruising and abnormal bleeding is noted from the time they begin to walk and fall over.

In later life, recurrent soft tissue, muscle, and joint bleeding are the main problems. Haemarthroses cause pain and swelling of the affected joint and repeated haemorrhage may lead to chronic joint disease. Life-threatening internal haemorrhage (e.g. intracranial) may follow trauma.

Diagnosis

Diagnostic evaluation reveals a prolonged activated partial thromboplastin time (APTT), indicating a defect in the intrinsic pathway; Factor VIII assay confirms the diagnosis.

Management

Bleeding is treated by replacement of the missing clotting factor with intravenous infusion of factor VIII concentrate. The amount required depends on the site and severity of the bleed. Prompt and adequate therapy is important to avoid chronic arthropathy; home therapy may avoid delay and minimize inconvenience.

Recombinant DNA technology is now used to produce factor VIII that is safer than the blood products previously used. In the past, infection with Hepatitis B and C, and HIV has occurred from contaminated blood products. Antibodies to factor VIII may develop.

Mild haemophilia can be managed with infusion of desmopressin that releases factor VIII from tissue stores.

Haemophilia B (factor IX deficiency, Christmas disease)

This is an X-linked recessive disorder caused by deficiency of Factor IX. It is clinically similar to

Factor VIII levels in haemophilia A	
mild	5–25% of normal
moderate	1–4% of normal
severe	no detectable factor VIII activity

Fig. 21.6 Factor VIII levels in haemophilia A.

Haemophilia A, but much less common. Investigation reveals a prolonged APTT and reduced factor IX activity. Treatment is with prothrombin complex concentrate.

von Willebrand disease

This is due to a deficiency of von Willebrand factor (VWF; VIII:R) which has two major roles:

- Carrier protein for factor VIII:C (preventing it from breakdown).
- Facilitates platelet adhesion.

Inheritance is usually autosomal dominant. The clinical hallmark is bleeding into the skin and mucous membranes (gums and nose).

Disseminated intravascular coagulation (DIC)

Intravascular activation of the coagulation cascade may be secondary to various disease processes:

- Damage to vascular endothelium—sepsis, renal disease.
- Thromboplastic substances in the circulation—e.g. in acute leukaemia.
- Impaired clearance of activated clotting factors—e.g. in liver disease.

There is fibrin deposition in small blood vessels with tissue ischaemia, consumption of labile clotting factors and activation of the fibrinolytic system.

Clinical features

Clinical features are:

- A diffuse bleeding diathesis, with oozing from venepuncture sites.
- Bleeding from the lungs.
- Bleeding from the gastrointestinal tract.

Diagnosis and treatment

Investigations reveal:

- Prolonged prothrombin type (INR), activated partial thromboplastin time (APTT), and thrombin time ((TT).
- Thrombocytopenia and microangiopathic red cell morphology.
- Hypofibrinogenaemia.
- Elevated fibrinogen degradation products.

Supportive treatment includes replacement of platelets and fresh frozen plasma.

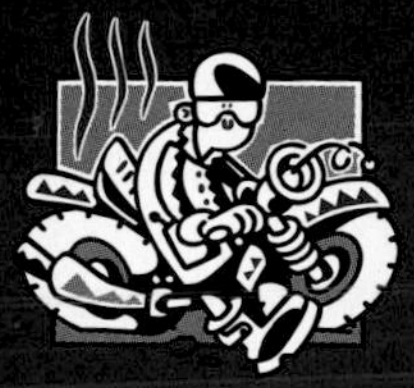

22. Malignant Disease

Cancer in childhood is uncommon. Approximately 1 out of 600 children between the ages of 1 and 15 years will develop cancer. Despite the dramatic increases in survival rate due to new treatments, it remains an important cause of death in childhood. The spectrum of cancer in childhood is very different from that in adults (Fig. 22.1). Leukaemia accounts for over one third of cases.

The aetiology, clinical features, investigation, and management of malignant disease in childhood are considered below, before the individual diseases are described.

Aetiology

Most childhood cancers are of uncertain cause and occur sporadically in otherwise healthy children. Risk is increased by a combination of:

- Genetic predisposition: genetic factors are often more evident in childhood than adult malignancy.
- Environmental factors.

Malignant cells proliferate and develop abnormally because they have escaped normal control mechanisms. In younger children in particular, the malignant cells may be immature precursor cells that fail to mature into normal, differentiated functional cells.

Important causative factors in childhood malignancy include:

- Genetic.
- Infections.
- Environmental.

Relative frequencies of childhood cancer	
Type	**% childhood cancer**
leukaemia	35
CNS tumours	23
lymphomas	12
Wilms tumour	7
neuroblastoma	7
bone tumours	6
other	10

Fig. 22.1 Relative frequencies of childhood cancer.

Genetic causes of childhood cancer

During periods of rapid proliferation, a normal cell may undergo a genetic alteration that transforms it into a malignant cell. Two important mechanisms of transformation are:

- Activation of oncogenes.
- Loss of tumour suppressor genes.

Examples of childhood cancer with an identifiable genetic aetiology are shown in Fig. 22.2.

Infections

Two viruses that infect the cells of the human immune system are associated with malignancy:

- Epstein–Barr virus: the virus transforms human B cells. If not limited by an effective immune response, a translocation disrupts the *c-myc* oncogene on chromosome 8 leading to malignant change, e.g. Burkitt's lymphoma.
- Human immunodeficiency virus (HIV): this retrovirus targets the human helper T cells. Children who develop AIDS are susceptible to lymphoid malignancies.

Environmental

Carcinogens and toxins are less often a cause of childhood cancer. One important risk factor, sadly, is previous treatment of malignancy in a child.

Clinical features

Cancer in childhood presents in a limited number of ways, some of which are non-specific (Fig. 22.3).

Genetic childhood cancer syndromes
retinoblastoma
Wilms tumour
DNA repair defects, e.g. ataxia telangiectasia
aneuploidies, e.g. Down syndrome
neurocutaneous syndromes, e.g. neurofibromatosis type 1

Fig. 22.2 Genetic childhood cancer syndromes.

Childhood cancer—clinical features at presentation	
Clinical feature	**Type of cancer**
constitutional symptoms: fever, weight loss, night sweats	lymphomas
a localized mass in: • abdomen • thorax • soft tissue	 Wilms tumour, neuroblastoma non-Hodgkin lymphoma rhabdomyosarcomas
lymph node enlargement	lymphomas
bone marrow failure	acute leukaemia
bone pain	leukaemia, bone tumours
signs of raised ICP	primary CNS tumours

Fig. 22.3 Childhood cancer—clinical features at presentation.

Classification systems employ numerical staging for solid tumours based on the extent of dissemination:

- Stage I: localized.
- Stage II & III: advanced, localized disease.
- Stage IV: disseminated disease with metastases.

Investigations

Histological confirmation is the cornerstone of diagnosis. This is provided by biopsy (of course, initial biopsy is not possible at some sites, e.g. brain tumours) or bone marrow aspiration.

Imaging is a vital aid and all modalities may be useful: ultrasound, X-ray, computed tomography (CT), and magnetic resonance imaging (MRI) scans. Tumour markers are useful in certain tumours, e.g. α-fetoprotein in liver tumours, urinary catecholamines in neuroblastoma.

Management

The main therapeutic strategies available are:

- Surgery—required for biopsy, total or partial removal of solid tumours (debulking), or for removal of residual disease after chemotherapy or radiotherapy.
- Radiotherapy—has an important role in specific circumstances, e.g. brain tumours.
- Chemotherapy—has a prominent role. A number of highly effective antineoplastic agents have been developed in the last 4 decades. Their use is based on a number of principles (see Hints & Tips).

Chemotherapy may be used as:

- Primary therapy for disseminated malignancy, e.g. the leukaemias.
- To shrink bulky primary or metastatic disease before local treatment.
- Adjunctive treatment for micrometastases.

Bone marrow toxicity is the limiting factor for many therapeutic regimens. This can be circumvented by using bone marrow transplantation to 'rescue' patients after administering potentially lethal, but potentially curative, doses of chemotherapy or radiation.

Supportive care

Treatment produces many predictable and often severe side effects in many systems. Supportive care is a vital part of treatment (Fig. 22.4). Indwelling central venous catheters allow pain-free blood sampling and injections.

Psychosocial support is very important. Diagnosis of

Supportive care in treatment of cancer	
infection	immunosuppression places children at risk of: • Gram-negative septicaemia from neutropenia • opportunistic infection with *Pneumocystis carinii* and fungi • viral infections—measles or chickenpox may be life-threatening treatment with appropriate antibiotics and antiviral agents is required
anaemia	blood transfusion
nausea and vomiting	antiemetic agents

Fig. 22.4 Supportive care in treatment of cancer.

a potentially fatal illness provokes enormous anxiety, guilt, fear, and sadness. Children and their siblings need an explanation of the illness tailored to their age. The severe stress may give rise to relationship problems in the parents and behavioural difficulties in siblings. Help with practical difficulties such as transport and finances may be required.

For some children, a time comes when further treatment represents postponement of inevitable death rather than prolongation of life. A definite decision to concentrate on palliative care is then appropriate. For survivors, long-term follow-up is required to detect and manage long-term sequelae (Fig. 22.5).

Long-term problems in survivors of childhood cancer	
growth/endocrine problems	GH deficiency from pituitary irradiation
infertility	gonadal irradiation chemotherapy
second malignancy	<10%
educational disadvantage	school absence, cranial irradiation

Fig. 22.5 Long-term problems in survivors of childhood cancer.

Chemotherapy in childhood cancer:

- **Chemotherapy is most likely to effect a cure when the malignant cell burden is small.**
- **Adverse effects are produced on rapidly dividing normal cells, e.g. those of the bone marrow, gastrointestinal tract, and hair follicles.**
- **Drugs with different toxicities can be used in combination.**

THE LEUKAEMIAS

Leukaemia is a disease characterized by proliferation of immature white cells and is the most common malignancy of childhood. Acute leukaemias account for the majority (97%) of cases. The malignant cells are termed 'blasts'.

The leukaemias are classified according to the white blood cell line involved:

- Acute lymphocytic (lymphoblastic) leukaemia (ALL)—cells of lymphoid lineage.
- Acute non-lymphocytic leukaemia (ANLL)—cells of granulocytic or monocytic lineage.

Clinical features

In most children with acute leukaemia, there is an insidious onset of symptoms and signs arising from infiltration of the bone marrow or other organs with leukaemic blast cells. Most will have one or more of the following:

- Pallor and malaise—anaemia.
- Haemorrhagic diathesis—purpura, easy bruising, epistaxis due to thrombocytopenia.
- Hepatosplenomegaly, lymphadenopathy—reticuloendothelial cell infiltration.
- Bone pain—due to expansion of marrow cavity.
- Infection—due to neutropenia.

Investigations

Peripheral blood investigations reveal:

- Anaemia—normocytic, normochromic.
- Thrombocytopenia.
- Neutropenia—total WBC may be low, normal, or high.
- Blast cells.

Bone marrow examination reveals:

- Replacement of normal elements by leukaemic cells.

A diagnosis of leukaemia should always be confirmed by bone marrow aspiration.

Acute lymphocytic leukaemia (ALL)

This accounts for 80% of childhood leukaemia and has a peak incidence between age 3 and 6 years. It is slightly more common in boys than girls. Lymphoblasts in these children do not successfully complete the rearrangement of immunoglobulin and T cell receptor genes necessary for full maturation. Coupled with genetic alterations, which permit them to survive and proliferate, the lymphoblasts remain 'frozen' at an early stage of development.

ALL can be classified according to cell-surface antigens (immunophenotype) into:

- Non-T, non-B cell (common) ALL: 75% are mostly early B cell clone.
- T cell ALL: 15%.
- B cell ALL: 1%.

Clinical features

Prognosis and clinical presentation varies with subtype. T cell ALL tends to occur in older children and teenagers, with a high peripheral white cell count and mediastinal mass. The prognosis is related to tumour load and can be defined according to certain clinical and laboratory features (Fig. 22.6).

Management

Overall, at least 65% of patients with ALL can now expect to be cured. Children with null cell (common) ALL have the best prognosis:

- 75% will go into remission.
- 75% survive beyond 5 years.

A typical treatment regimen can be divided into three phases:

- Induction—4 weeks of combination chemotherapy with vincristine, prednisolone and asparaginase, and intrathecal methotrexate.
- Consolidation—continued systemic therapy with blocks of 'intensification' therapy for selected patients.
- Maintenance—chemotherapy continues for 2 years from diagnosis with oral 6-mercaptopurine (daily), oral methotrexate (weekly), vincristine and prednisolone (monthly).

Prognostic groups in acute lymphocytic leukaemia		
Factors	**Good >70% cure (all factors required)**	**Poor <60% cure (any factor sufficient)**
age	2–9 years	<1 year
WBC	$<50 \times 10^9$ g/L	$>50 \times 10^9$ g/L
lineage	non-T, non-B cell	T cell or B cell

Fig. 22.6 Prognostic groups in acute lymphocytic leukaemia.

Initial preparation involves:

- Blood transfusion.
- Treatment of infection.
- Allopurinol to protect the kidneys against the effects of rapid cell lysis.

Additional treatment is given for leukaemic cells in the CNS in the form of intrathecal chemotherapy and cranial irradiation.

Relapses may occur in bone marrow, CNS, or testes. Then, prognosis is poor and high-dose chemotherapy with total body irradiation and bone marrow transplantation may be necessary for survival.

LYMPHOMAS

These can be classified into:

- Non-Hodgkin's lymphoma (NHL)—more common in young children.
- Hodgkin's disease—more common in adolescents and young adults.

Non-Hodgkin's lymphoma (NHL)

NHLs are a heterogeneous group of lymphomas with different characteristics and cells of origin. They may develop in immunocompromised children with HIV infection, severe combined immunodeficiency, or other severe inherited immunodeficiencies.

Clinical features

They tend to be aggressive and rapidly growing and may present with:

- Peripheral lymph node enlargement—usually B cell origin.
- Intrathoracic mass—usually T cell origin.
- Mediastinal mass or pleural effusion.
- Abdominal mass—usually advanced B cell disease.
- Gut or lymph node masses.

Subtypes of ALL and NHL may represent a continuation of the same disease.

Treatment

Chemotherapy is the mainstay of treatment, but

extensive surgical debulking may be required for abdominal tumours.

Hodgkin's disease

This is characterized histologically by the Reed–Sternberg cell. It is relatively uncommon in prepubertal children and usually presents in adolescence or young adulthood with a slight preponderance in females.

Clinical features

The usual presentation is with painless cervical or supraclavicular lymphadenopathy. Systemic symptoms are uncommon. Metastatic disease occurs in the lungs, liver, and bone marrow.

Diagnosis

Diagnosis is confirmed by histiological examination of a lymph node biopsy. Classification based on histopathology identifies four subtypes of different prognosis:

- Lymphocyte predominance—best prognosis.
- Mixed cellularity.
- Nodular sclerosing—most common in children and adolescents.
- Lymphocyte depletion—least common, worst prognosis.

Treatment

The disease is staged to determine treatment using imaging of chest, mediastinum, and abdomen. (Staging laparotomy is no longer performed in the UK.) Treatment is combination chemotherapy for all except patients with localized disease who may be treated with radiotherapy. The overall prognosis is good and 80% of patients are cured overall.

BRAIN TUMOURS

Brain tumours are the second most common form of childhood cancer and the most common solid tumour of childhood. Most are located infratentorially and present with signs and symptoms of raised intracranial pressure and cerebellar dysfunction.

A classification based on histology is shown in Fig. 22.7. An example of a posterior fossa tumour with hydrocephalus is shown in Fig. 22.8.

Classification of brain tumours in childhood

Astrocytic tumours
- high-grade astrocytomas
  - supratentorial
- low-grade astrocytomas
  - cerebellar
- brainstem gliomas

Neuroepithelial tumours
- primitive neuroectodermal tumours (PNET) (includes cerebellar medulloblastoma)

Fig. 22.7 Classification of brain tumours in childhood.

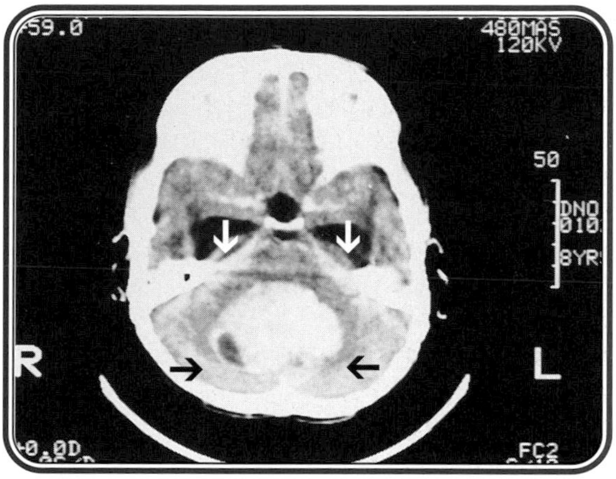

Fig. 22.8 CT of an enhancing posterior fossa tumour (black arrows) with hydrocephalus demonstrated by dilated temporal horns (white arrows).

Astrocytomas (40%)

Cerebellar astrocytomas are usually low-grade, slow-growing, cystic gliomas occurring between the ages of 6 and 9 years. Presentation may be with:

- Headache and vomiting: caused by obstructive hydrocephalus; papilloedema may be present.
- Cerebellar signs: ataxia, nystagmus, and uncoordination.
- Diplopia, squint: sixth nerve palsy.

Supratentorial astrocytomas and gliomas are less common and present with focal neurological signs and seizures.

Brainstem gliomas (6%) present with cranial nerve palsies, ataxia, and pyramidal tract signs.

Diagnosis is usually based on clinical findings and MR imaging as biopsy is hazardous. Prognosis is poor with median survival less than 1 year after diagnosis despite radiotherapy.

Primitive neuroectodermal tumours (medulloblastomas) (20%)

These are the most common malignant brain tumours of childhood, with a peak incidence between the ages of 2 and 6 years, with a preponderance in boys. They usually arise in the midline and invade the fourth ventricle and cerebellar hemispheres. They seed through the CNS and up to 20% have spinal metastases at diagnosis.

Presentation is usually with headache, vomiting, and ataxia.

Treatment is surgical removal and whole CNS irradiation (5-year survival rates are 50%). Adjuvant chemotherapy may be added for children with higher than average risk of recurrence.

Craniopharyngioma (4%)

These arise from the squamous remnant of Rathke's pouch and are locally invasive. They present with:

- Visual field loss—due to compression of the optic chiasm.
- Pituitary dysfunction—growth failure, diabetes insipidus.

Most are calcified and are visible on skull radiographs. Treatment is surgical excision. Prognosis is good but sequelae include visual impairment and endocrine deficiency.

Brain tumours are the most common solid tumour of children. Two-thirds arise below the tentorium.

NEUROBLASTOMA

Neuroblastoma is a malignancy of neural crest cells that normally give rise to the paraspinal sympathetic ganglia and the adrenal medulla.

It is the second most common solid tumour of childhood, occurring predominantly in infants and preschool children with a median age at diagnosis of 2 years. It is unusual in that it may regress spontaneously in very young children.

Clinical features

The clinical features depend on the location and may include:

- Abdominal mass: a firm, non-tender abdominal mass is the most common mode of presentation
- Systemic signs: pallor, weight loss, bone pain from disseminated disease.
- Hepatomegaly or lymph node enlargement.
- Unilateral proptosis: periorbital swelling and ecchymosis from metastasis to the eye.
- Opsoclonus–myoclonus: 'dancing-eye' syndrome caused by an immune response.
- Watery diarrhoea due to secretion of vasoactive intestinal peptide.

Diagnosis

Diagnosis is usually made from the characteristic clinical and radiological features (Fig. 22.9).

- Raised urinary catecholamines (vanillylmandelic acid, homovanillic acid) are useful in diagnosis and monitoring response to therapy.

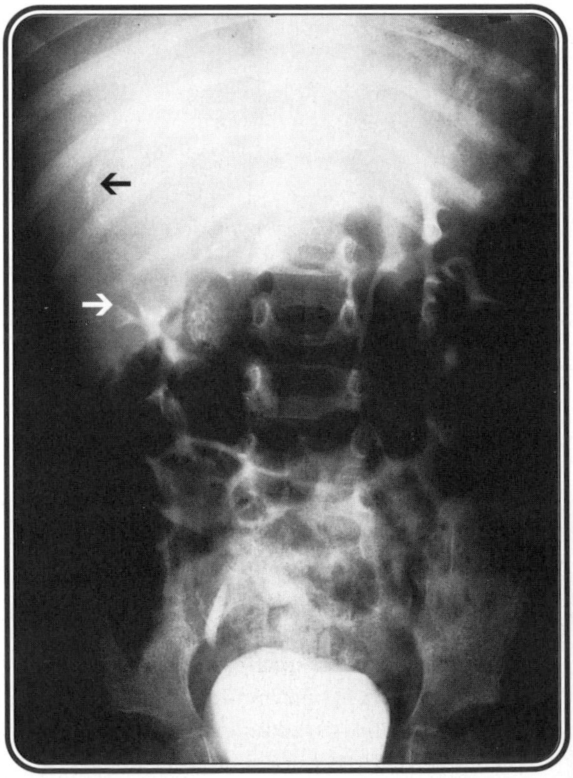

Fig. 22.9 IVU of neuroblastoma. Extensive calcification in soft tissue mass (black arrow) displacing the right kidney inferiorly (white arrow).

- Confirmatory biopsy is usually possible and scanning using MIBG (meta-iodobenzyl guanidine), a radiolabelled tumour-specific agent, is useful to measure disease extent.

Treatment

Treatment of neuroblastoma includes:

- Surgical resection.
- Chemotherapy.
- Irradiation.

Prognosis is worse for older children and those with metastatic disease. Over expression of the N-myc oncogene in tumour material is associated with a poor prognosis.

WILMS TUMOUR (NEPHROBLASTOMA)

Wilms tumour arises from embryonal renal cells of the metanephros. It is predominantly a tumour of the first 5 years of life with a median age of presentation of 3 years of age. Sporadic and familial forms occur. Most tumours are unilateral.

Clinical features

The most common clinical presentation is an asymptomatic abdominal mass that does not cross the midline. Other features may include:

- Abdominal pain—due to haemorrhage into the tumour.
- Haematuria.
- Hypertension—in 25%. May be caused by compression of the renal artery or renin production by tumour cells.

Wilms tumour:

- **Arises from embryonic renal cells.**
- **Usually presents as an abdominal mass in a child under 5 years old.**
- **Bilateral in 5% of cases.**
- **Association with aniridia (absent iris).**

A Wilms tumour susceptibility gene has been recognized from the rare association of Wilms tumour, sporadic aniridia, and deletions of part of chromosome 11. Associated abnormalities found in some children include:

- Hemihypertrophy.
- Genitourinary tract abnormalities.
- Mental retardation.
- Aniridia.

Diagnosis

Diagnosis is normally made from the characteristic appearance on CT (Fig. 22.10), which shows an intrinsic renal mass with mixed solid and cystic densities, and from biopsy. A search for distant metastases, which are most common in lungs and liver, should be made.

Treatment

Treatment involves surgical resection of the primary tumour, chemotherapy tailored to the stage and histology, and radiotherapy for those with advanced disease. Overall, the prognosis is good with an 80% chance of cure.

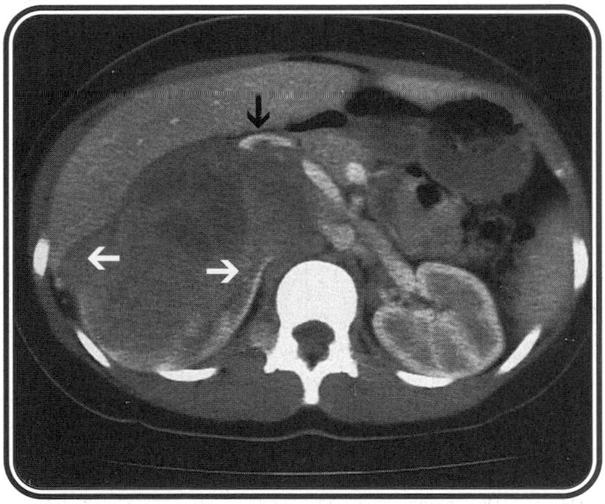

Fig. 22.10 CT scan of nephroblastoma. Wilms tumour mass arising out of right kidney (white arrows) displacing the inferior vena cava (black arrow).

SOFT TISSUE SARCOMAS

These arise from primitive mesenchyme. The most important is rhabdomyosarcoma, but even rarer forms include fibrosarcomas and liposarcomas.

BONE TUMOURS

Primary malignant bone tumours account for 4% of childhood cancer. They are uncommon before puberty and are most common in adolescents with a preponderence in boys. The two main types are:

- Osteogenic sarcoma—older children, most common.
- Ewing's sarcoma—younger children, less common.

Osteogenic sarcoma

This is a malignant tumour of the bone-producing mesenchyme, which is twice as common in males as females.

Clinical features

The usual presenting feature is local pain and swelling. Persistent bone pain precedes the detection of a mass. Half of all cases occur around the knee joint in the metaphysis of the distal femur or proximal tibia. Systemic symptoms are rare. Metastases are mainly to the lungs and are often asymptomatic.

Diagnosis

Bone X-ray shows destruction and a characteristic 'sunburst' appearance as the tumour breaks through the cortex and spicules of new bone are formed.

Treatment

Treatment involves surgery. En bloc resection may allow amputation to be avoided. Aggressive adjuvant chemotherapy is important to treat metastatic disease. Survival has improved and is greater than 50%.

Ewing's sarcoma

This is less common than osteogenic sarcoma and is very rare in Afro-Carribean children. It is an undifferentiated sarcoma of uncertain tissue of origin that arises primarily in bone, but occasionally in soft tissues.

It most commonly affects the long bones, especially mid to proximal femur, but may also affect flat bones such as the pelvis.

Clinical features and diagnosis

Pain and localized swelling are the usual presenting complaints. X-ray demonstrates a destructive lesion with periosteal elevation or a soft tissue mass (so called 'onion skin' appearance). Metastases occur to the lungs and other bones.

Treatment

Radiotherapy to the primary tumour is combined with chemotherapy for the prevention or treatment of metastases.

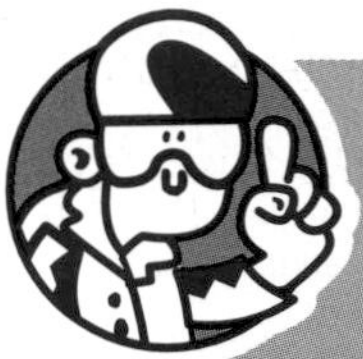

Bone tumours:

- **Are most common in adolescence.**
- **Are more common in boys.**
- **Most commonly affect the long bones.**

LANGERHANS CELL HISTIOCYTOSIS

Formerly called histiocytosis X, this term encompasses a group of relatively rare diseases characterized by the clonal proliferation of Langerhans cells (components of the bone marrow derived mononuclear phagocytic system). It is not now considered a true malignancy, but the potentially aggressive course and response to chemotherapy brings it within this sphere of clinical practice.

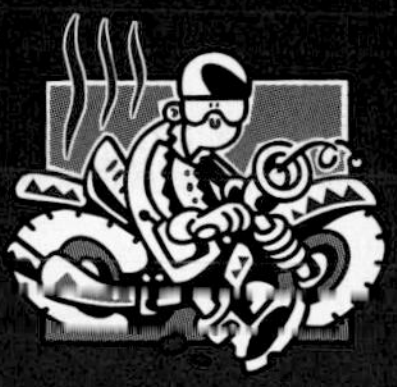

23. Endocrine and Metabolic Disorders

The most common and important of this group of disorders is insulin-dependent diabetes mellitus type 1 with an incidence of 1 out of 500 children and adolescents. Although less common, a host of other childhood endocrine and metabolic diseases exist which affect such vital processes as growth, sexual maturation, and calcium metabolism. Lastly, there are several hundred inborn errors of metabolism which are individually rare but important to recognize as many are treatable and genetic counselling for parents is often required.

DISORDERS OF CARBOHYDRATE METABOLISM

Diabetes mellitus

This is a heterogeneous group of disorders characterized by hyperglycaemia caused by reduced or absent insulin secretion or action. Insulin-dependent diabetes mellitus (IDDM, or Type 1 diabetes) is the most common form of childhood diabetes, although other varieties may be encountered. Further discussion refers to IDDM.

Aetiology

There is good evidence that IDDM results from auto-immune destruction of β cells in the pancreatic islets of Langerhans perhaps triggered by environmental factors (e.g. viruses) in people with a genetic predisposition (Fig. 23.1).

Pathophysiology

The pathophysiological pathways are described in Fig. 23.2. Key features include:

- Insulin deficiency becomes clinically significant when 90% of β cells are destroyed.
- Osmotic diuresis ensues when blood glucose concentration exceeds renal threshold.
- Ketoacidosis develops when insulin deficiency is severe.

Clinical features

IDDM may present at any age, but the most common age of onset is early adolescence (11–14 years). Increasingly, IDDM is diagnosed at an early stage, when the principal features are:

- Polyuria—increased frequency of urination (may be enuresis).
- Polydipsia—increased thirst.
- Weight loss.

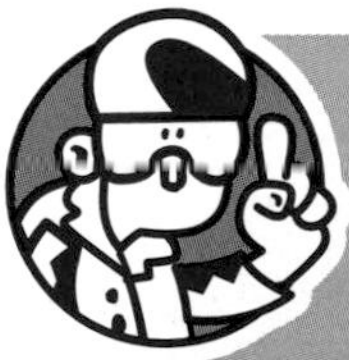

Always check for glycosuria in a child with a history of polyuria and polydipsia. Never ascribe frequency of micturition to urinary tract infection without checking for glycosuria and culturing urine.

Aetiology of insulin-dependent diabetes mellitus

Genetic factors
inherited susceptibility is demonstrated by increased incidence of IDDM in first-degree relatives: 2–5% in siblings and offspring. Concordance for identical twins is 30%. There is an 8–10 times risk for IDDM in people who are HLA-DR3, HLA-DR4, or both
Auto-immune factors
auto-immune basis is supported by:
- anti-islet cell antibodies
- lymphocytic infiltration of pancreas
- association with other auto-immune endocrine diseases, e.g. thyroiditis, Addison disease

Environmental factors
triggers may include viruses and dietary proteins

Fig. 23.1 Aetiology of insulin-dependent diabetes mellitus.

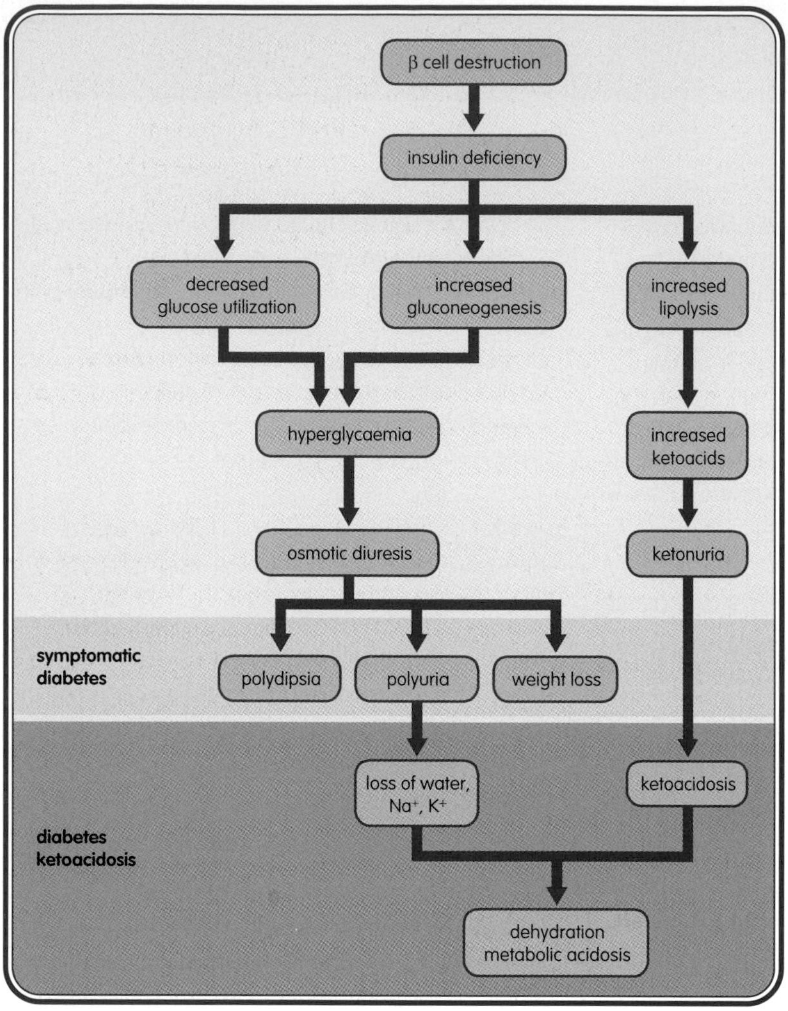

Fig. 23.2 Pathophysiology of insulin-dependent diabetes mellitus.

Diabetic ketoacidosis supervenes at a late stage over a short period and is characterized by abdominal pain, vomiting, features of severe dehydration, and ketoacidosis (see Hints & Tips).

Diagnosis

Diagnosis is confirmed in a symptomatic child by documenting hyperglycaemia, a random plasma glucose level greater than 11 mmol/L. If there is doubt, as may occur very early in the disease process, a fasting plasma glucose above 8 mmol/L or a raised glycosylated haemoglobin level will clarify the situation. Oral glucose tolerance tests are rarely needed in children.

Management

The discovery of insulin in 1922 transformed type 1 diabetes mellitus from a fatal disease into a treatable one. Initial management depends, of course, on the child's clinical condition. Long-term management of this life long condition rests on:

- Insulin replacement.
- Diet.
- Exercise.
- Monitoring.
- Education and psychological support.
- Management of complications—hypoglycaemia and diabetic ketoacidosis.

These are considered in turn.

Insulin replacement

The important features of insulin replacement are:

- Average requirement is 1.0 unit/kg/day. During the 'honeymoon' or remission phase, which may last for weeks or months after presentation, temporary return of function in residual islet cells causes a reduction in insulin requirements.

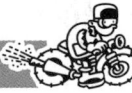

- The total daily dose is divided in a 1:3 proportion between short-acting (regular, soluble) insulin and medium-acting (isophane) insulin. Two-thirds is usually given before breakfast and one-third before the evening meal.
- Recombinant human insulin (rather than insulin from animal sources, e.g. pork or beef) is used.
- Injections are given subcutaneously and can be given in upper arms, outer thighs, or abdomen. The site must be rotated to avoid local complications such as fat atrophy.

Diet and exercise

Food intake needs to match the time course of insulin absorption and be adjusted for unusual heavy exercise. Dietary management therefore encompasses:

- High fibre, complex carbohydrates. This provides sustained release of glucose and avoids rapid swings in blood glucose generated by refined carbohydrates (e.g. sweets or ice creams).
- Food intake is divided between the three main meals and intervening snacks.
- Food intake is increased before or after heavy exercise to avoid hypoglycaemia.

Monitoring

Monitoring of blood glucose concentrations is necessary to evaluate the management and control. This is done using 'finger prick' devices together with dextrostix and a reflectometer which reads the colour change on the stick.

Twenty-four hour profiles are more useful than single daily records. Urine testing is more indirect, does not detect unacceptably low levels of glucose, and is often less popular, especially with teenagers. However, urine testing for ketones is important if ketoacidosis is suspected.

Education and psychological support

Children and their families require an educational programme that covers:

- A basic understanding of diabetes in lay language.
- The influence of diet and exercise on blood glucose levels.
- Practical aspects of insulin injection and blood glucose monitoring.

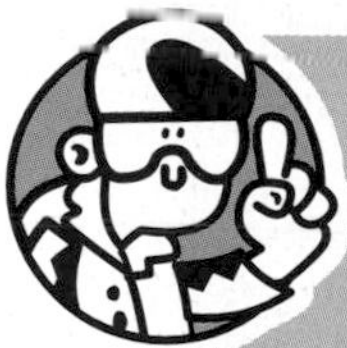

Traps for the unwary regarding diabetic ketoacidosis include mistaking the abdominal pain for acute appendicitis and mistaking the hyperventilation for pneumonia.

- Recognition and treatment of hypoglycaemia.
- Adjustments for intercurrent illness, significance of ketonuria.
- The importance of good control.

The diagnosis of IDDM provokes strong emotional responses in the child and family, including anger, guilt, resentment, and fear. Adjustment to these normal responses is facilitated by open discussion. Voluntary groups (e.g. British Diabetic Association) are important sources of support.

Management of complications

These may be divided into immediate complications, which include hypoglycaemia and diabetic ketoacidosis, and late complications.

Hypoglycaemia

A low blood glucose concentration may occur when there is inadequate carbohydrate intake or excessive exercise in relation to the insulin administered.

Symptoms usually occur at blood glucose levels below 4 mmol/L. Initial symptoms reflect the compensatory sympathetic discharge and include feeling faint, dizzy or 'wobbly', sweating, tremulousness, and hunger. More severe symptoms reflect glucose deprivation to the central nervous system and include lethargy, bizarre behaviour, and ultimately coma or seizures.

Treatment of a 'hypo' is easily achieved at an early stage by administration of a sugary drink, glucose tablet, or glucose polymer gel which is well absorbed via the buccal mucosa. At a later stage, if consciousness is impaired or there is lack of cooperation, IV glucose, or 1 mg of glucagon is administered.

Diabetic ketoacidosis

This may occur at presentation or complicate established diabetes (e.g. if there is poor compliance or intercurrent illness). It is considered in Chapter 28.

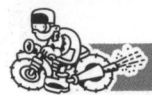

Adolescence and diabetes mellitus:

- **Adolescence is often a difficult time for the diabetic.**
- **There may be conflict at home and with health care professionals.**
- **Problems occur with self-image, self-esteem, and desire for independence.**
- **Denial or indifference may lead to poor compliance.**
- **'Feeling well' is equated with good control and long-term risks are often ignored.**
- **Helpful strategies include: a united team approach, clear guidelines plus short-term goals, and peer group pressure**

Hypoglycaemia

This is a common problem in the newborn (see Chapter 27), but is still seen occasionally in infants and children. It is important to diagnose as it is easy to treat and has serious consequences if unrecognized.

The various causes are best understood in relation to the normal factors determining glucose homeostasis. The major causes are listed in Fig. 23.3.

Clinical features

Early symptoms reflect the compensatory sympathetic response and include dizziness, faintness, and hunger. Signs include sweating and pallor. Late features are those of neuroglycopenia: behavioural changes, altered consciousness, and seizures.

Diagnosis

The precise definition of hypoglycaemia is problematic, but a useful working definition is a blood glucose less than 2.6 mmol/L. Measurements made using a glucose sensitive strip should always be verified by a laboratory measurement.

Ketotic hypoglycaemia

The most common cause of hypoglycaemia in children 1–4 years of age, this ill-defined entity is the result of diminished tolerance of normal fasting. The typical child is short and thin and becomes hypoglycaemic after a short period of starvation, for example, in the early morning. Insulin levels are low and there is ketonuria. Treatment is with frequent snacks and extra glucose drinks during intercurrent illness. Spontaneous resolution occurs by the ages of 6–8 years.

Regarding hypoglycaemia, at the time of blood glucose measurement, samples should be sent for measurement of:

- **Plasma insulin, growth hormone, and cortisol.**
- **β-hydroxybutyrate.**
- **Urine should be tested for ketones.**

Causes of hypoglycaemia beyond the neonatal period

Metabolic
- ketotic hypoglycaemia
- liver disease
- inborn errors of metabolism, e.g. glycogen storage disorders

Hormonal
- deficiency
  - adrenocortical insufficiency, e.g. Addison disease, congenital adrenal hyperplasia
  - panhypopituitarism
  - growth hormone deficiency
- hyperinsulinism
  - islet cell adenoma
  - exogenous insulin-treated IDDM

Fig. 23.3 Causes of hypoglycaemia beyond the neonatal period.

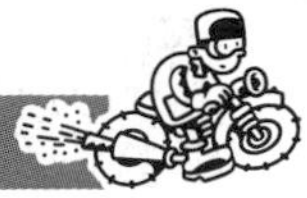

THYROID DISORDERS

Thyroid hormone is critical for normal growth and neurological development in infants and children. Conditions causing hypothyroidism and hyperthyroidism occur, and the gland may also be the site of benign and malignant tumours. Worldwide, the most important condition affecting the thyroid gland is iodide deficiency, estimated to affect at least 800 million people.

- **Slow linear growth is the hallmark of hypothyroidism in childhood.**
- **Children with Down syndrome have an increased incidence of hypothyroidism and hyperthyroidism.**

Hypothyroidism

This may be present at birth (congenital hypothyroidism) or may develop at any time during childhood or adolescence (juvenile hypothyroidism).

Congenital hypothyroidism

This has an incidence of 1 in 4000 live births. The causes include:

- Developmental defects: thyroid agenesis or failure of migration.
- Dyshormonogenesis: inborn error of thyroid hormone synthesis (accounts for 15%, a goitre usually occurs).
- Transient congenital hypothyroidism: (e.g. ingestion of maternal goitrogens).
- Congenital pituitary lesions (rare).
- Maternal iodide deficiency: the most common cause worldwide.

Clinical features

Infants may appear clinically normal at birth. The classical clinical features that develop include:

- Prolonged neonatal jaundice.
- Feeding problems.
- Constipation.
- Coarse facies, large tongue, umbilical hernia.

Diagnosis and treatment

As congenital hypothyroidism is common and treatable, neonatal screening is undertaken in the UK. Most laboratories test for raised levels of thyroid stimulating hormone (TSH) (although some measure both TSH and T_4). With neonatal screening and early treatment with oral thyroxine, neurological function and intelligence are within the normal range.

Hyperthyroidism

Neonatal hyperthyroidism may occur in the infants of mothers with Graves' disease from the transplacental transfer of thyroid-stimulating immunoglobulins (see Chapter 28).

Juvenile hyperthyroidism

This is most commonly caused by Graves' disease, an auto-immune condition in which one type of antibody mimics TSH by binding and activating the TSH receptor. It usually presents during adolescence and is much more common in girls than boys.

The clinical features are similar to those seen in adults.

On laboratory testing, serum levels of thyroxine (T_4) and triiodothyronine (T_3) are elevated and TSH levels are depressed. Antimicrosomal antibodies are often present.

Medical therapy with carbimazole or propylthiouracil is the first line of treatment. β-blockers can be added for relief of severe symptoms. Subtotal thyroidectomy or radioiodine treatments are options for relapse after medical treatment.

ADRENAL DISORDERS

Disorders of the adrenal cortex may result in deficiency or excess of adrenocortical hormones. The latter causes Cushing syndrome the most common cause of which is chronic administration of corticosteroids. Disorders of the medulla (e.g. phaeochromocytoma) are exceedingly rare.

Cortisol, the major glucocorticoid is stimulated by pituitary adrenocorticotrophic hormone (ACTH) under a negative feedback loop. Aldosterone is the principal mineralocorticoid and is controlled by the renin–angiotensin system. The major sex steroids produced by the adrenal glands are androgens.

Adrenocortical insufficiency

Diminished production of adrenocortical hormones may arise from:

- Congenital adrenal hyperplasia (CAH): an inherited inborn error of metabolism in biosynthesis of adrenal corticosteroids.
- Primary adrenal cortical insufficiency: Addison's disease.
- Secondary adrenal insufficiency: ACTH deficiency due to pituitary disease or long-term corticosteroid therapy.

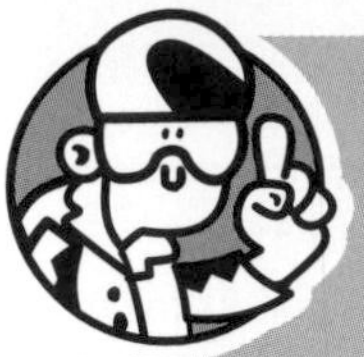

Congenital adrenal hyperplasia is a potentially lethal but treatable cause of vomiting and dehydration in young infants.

Congenital adrenal hyperplasia (CAH)

This is an autosomal recessive inborn error of metabolism causing defective synthesis of adrenal corticosteroids. Five different enzyme defects in the biosynthetic pathways have been described, but 95% of cases are caused by a deficiency in 21-hydroxylase.

Clinical features

The deficiency in cortisol production causes an increased secretion of ACTH which leads to adrenal hyperplasia (hence the name). In about three-quarters of affected cases, 'salt wasting' occurs due to mineralocorticoid deficiency. These 'salt losers' present within the first few weeks of life with:

- Failure to thrive.
- Vomiting and dehydration.
- Volume depletion, shock, and death.

Serum electrolytes show low levels of sodium and chloride with hyperkalaemia and hypoglycaemia.

The enzymatic block leads to increased levels of 17 α-hydroxyprogesterone, which is converted to testosterone. In girls, virilism occurs which may vary in severity from mild clitoral hypertrophy and labial fusion to true ambiguous genitalia. In boys, no genital abnormality may be evident or isosexual precocity may develop in the first few months of life.

Diagnosis

Diagnosis rests on the demonstration of markedly elevated levels of 17α-hydroxyprogesterone in the serum. In the 'salt losing' form, the characteristic electrolyte disturbance of hyponatraemia, hypochloridaemia, and hyperkalaemia provides a clue to the diagnosis.

Management

Initial management of a 'salt losing' crisis involves volume replacement with normal saline and systemic steroids.

Long-term treatment involves:

- Cortisol replacement—to suppress ACTH and androgen overproduction.
- Mineralocorticoid replacement—fludrocortisone, if there is salt wasting.
- Surgical correction of female genital abnormalities.

Primary adrenal insufficiency

Addison's disease is rare in children but may be caused by:

- Autoimmune disease.
- Haemorrhage and infarction (Waterhouse–Friderichsen syndrome).
- Tuberculosis (rare).

Physical findings include postural hypotension and increased pigmentation. Intercurrent illness or trauma may trigger an adrenal crisis (characterized by vomiting, dehydration, and shock).

Cushing syndrome

This is a cluster of symptoms and signs caused by glucocorticoid excess, due either to endogenous overproduction of cortisol or exogenous treatment with pharmacological doses of corticosteroids. The causes are listed in Fig. 23.4

Causes of Cushing syndrome
Endogenous overproduction
adrenal tumours (adenomas or carcinomas)
bilateral adrenal hyperplasia secondary to ACTH production by a pituitary microadenoma (Cushing disease)
Exogenous administration
long-term glucocorticoid treatment, e.g. for nephrotic syndrome, asthma, bronchopulmonary dysplasia

Fig. 23.4 Causes of Cushing syndrome.

Clinical features

The clinical features include

- Short stature.
- Truncal obesity, 'buffalo' hump.
- Rounded 'moon' facies.
- Signs of virilization, striae.
- Hypertension.

Diagnosis

Elevated serum cortisol levels are found with absence of the normal diurnal rhythm (high midnight levels). A prolonged dexamethasone suppression test may be required to distinguish Cushing's disease (ACTH-driven bilateral adrenal hyperplasia—suppressible by dexamethasone) from Cushing syndrome (adrenal tumour—cortisol levels not suppressed by dexamethasone). Computed tomography or magnetic resonance imaging of the adrenals and pituitary may identify an adrenal tumour or pituitary adenoma. Treatment depends on the cause and may involve surgical resection and radiotherapy.

Disorders of the pituitary gland

The pituitary gland has two distinct portions, the anterior and posterior lobes. These have different embryonic origins and separate hormonal functions. Pituitary disorders in childhood are rare.

Anterior pituitary disorders

A deficiency of the anterior pituitary hormones is more common than an excess of these and may involve individual hormones or all (panhypopituitarism).

Hypopituitarism in children may be caused by:

- Cranial defects, e.g. septo–optic dysplasia.
- Craniopharyngiomas.
- Langerhans cell histiocytosis.
- Cranial radiotherapy.

Growth retardation is a common feature, together with thyroid, adrenal, and gonadal dysfunction depending on the pattern of deficiency. Isolated idiopathic growth hormone (GH) deficiency accounts for most cases of GH deficiency.

Posterior pituitary disorders

The posterior lobe (neurohypophysis) secretes arginine vasopressin (antidiuretic hormone, ADH) and oxytocin.

Diabetes insipidus

This results from deficiency of ADH. It may occur as an isolated idiopathic defect or in association with anterior pituitary deficiency (e.g. due to tumours, infections, or trauma).

It presents with polydipsia and polyuria. Several conditions mimic diabetes insipidus including hypercalcaemia, chronic renal disease, and psychogenic water drinking.

Syndrome of inappropriate ADH (SIADH)

This is associated with expansion of the vascular volume and low serum sodium levels, which may cause neurological symptoms including lethargy, irritability, and seizures.

SIADH may be caused by several underlying conditions including:

- CNS disease: meningitis, brain tumours, or head trauma.
- Lung disease: pneumonia or TB.

DISORDERS OF THE GONADS

These cause abnormalities of sexual differentiation (which usually present in the newborn) and disorders of puberty which may be precocious or delayed.

Disorders of sexual differentiation

Abnormal sexual differentiation results in a newborn with ambiguous genitalia (intersex). Congenital adrenal hyperplasia leading to a virilized female is the most common cause. The causes can be classified as shown in Fig. 23.5.

Complete diagnostic evaluation should be undertaken as soon as possible. A definite sex cannot and should not be assigned immediately. It is worth remembering that 'sex' is determined at many different

Causes of abnormal sexual differentiation

46XY males with testes and incomplete masculinization due to:
- defects in testosterone synthesis
- defects in androgen action, e.g. 5α-reductase deficiency
- androgen resistance (testicular feminization syndrome)

46XX females with ovaries who are masculinized due to:
- congenital adrenal hyperplasia
- maternal androgen exposure

Fig. 23.5 Causes of abnormal sexual differentiation.

levels (Fig. 23.6). Naming and announcement of the child's sex should be delayed until the diagnostic work-up is complete.

Investigations may include:

- Chromosomal analysis.
- Hormone levels: testosterone, luteinizing hormone, follicle stimulating hormone, 17-hydroxyprogesterone.
- Pelvic ultrasonography.

Disorders of puberty

During normal puberty, secondary sex characteristics are acquired and reproductive capacity is attained. Features of normal puberty in males and females are listed in Fig. 23.7. Puberty may be precocious or delayed.

Precocious puberty

This refers to the development of secondary sexual characteristics before the age of 8 years in girls or 9 years in boys. There is an associated growth spurt. It should be differentiated from:

- Premature thelarche: isolated breast development in a very young girl. A non-progressive, benign condition.
- Premature adrenarche: isolated early appearance of pubic hair in either sex. A benign self-limiting condition due to early maturation of adrenal androgen secretion, but an adrenal tumour may need to be excluded.

The causes of precocious puberty are shown in Fig. 23.8. In females, it is usually due to early onset of normal puberty. In boys, it is usually due to an intracranial tumour.

Treatment depends on cause. It may be necessary to attempt to reduce the rate of skeletal maturation to avoid early cessation of growth and a reduction in adult height.

Delayed puberty

This may be defined as the absence of secondary sex characteristics at 14 years of age in girls or 15 years of age in boys. The problem is more common in boys in whom it is usually due to constitutional delay. The causes are listed in Fig. 23.9.

Assessment should include pubertal staging and examination to exclude systemic disease. If indicated, helpful investigations are:

- Chromosomal analysis.
- Measurement of gonadotrophin levels.

Treatment is often not required for constitutional delay, but hormone therapy (e.g. oxandrolone or low-dose testosterone) can be used to accelerate growth and induce secondary sexual characteristics.

- **Precocious puberty is more common in girls.**
- **Delayed puberty is more common in boys.**

Sex determination

An individual's sex is determined at many different levels:
- chromosomal
- gonadal (testis, ovary)
- anatomical (internal and external genitalia)
- hormonal
- psychological
- sex of rearing

Fig. 23.6 Sex determination.

Features of puberty

Females
- breast development is first sign
- height spurt reaches maximum before menarche
- menarche occurs between 11 and 15 years

Males
- testicular growth is first sign
- maximum height spurt reached 2 years after females

Fig. 23.7 Features of puberty.

Causes of precocious puberty

Gonadotrophin-dependent
- idiopathic, familial
- CNS lesions, e.g. postirradiation, surgery, tumours, hydrocephalus

Gonadotrophin-independent
- McCune–Albright syndrome (polyostotic fibrous dysplasia of bone)
- tumours of adrenals or gonads

Fig. 23.8 Causes of precocious puberty.

Causes of delayed puberty

Central causes—gonadotrophins low
constitutional delayed puberty
hypothalamo-pituitary disorders, e.g. panhypopituitarism, intracranial tumours, isolated gonadotrophin deficiency
severe systemic disease, e.g. cystic fibrosis, severe asthma, starvation
Gonadal failure—gonadotrophins high
chromosomal abnormalities, e.g. Klinefelter syndrome (47, XXY), Turner syndrome (45, XO)

Fig. 23.9. Causes of delayed puberty.

INBORN ERRORS OF METABOLISM

This term is used to describe any of the inherited disorders that result in a defect in normal biochemical pathways. Several hundred of these conditions have been described. Individually they are rare, although certain ethnic groups may be at increased risk for specific diseases.

Inborn errors of metabolism are usually autosomal recessive, although some are X-linked. The main categories are listed in Fig. 23.10.

Many of these disorders present in the neonatal period, but some present later. The clinical effects may be caused by accumulation of excess precursors, toxic metabolites of the excess precursors, or deficiency of products needed for normal metabolism.

Features in the neonate that should raise the suspicion of a metabolic error include:

- Vomiting after initiation of milk feeds, especially if persistent or recurrent
- Lethargy, coma, or seizures.
- Jaundice.
- Hepatosplenomegaly.
- Unusual odour of urine or sweat.

Investigations may reveal severe metabolic acidosis, hypoglycaemia, or hyperammonaemia.

In older children, they should be considered as a cause of:

- Progressive learning difficulties.
- Developmental delay.
- Seizures.
- Failure to thrive.
- Coarse facies.
- Hepatosplenomegaly.

A family history of unexplained early infant death and parental consanguinity should suggest the possibility of an inborn error of metabolism. Investigations that should be undertaken for an initial screen include:

- Urea and electrolytes, and ammonia levels.
- Acid–base status.
- Blood levels of glucose and amino acids.
- Urine amino acids and organic acids.

Examples of individual inborn errors of metabolism are considered briefly in turn.

Categories of inborn errors of metabolism

Category	Examples
amino acid metabolism	phenylketonuria
organic acid metabolism	maple syrup urine disease
urea cycle disorders	ornithine transcarbamylase deficiency
carbohydrate metabolism	galactosaemia glycogen storage diseases
mucopolysaccharidosis	Hurler syndrome

Fig. 23.10 Categories of inborn errors of metabolism.

Phenylketonuria (PKU)

This autosomal recessive trait has an incidence of 1 in 12 000 live births. In most cases, the defect lies in the enzyme phenylalanine hydroxylase, which normally converts phenylalanine to tyrosine. Hyperphenylalaninaemia occurs with build up of toxic by-products, such as phenylacetic acid, which are excreted in the urine (hence phenylketonuria).

As PKU is relatively common and is treatable, newborn screening is carried out by the Guthrie test.

This is carried out at several days of age, because it is necessary for the infant to have been fed milk, which contains phenylalanine.

Infants with PKU are clinically normal at birth. Symptoms and signs appear later in infancy and childhood if the disorder is undetected and untreated. These include:

- Neurological manifestations: moderate to severe mental retardation, hypertonicity, tremors, behaviour disorders, and seizures.
- Growth retardation.
- Hypopigmentation: fair skin, light hair (due to the block in tyrosine formation that is required for melanin production).

Treatment consists of dietary manipulation. The phenylalanine content of the diet is reduced. This should start early in infancy and is continued until at least 6 years of age. Some authorities recommend lifelong dietary restriction, but the diet is unpalatable.

Females with PKU must be on dietary restriction if planning a pregnancy, as maternal hyperphenylalaninaemia is associated with spontaneous abortion, microcephaly, and congenital heart disease.

Glycogen storage diseases

This is a group of conditions caused by defects in the enzymes involved in glycogen synthesis or breakdown. There is an abnormal accumulation of glycogen in tissues. The pattern of organ involvement depends on the enzyme defect and may include liver, heart, brain, skeletal muscle, or other organs. There are at least six varieties, some of which have eponyms, e.g.

Type 1A: von Gierke's disease (glucose-6-phosphatase deficiency)

Affected children have growth failure, hypoglycaemia and hepatomegaly.

Mucopolysaccharidoses (MPS)

This group of disorders is caused by defects in enzymes involved in the metabolism and storage of mucopolysaccharides. They are progressive multisystem disorders that may affect the central nervous system, eyes, heart, and skeletal system. Characteristic features are:

- Hepatosplenomegaly.
- Coarse facies—develop in most cases.

There are numerous types, many of which have eponymous designations, e.g.

MPS I: Hurler syndrome (autosomal recessive)

Affected children develop coarse facial features, corneal opacities, hepatosplenomegaly, kyphosis, and mental retardation.

Diagnosis is made by identifying the enzyme defect, and identifying the excretion in the urine of the major storage substances, the glycosaminoglycans.

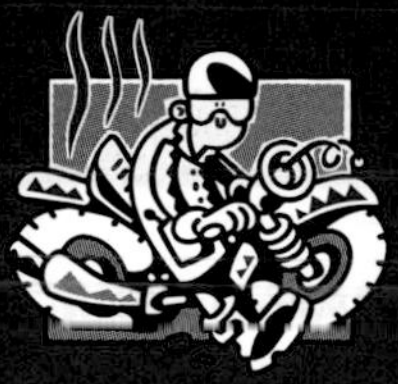

24. Disorders of Emotion and Behaviour

Major psychoses rarely present during childhood, but disturbed emotions and behavioural problems are very prevalent. The conditions encountered are, not surprisingly, age-related and range from the toddler who will not sleep to deliberate self-harm in an adolescent.

A child's personality, behaviour patterns, and emotional responses are determined by an interplay between nature (genetic endowment) and nurture (predominantly provided by parents). The relative importance of genes and environment remains the subject of debate and current research.

An infant's first relationship is usually with the mother and separation anxiety typically becomes evident at about 6 months to 1 year. By the second year, emotional attachments are extended to the father and other family members, and by the age of 4–5 years, separation from parents can be tolerated for several hours as occurs with school attendance.

With entry into school the importance of others, such as teachers and fellow school children, in shaping the child's psychosocial development increases.

Early, strong, emotional bonding underpins normal emotional development.

Nature

Some children have a temperament, which in itself may make it difficult for the parents to maintain a positive, loving relationship. Features may include:

- Predominantly negative mood.
- Intense emotional reactions.
- Poor and slow adjustment to new situations.

Developmental delay, for example, slow language development, may also cause problems.

Nurture

Families are the most powerful environmental influence on a child's emotional and behavioural development. Adequate parents will endeavour to:

- Provide love and affection.
- Provide food and shelter and protect children from physical harm.
- Exert authority to establish reasonable limits on behaviour.

Risk factors with an adverse influence are shown in Fig. 24.1.

PROBLEMS OF EARLY CHILDHOOD

Behavioural problems may relate to sleeping or eating, and tantrums are common. The rare disorder of autism may present at this time.

Sleep-related problems

Babies

An average baby sleeps for 15 hours a day in the first 2–3 months of life, sleeping for about 4 hours and waking for 3 hours at a time. At about 4 months, night-time breastfeeds are often discontinued and the baby may sleep through for 8 hours. Some babies are 'quiet wakeners', some are not, and appear to sleep less.

Factors associated with disturbed emotional and behavioural development
Parental factors
maternal depression
marital discord
divorce or bereavement
intrusive overprotection or emotional rejection
inconsistent discipline
Socio-economic factors
poverty, poor housing

Fig. 24.1 Factors associated with disturbed emotional and behavioural development.

Urinary continence (dryness) is achieved by most girls by age 5 years and boys by age 6 years.

suggests an underlying cause. A family history may be present and an assessment made of any emotional stresses either at school or at home.

Physical examination must include:

- A review of growth and measurement of blood pressure to identify unrecognized renal failure.
- Careful abdominal palpation to exclude an enlarged bladder.
- Inspection of the genitalia.

The spine and overlying skin should be inspected for any deformity, hairy patch, or sinus and the neurology of the lower limbs thoroughly examined.

Investigation should include:

- Urinalysis—tests for proteinuria and glycosuria.
- Microscopy and culture of a clean catch midstream urine.

Management

Important general measures include the establishment of a supportive and trusting relationship with the child and parents. A simple explanation of how the bladder works as a muscular balloon and the problem of being unaware of a full bladder during sleep should be given. Parental intolerance should be discouraged (by reminder of how common enuresis is) and 'functional payoffs' (e.g. sleeping in parents' bed) should be identified and stopped. A diary of wetting should be kept for at least 4 weeks and frequent, regular supervision by the doctor should be arranged.

Further management is age-dependent:

- Under 5 years: The situation may improve with reassurance, waterproof sheets, support from Social Services, and a scheduled lifting regimen. The latter is designed to increase bladder capacity. Initially the child is woken 1 hour after sleep and the interval increased by 30 minutes every 3–5 nights.
- Over 5 years: in addition to the above methods, star charts may be of value.
- Over 7 years: in addition to the above methods, alarms may be used. A choice of body-worn or pad and buzzer type alarm should be offered. The alarm rings when urination begins, causing the child to wake up and 'hold-on' to the sensation of a full bladder. A high degree of compliance and motivation is required and 60–70% of children will attain dryness after a few months.

Tricyclic antidepressants are no longer used in the treatment of enuresis. Desmopressin (a synthetic analogue of antidiuretic hormone) is available in tablet form and provides effective short-term relief. A percentage of patients who attain dryness on desmopressin remain dry when it is stopped.

Encopresis (faecal soiling)

Encopresis is involuntary faecal soiling at an age beyond which continence should have been achieved (normally about 4 years).

Children with encopresis fall into two main groups:

- Retentive: those with a rectum loaded with faeces. There is overflow incontinence (the majority).
- Non-retentive: children without constipation and a loaded rectum who have a neurogenic sphincter disturbance or psychiatric illness.

A number of factors predispose to chronic stool retention. These include:

- Environmental problems—lack of toilet facilities, harsh toilet training.
- Idiopathic—some children's rectums only empty occasionally, perhaps due to poor coordination with anal sphincter relaxation.
- Transient constipation—an episode of constipation due to dehydration or an anal fissure may lead to chronic retention.
- Organic constipation—associated with Hirschsprung's disease, drugs, or hypothyroidism.

Once established, a large bolus of faeces in the rectum may be impossible for the child to expel. The loaded rectum becomes dilated and may habituate to distension so the child is unaware of the need to empty it. Psychological factors may be both a cause and a result of encopresis. Soiling disturbs the child and can have a profound impact in school, socially, and in the family.

Onset of soiling in middle childhood, without a previous history of constipation suggests a primary psychiatric cause. It may occur in the setting of a chaotic family with high levels of emotional deprivation, neglect, and disturbed behaviour.

Diagnosis

Assessment must include a full bowel history, assessment of the family's psychological functioning, and careful examination of the neurological system and abdomen. Rectal examination and abdominal palpation will determine whether there is faecal retention.

Management

The key objective in management of encopresis due to faecal retention is to empty the rectum as soon as possible. This may require an enema but can often be achieved by a combination of stool softener (e.g. lactulose) and laxative (e.g. senna).

Regular defecation should then be encouraged by:

- Regular laxatives.
- Star charts.
- Sitting on the toilet after meals.
- Dietary changes—increased roughage.

The distended rectum will take several weeks to shrink to normal size.

Attention-deficit hyperactivity disorder (ADHD)

The three hallmarks of ADHD are:

- Inattention.
- Hyperactivity.
- Impulsiveness.

Incidence and aetiology

In the USA, this diagnosis is applied if either inattention or hyperactivity and impulsiveness persist in two or more situations. In the UK, the diagnosis of hyperkinetic syndrome is made only if all three features:

- Are present from an early age.
- Persist in more than one situation (home and school).
- Impair function.

This identifies a more severe subtype of ADHD with prevalence of 1 in 200 (ADHD affects 2–4% of school children). Hyperkinetic syndrome is four times more common in boys than girls.

Twin studies suggest a genetic contribution to aetiology. Perinatal problems and delays in early development appear to be more common in hyperkinetic syndrome. Disturbed relationships such as may occur with an emotionally rejecting parent or institutional upbringing may exacerbate it.

Hyperkinetic syndrome is a severe subtype of ADHD. It is more common in boys than girls.

Clinical features

Features of ADHD:

- Inattention—manifests as an easily distracted child who changes activity frequently and does not persist with tasks.
- Hyperactivity—an excess of movement with persistent fidgeting and restlessness that can be distinguished from normal high-spirited, energetic behaviour by the interference with normal social functioning.
- Impulsiveness—acting without reflection: affected children act impetuously and erratically.

Although these features may be present in the preschool years, they often come to clinical attention with the increased demands of the classroom.

Physical examination should include a search for:

- Developmental delay, clumsiness.
- Deficits in hearing or vision and specific learning difficulties.
- Dysmorphic features.

Most children do not have a sudden onset or an identifiable brain disorder and do not need special investigations such as electroencephalography or brain imaging.

Management

A behaviour-modifying and educational approach is the mainstay of treatment but drug treatment should be considered if these strategies fail. It is important to explain the nature of the disorder to the parents and school staff. Parent support groups may provide reassurance and help.

Behavioural therapy

About 50% of children respond to behavioural therapy comprising:

- A structured environment.
- Positive reinforcement.
- Cognitive approaches emphasizing relaxation and self-control.

Extra help in the classroom and modification of the curriculum may be required.

Drug therapy

Drug therapy is usually reserved for children who have failed to benefit from behavioural approaches applied consistently for 3 months. Paradoxically, central stimulant drugs are most effective in promoting attentiveness and reducing hyperactivity. Those most studied are:

- Dexamphetamine.
- Methylphenidate.

The effect may be dramatic and the best responses are seen in children aged 5–10 years. A 1-month trial is usually sufficient to determine whether a worthwhile effect has been achieved.

Alternative therapies

Numerous alternative therapies have been advocated. Diets may have a role in a minority of children and the parents' observations that a particular food aggravates hyperactivity should be heeded. A trial of an exclusion diet may be warranted. (Few children react to additives alone and a diet just excluding foods with synthetic dyes or preservatives is unlikely to be helpful.)

Hyperactivity itself does not usually persist as a predominant feature into adulthood. However, affected children tend to do poorly at school and low self-esteem together with antisocial traits may turn them into disadvantaged adults.

Recurrent pain syndromes

Recurrent pain without an organic cause is not uncommon in children. The usual sites are the abdomen, head, or limbs.

A strict dichotomy between organic and psychological causation for recurrent pain is unhelpful and explains only a minority of cases. In most cases the pain is best explained as dysfunctional, a result of mild individual differences in physiology that render the child vulnerable to pain in response to stress.

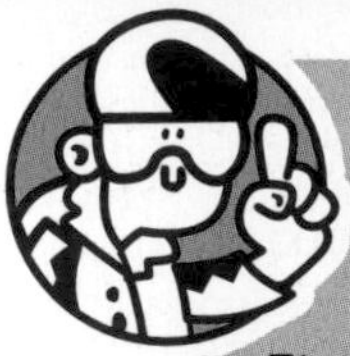

- **Apley's law: the further the pain is from the umbilicus, the more likely it is to be organic.**
- **The more localized limb pain is, the less likely it is to be 'growing pains'.**
- **Measure the blood pressure and examine the fundi in a child with recurrent headaches.**

Clinical features and diagnosis

The history should establish:

- Onset, frequency, and duration of the pain and associated symptoms.
- Family functioning.
- Existence of stressors, e.g. bullying at school.

Physical examination is directed towards excluding an organic cause (Fig. 24.3). Investigations have a low yield if physical examination is normal and should be kept to a minimum. Full blood count, erythrocyte sedimentation rate, and urinalysis may be indicated.

Management

For dysfunctional pain, normal activity should be encouraged. Symptomatic relief should be offered (e.g. mild analgesics) and the patient should be encouraged to keep a symptom diary.

School refusal

Repeated absence from school may be due to illness or truancy, but in a few cases it is due to school refusal, i.e. an unwillingness to attend because of anxiety. School refusal may be associated with:

- Separation anxiety (under 11 years).
- Adverse life events (bereavement, moving).
- Stressors (bullying).

True school phobia is seen in older, anxious children, who typically have problems beginning school in the

Organic causes of recurrent pain	
Site	**Cause**
abdominal pain	genitourinary problems: UTI, obstructive uropathy gastrointestinal disorders: inflammatory bowel disease, peptic ulcer
headache	refractive disorders migraine hypertension raised intracranial pressure
limb pain	neoplastic disease, e.g. leukaemia, bone tumour orthopaedic: Osgood–Schlatter disease

Fig. 24.3 Organic causes of recurrent pain.

autumn and returning to school after weekends and holidays.

Management

Management requires an early, graded return to school with support for the parents and treatment of any underlying emotional disorder.

PROBLEMS OF ADOLESCENCE

This is a period during which a number of important disorders may present, including emotional disorders such as anxiety and depression, conduct disorders, and disorders of eating.

Eating disorders

Anorexia nervosa

This eating disorder is characterized by:

- Refusal to maintain an expected bodyweight for height with weight less than 85% of expected bodyweight.
- Intense fear of gaining weight or being fat.
- Disturbed body image: feeling fat when actually emaciated.
- Amenorrhoea for at least three cycles (in women).

The prevalence rate is 1% with a peak age of onset of 14 years (and girls outnumbering boys by 20 to 1). The aetiology is unknown. The patient often displays obsessive, overachieving, perfectionist, and controlling personality traits.

Clinical features and diagnosis

Physical examination may reveal:

- Emaciation and muscle wasting.
- Fine lanugo hair over trunk and limbs.
- Bradycardia and poor peripheral perfusion.
- Slowly relaxing tendon reflexes.

Laboratory investigations may reveal:

- Reduced plasma proteins, vitmain B_{12}, and ferritin.
- Endocrine abnormalities: elevated cortisol, reduced T_4, luteinizing hormone, and follicle stimulating hormone.

In boys, cranial computed tomography should be undertaken to exclude a brain tumour.

Management and prognosis

The immediate goal is to make a therapeutic alliance with the patient to restore normal bodyweight by re-feeding. This can be attempted initially as an outpatient, aiming at a gain of 500 g per week. Failure to meet this target necessitates hospital admission for re-feeding under nursing supervision. This may be difficult. Affected girls may hide food and lie about their weight. Tube feeding may be required if there is continued weight loss in hospital.

Once weight gain is achieved, psychotherapeutic approaches are adopted. This aims to provide counselling on handling conflict, relationships, and personal autonomy.

Prognosis is variable with an eventual 5% mortality rate from malnutrition, infection, or suicide. Fifty per cent make a good recovery, 30% show partial improvement and 20% have a chronic relapsing course.

Emotional disorders

Depression

Depression as a clinical syndrome is more than just a transitory low mood or misery in response to adverse life circumstances. It is characterized by:

- Persistent feelings of sadness or unhappiness.
- Ideas of guilt, despair, and lack of self-worth.
- Social withdrawal.
- Lack of motivation and energy.
- Disturbances of sleep, appetite, and weight.

It is increasingly recognized in prepubertal children, but is predominantly a problem of adolescence. Aetiology is multifactorial but there is a clear genetic contribution. Dysfunctional families or adverse life events may contribute.

Management

Treatment may also include antidepressant medication or psychological approaches.

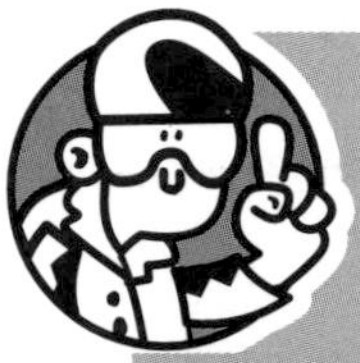

- **Suicide is the third most common cause of death in adolescents and young adults.**
- **Most intentional overdoses are not taken with suicidal intent, but an important minority are—so psychiatric evaluation is important in all cases.**

Conduct disorder

This is a syndrome characterized by the persistent (6–12 months) failure to control behaviour within socially defined rules. This involves three overlapping domains of behaviour:

- Defiance of authority.
- Aggressiveness.
- Antisocial behaviour: violating other people's property, rights, or person.

This is one of the most common child psychiatric problems. The aetiology is multifactorial with genetic and environmental contributions. It is more common in boys. In many children, it is preceded by the so-called oppositional defiant disorder, i.e. children who demonstrate a persistent pattern of angry, negative, vindictive, and defiant behaviour.

Management and prognosis

Psychological intervention, working with the child and family, is the mainstay of treatment.

A significant number (40%) of children with conduct disorder become delinquent young adults with ongoing behaviour problems and disrupted relationships. Those with onset before adolescence are most at risk.

Chronic fatigue syndrome

This refers to persistent (longer than 6 months) subjective fatigue causing rapid exhaustion on physical or mental exertion.

It appears to arise from both physical and psychological factors. Parents often insist on a physical cause being more likely and an agnostic stance by the physician is probably most useful.

Chronic fatigue syndrome encompasses myalgic encephalomyelitis (ME) and post-viral fatigue syndrome and there is sometimes serological evidence of preceding viral infection.

Management and prognosis

Graded rehabilitation approaches with physiotherapy to increase exercise tolerance may be beneficial. Most cases remit spontaneously with time, but this may take many months or even years.

Psychosis

Chronic disorders such as schizophrenia and bipolar affective disorder may present in adolescence. The prevalence of drug abuse in this age group renders drug-induced psychosis an important problem.

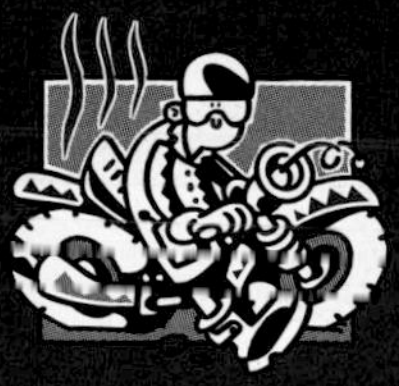

25. Social and Preventative Paediatrics

This includes all aspects of promoting health and preventing illness such as child health surveillance, immunization, health education, and accident prevention. In addition, Community Paediatric services are closely involved with the problems of child abuse, adoption and foster care, and children with special needs. Important legislation concerning children and health in the UK exists, in particular the Children Act and the Education Act.

PREVENTION IN CHILD HEALTH

There remains a high level of morbidity from preventable conditions including:

- Infectious diseases.
- Congenital disorders.
- Accidents.
- Malnutrition.
- Smoking in teenagers.

Strategies for prevention include:

- Immunization.
- Screening.
- Child health surveillance.
- Health promotion and education.

Immunization

Immunization has probably conferred more benefit on the world's children than any other medical advance or intervention. It has allowed the prevention of many major diseases such as diphtheria and polio, which killed or crippled millions of children, and the complete eradication of small pox. In recent times, the highly successful introduction of immunization against *Haemophilus influenzae* Type B (Hib) has dramatically reduced the incidence of invasive infections such as Hib meningitis and epiglottitis.

Immunization is effective against major bacterial diseases, such as diphtheria and TB, and viral diseases, such as measles, mumps, rubella, and hepatitis. bacille Calmette-Guérin (BCG) vaccination against TB is effective in some parts of the world. However, a vaccine has yet to be developed against the important parasitic disease, malaria.

Immunity—active and passive

Immunity can be induced either actively (long-term) or provided by passive transfer (short-term) against a variety of bacterial and viral agents.

Active immunity is induced by using:

- A live, attenuated form of the pathogen, e.g. oral poliomyelitis vaccine (OPV), measles, mumps, rubella vaccine (MMR), BCG vaccine for TB.
- An inactivated organism, e.g. inactivated poliomyelitis vaccine (IPV), pertussis.
- A component of the organism, e.g. Hib, pneumococcal vaccine, hepatitis B.
- An inactivated toxin (toxoid), e.g. tetanus vaccine, diphtheria vaccine.

In many individuals, live, attenuated viral vaccines promote a full, long-lasting antibody response after one dose. Several doses of an inactivated version or toxoid are usually required.

Passive immunity is conferred by the injection of human immunoglobulin. There are two main types:

- Human normal immunoglobulin (HNIG).
- Specific immunoglobulins for tetanus, hepatitis B, rabies, and varicella zoster (VZIG).

Routes of administration may be:

- By mouth: oral polio vaccine.
- Intradermal: BCG.
- Subcutaneous or intramuscular injection: all other vaccines.

In infants, the upper outer quadrant of the buttock or the anterolateral aspect of the thigh are the recommended sites for the injection of vaccines.

Immunization schedule

In the UK, the schedule for primary immunization with DTP (diphtheria, tetanus, pertussis), Hib, and polio starts at 2 months with an interval of 1 month between doses. This accelerated schedule was adopted to provide earlier and more effective protection against haemophilus and pertussis infections, which are more dangerous to the very young. Added benefits have included fewer side effects and better completion of the full course.

The schedule is shown in Fig. 25.1.

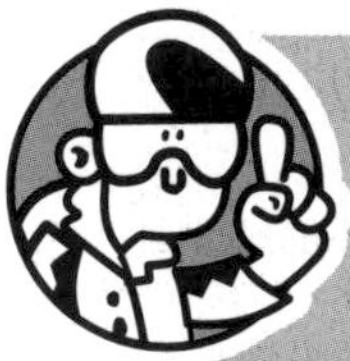

The timing of childhood immunization is critical: too early and the immune response may be inadequate, too late and the child may acquire the disease before being protected.

Indications and contraindications to immunization

Every child should be protected against infectious diseases, and a denial of immunization should not be allowed without serious consideration of the consequences.

Special risk groups can be identified for whom the risk of complications from infectious disease is high and who should be immunized as a priority. These include children with:

- Chronic lung and congenital heart disease.
- Down syndrome.
- HIV infection.
- Low birth weight.
- No spleen or hyposplenism.

In addition to the routine schedule, these children should have vaccines against pneumococcus and meningococcus (A and C).

General contraindications

These include:

- Acute illness with fever >38°C: postpone until recovery has occurred.
- A definite history of a severe local or general reaction to a preceding dose.

Live vaccines—special risk groups

Live vaccines pose a risk for certain individuals whose immunity is impaired. These include children:

- Being treated with chemotherapy or radiotherapy for malignant disease.
- On immunosuppressive treatment after organ or bone marrow transplant.
- On high-dose systemic steroids.
- With impaired cell-mediated immunity, e.g. severe combined immunodeficiency syndrome or acquired immune-deficiency syndrome (AIDS).

Children positive for antibodies to HIV, with or without symptoms, should be given all vaccines except BCG (there have been reports of dissemination of BCG in HIV-positive individuals).

Specific contraindications

Particular vaccines are contraindicated in certain circumstances:

- Measles vaccination is contraindicated if there is allergy to neomycin. Data indicate that over 99% of

UK immunization schedule		
Vaccine	**Age**	**Comments**
DTP, Hib, and polio (primary course)	first dose second dose third dose	2 months 3 months 4 months
measles, mumps, and rubella (MMR)	12–15 months	can be given at any age over 12 months
DT, polio (booster) MMR second dose	3–5 years	3 years after completing primary course
BCG	10–14 years or infancy	
Td, polio (booster)	13–18 years	

Fig. 25.1 UK Immunization schedule.

children who are allergic to eggs can safely receive MMR vaccine. If there is concern, immunization should be given under hospital supervision.

- Pertussis. It has never been conclusively demonstrated that this vaccine ever causes permanent brain damage. There are no specific contraindications (in particular, a family or personal history of epilepsy is not a contraindication). Immunisation is best delayed in patients with progressive neurological disease until the condition is stabilized.

'False' contraindications

The following are *not* contraindications to immunization:

- Family history of adverse reaction to immunization.
- Prematurity.
- Stable neurological conditions, e.g. cerebral palsy.
- Asthma, eczema, hay fever.
- Under a certain weight.
- Over the age recommended in standard schedule.
- Minor afebrile illness.
- Child's mother being pregnant.

Adverse reactions associated with specific vaccines are shown in Fig. 25.2.

Screening

An effective and worthwhile screening programme should satisfy certain criteria:

- The condition screened for should be an important health problem.
- There should be a sensitive and specifc test.
- Treatment should improve the condition.
- Screening should be cost-effective.
- The screening method should be acceptable to child and parents.

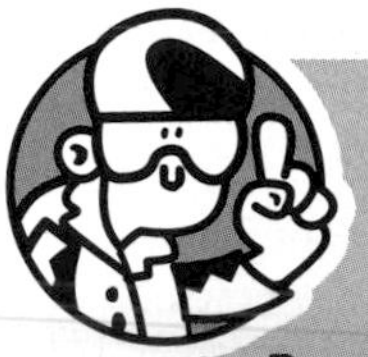

- **Immunization should be postponed if the child has an acute febrile illness.**
- **Premature babies can be immunized following the recommended schedule according to chronological age, i.e. immunization should not be postponed.**
- **Live vaccines are contraindicated in immunocompromised children.**

Screening may be targeted at a 'high-risk' population, or carried out opportunistically when a patient presents for some other reason at the relevant age.

Child health promotion

A programme of health surveillance is undertaken to identify important conditions that have a better outcome if diagnosed and treated early (e.g. congenital dislocation of the hip and deafness).

This programme includes:

- Neonatal examination.
- 6-week check.
- 6–9 month check.
- 18–24 month check.
- 36–42 month check.

Adverse reactions associated with specific vaccines

Vaccine	Minor reaction	Major reaction
diphtheria/tetanus	local	neurological (very rare)
pertussis	fever, crying	convulsions (1:300 000) encephalopathy (very rare)
polio	—	vaccine-associated polio (1 in 2 million)
MMR	fever, rash, arthropathy	encephalopathy (very rare) thrombocytopenia
BCG	local abscess	adenitis

Fig. 25.2 Adverse reactions associated with specific vaccines.

Neonatal examination

Full physical examination looking for congenital anomalies such as congenital dislocation of the hips, undescended testes , and absence of the red reflex. A test of hearing (otoacoustic emission test) is planned for introduction.

Guthrie test: on day 6 a heel prick blood sample is taken to screen for phenylketonuria and hypothyroidism.

Six-week check

Physical examination with emphasis on:

- Surveillance for congenital anomalies, e.g. cardiac, undescended testes ,and dislocated hips.
- Growth: weight, length, and head circumference.
- Development: alert, makes eye contact, smiling in response.
- Vision and hearing (explore parental concerns).

Assessment should also be made of the family's adjustment to the new infant, quality of parent–child interactions, and signs of maternal depression.

Six to nine months

- Check for congenital dislocation of the hips.
- Distraction test for hearing (for those not screened in neonatal period).
- Assess development.
- Anticipatory guidance on feeding, safety and injury prevention, sleep habits.

Eighteen to twenty-four months

- Assess development: confirm walking with normal gait and age-appropriate vocalization and language.
- Growth: height and weight.
- Anticipatory guidance on toilet training, temperament, and behaviour.

Thirty-six to forty-two months

- Growth: height and weight.
- Hearing and vision tests.
- Developmental tests.

CHILD ABUSE

Although it is probable that children have been abused throughout history, it is only in the last few decades that the extent to which children may be abused by their parents or carers has been recognized. In the UK, one child in 1000 suffers severe physical abuse, and as many as 150 children are killed each year. Several types of abuse are recognized and these often occur together (Fig. 25.3).

Diagnosis

Certain families and children are at particular risk. Adults who abuse are often young, immature, isolated, poor, and subject to social or marital stress. Alcoholism, drug abuse, and personality or psychiatric disorders (e.g. postnatal depression) may be contributory. Young children under the age of 3 years, and babies born prematurely are at particular risk.

Child abuse may present to the GP or hospital doctor directly, or the health visitor, social services, the police, the school, a relative or even a neighbour may raise a suspicion of abuse. Diagnosis is difficult and, of course, false accusations cause great anguish. Each type is considered in turn.

Types of abuse

Physical abuse or non-accidental injury (NAI)

Certain features in the history of a physical injury should raise the suspicion that it may be non-accidental (Fig. 25.4). Actual injuries may include bruises (Fig. 25.5), bite marks, burns or scalds, and head injuries or fractures. Accidental fractures of long bones are rare in babies but common in mobile children aged 3–4 years. Metaphyseal fractures and posterior rib fractures should raise suspicion of NAI. Direct blows to the mouth or forcing a bottle into the mouth may tear the frenulum. Violent shaking of a baby may tear the vessels that cross the subdural space leading to subdural haemorrhage (Fig. 25.6). This is associated with irritability, poor feeding, and signs of raised intracranial pressure (increasing head circumference, a tense fontanelle, and retinal haemorrhages).

Types of abuse
physical (non-accidental injury)
sexual
emotional
neglect
Munchausen by proxy (fictitious illness)

Fig. 25.3 Types of abuse.

Features of non-accidental injury

delay in reporting the injury
history not consistent with the injury
variable and inconsistent accounts from caregivers
history incompatible with child's age/developmental capacity
previous unexplained injuries

Fig. 25.4 Features of non-accidental injury.

Features of non-accidental bruises

any bruises in a (non-mobile) baby
bruises on face, back, buttocks as opposed to forehead and shins in toddler
bruises in pattern of finger-tips, hand-print, belt (follow shape and size of object used)
bruises of different ages

Fig. 25.5 Features of non-accidental bruises.

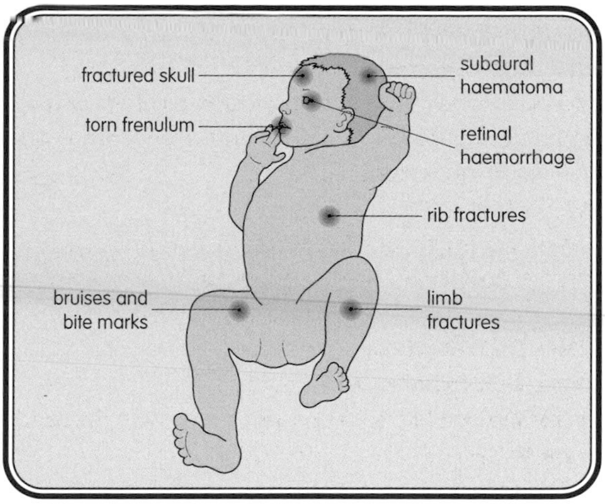

Fig. 25.6 Battered or shaken baby syndrome.

Neglect and emotional abuse

Neglect may manifest as failure to thrive, developmental delay, and poor hygiene. Emotional abuse includes rejection and withdrawal of love, and persistent malicious criticism or threats.

Munchausen syndrome by proxy (Meadow syndrome)

This extraordinary syndrome is a form of child abuse. The carer, usually the mother, fabricates illness in the child by inventing symptoms or faking signs (e.g. by putting blood or sugar in the urine, or contaminating microbiological specimens). The child may be deliberately poisoned and presents with bizarre, unexplained symptoms. Diagnosis is difficult.

Sexual abuse

Child sexual abuse (CSA) may involve either sex at any age, but is more common in girls. It has been defined as the involvement of dependent, immature children or adolescents in sexual activities that they do not fully understand and are unable to give informed consent to. It should be remembered that medical examination is rarely diagnostic. Physical findings such as tears or abrasions around genitalia, bruising around the genitalia or genital infection are present in less than 30% of abused children. Vulval soreness is very common in young girls and is rarely due to abuse.

Management

Extra care should be taken to record the history and physical findings in detail and with great accuracy. Physical findings should be measured, drawn, and if appropriate, photographed (with parental consent). As always, all notes should be dated, timed, and signed as this is particularly important in relation to any subsequent legal proceedings. If child abuse is suspected in the UK, the Social Services Child and Family department must be informed.

Treatment of any physical injury may be required and if abuse is suspected, a decision made as to whether the child needs immediate protection. This may mean hospital admission or placement in a foster home; if parental consent is not given, legal enforcement may be necessary. Senior staff should be involved from the beginning, as experience is required in handling what is always a very difficult situation.

Investigations may be indicated. In the presence of suspicious bruising it is advisable to do a platelet count and coagulation screen to exclude thrombocytopenia and other bleeding diatheses, which often present with multiple and excessive bruising. A skeletal survey by X-ray should be carried out in any infant with suspected physical abuse.

In most cases, further management will involve evaluation of the family by social workers and the convening of a Child Protection Conference. The conference may include the paediatrician, GP, health visitor, social workers, police, and nursing staff. Parents usually attend all or part of the conference. A decision will be made on whether to place the child's name on the Child Protection Register, whether court proceedings are required, and whether the child can safely be returned to the family. A child protection care plan will be produced and will define the level of supervision and medical follow-up.

CHILDREN AND THE LAW

The principal legislation concerning children and health in the UK is contained in:

- The Children Act (England and Wales 1989, Scotland 1995).
- The Education Act (1993).
- UN Convention on the Rights of the Child (1989).

The Children Act

This integrates the law relating to private individuals with the responsibilities of public authorities towards children. It aims to strike a balance between family independence and child protection. The essential components include:

- Parental responsibilities are defined. Responsibilities replace rights. Parents have the prime responsibility for their children and this is retained in all circumstances except adoption.
- The welfare of the child is paramount. The wishes and feelings of the child must be respected and courts should ensure that any orders made positively benefit the child or children concerned.
- Professionals are encouraged to work in partnership with parents.
- Defines responsibilities for 'children in need'. Local authorities are required to provide supportive services to assist parents in bringing up their children. A register must be kept of children with disabilities and special services provided for those whose health or development may be impaired.
- The court must consider the child's race, religion, culture, and language.
- A child should remain with his or her family whenever possible.
- Describes court orders in relation to custody and access, and child protection. The latter include: Emergency Protection Order, Child Assessment Order, Care and Supervision Order, Police Protection Order

Foster care

The purpose of foster care is to provide a safe, temporary placement for a child who is at physical, emotional, or social risk. Common reasons for foster placement include:

- Child abuse.
- Death or absence of parents.
- Severe neurodevelopmental problems.

Placement may be voluntary by a parent, voluntary with court ratification, or involuntary by a court order. Families which are more likely to have their children placed in foster care, are those with lower socio-economic status and a history of continuing multigenerational dysfunction.

Children placed in foster care are at risk of:

- Failure to thrive.
- Developmental delay, behavioural, and psychiatric problems.
- Discontinuity of primary health care.
- Higher incidence of conduct disorders in adolescence.

The benefits of foster placement include:

- Decrease of abuse and maltreatment.
- Improved school attendance.

Foster parents receive an allowance according to the age and needs of the child.

Adoption

The annual number of adoptions in the UK has fallen from 21 000 in 1975 to fewer than 6000 by 1995. Baby adoptions fell from 4500 to 300. This fall is partly attributable to wider use of contraception and abortion and greater social acceptance of single parenthood.

Most children available for adoption are in local authority care, either with foster parents or in a children's home. Unfortunately, the children available for adoption, many of whom are older, disabled, or have suffered abuse or neglect, are not always the kind that adopting couples are looking for.

Adoption is a legal procedure encompassing several important features:

- It is arranged by registered agencies. Adopters must be aged over 21 years.
- An adoption cannot be reversed except in exceptional circumstances.
- An adopted child loses all legal ties with his or her birth parents (has no claim to maintenance or inheritance) and becomes a full member of the new family taking on the nationality of the adoptive parents.
- The original parents have no right of access, but contact for older children is often maintained.

- The natural parents must give informed consent, unless they cannot be found or are judged unlikely to ever be able to look after the child adequately.
- The child lives with the adoptive parents for 3 months before the order is finalized.
- At age 18, an adopted child is entitled to his or her original birth certificate.

Consent to medical care

A person older than 16 years can legally give his or her own consent. Below the age of 16, the consent of a parent or guardian (person with parental responsibility for the child) is required unless:

- Emergency treatment is required.
- The child consents and the doctor considers that the child is of sufficient understanding to make an informed decision and the child will not consent to a parent being asked (the Gillick principle).

If the parent(s) of a child younger than 16 years refuse a life-saving treatment, a court can give consent.

Confidentiality

A person aged 16 years and over has full rights to confidentiality. However, the duty of confidentiality owed to a patient under 16 years old is as great as that owed to any other person. Information may be disclosed to parents if it is in the interests of the child.

THE CHILD WITH A DISABILITY

Many children have complex and long-lasting neurodevelopmental disabilities that require early identification and support in the community. It is useful to define some of the terms used:

- Impairment: any loss or abnormality of physiological or anatomical structure.
- Disability: any restriction or loss of ability in performing an activity in a way considered normal for a particular age which is caused by an impairment.
- Handicap: a disadvantage for an individual arising from a disability that prevents the achievement of desired goals.

For example, an intraventricular haemorrhage with periventricular leucomalacia (impairment of motor tracts) may cause a hemiparesis (the disability) resulting in difficulty playing the piano (handicap). The use of the term 'handicap' with its connotation of dependency has fallen out of favour.

Disabilities may give rise to 'special needs', which in the terms of the Education Act (1993) are educational needs not normally met by the normal provisions for a child of that age.

Presentation of children with disabilities

The kinds of conditions under consideration include, for example:

- Speech and language problems.
- Behavioural problems.
- Down syndrome.
- Cerebral palsy.
- Spina bifida.
- Hearing or visual impairment.
- Learning disability.

Examples of how different problems tend to present at different ages are shown in Fig. 25.7.

Telling parents about a disability

Diagnosis of a disability may be sudden and unexpected, or the culmination of protracted concern and investigation. In any event, the news is likely to provoke reactions of grief accompanied by anger, guilt, despair, or denial. The initial interview requires sensitive handling (see Hints & Tips).

Assessment

It is necessary to assess what a child is able to do and what the main difficulties are in several areas:

- Hearing, language, and communication.
- Vision and coordination.
- Physical health and mobility.
- Behaviour and emotions.
- Social interactions and self-care including continence.
- Learning disabilities.

Medical problems commonly encountered in children with disabilities are shown in Fig. 25.8.

Management—the multidisciplinary team

Management of a severe or complex disability requires a multidisciplinary clinical team working in concert with the social services, local education authorities, and voluntary agencies. The balance changes with age:

- Preschool children: community-led child development team, voluntary agencies.

Presentation of disabilities by age	
Age	**Disability**
neonatal period	chromosomal abnormality or syndrome, e.g. Down syndrome hypoxic–ischaemic encephalopathy
infancy	cerebral palsy severe visual or hearing impairment
preschool	speech and language delay abnormal gait global delay loss of skills from neurodegenerative disorder
school age	learning difficulties—specific or general

Fig. 25.7 Presentation of disabilities by age.

- School-age children: education authorities, community health services.
- School-leavers/young adults: Social Services, community disability teams.

Members of the child development team will usually include:

- Paediatricians.
- Physiotherapists.
- Occupational therapists.
- Speech and language therapists.
- Psychologists.
- Social workers.
- Nurses and health visitors.

Medical problems in children with neurodisability	
System	**Problem**
nervous system	vision and hearing impairment epilepsy behavioural disorders
skeleton	postural deformities, e.g. scoliosis
gastrointestinal trait	feeding difficulties gastro-oesophageal reflux constipation or faecal incontinence
respiratory system	recurrent aspiration pneumonia
genitourinary tract	renal failure urinary incontinence

Fig. 25.8 Medical problems in children with neurodisability.

Statementing

Education authorities have a duty to identify children with special needs and provide appropriate resources. A detailed assessment is undertaken with reports from the educational psychologist, members of the multidisciplinary team, and the parents. The resulting 'statement' sets out the child's educational and non-educational needs and the provision of services required to meet those needs. Regular reviews of the statement are also undertaken.

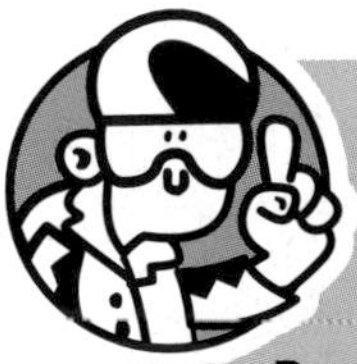

Breaking news to parents about a disability:

- **Parents should be told as soon as possible.**
- **Parents should be told together rather than separately.**
- **Tell them in a quiet place with a colleague, e.g. a nurse.**
- **An honest and direct approach is required.**
- **A period of privacy should be arranged after the initial interview.**
- **A second meeting is required to allow questions after the news has been assimilated.**

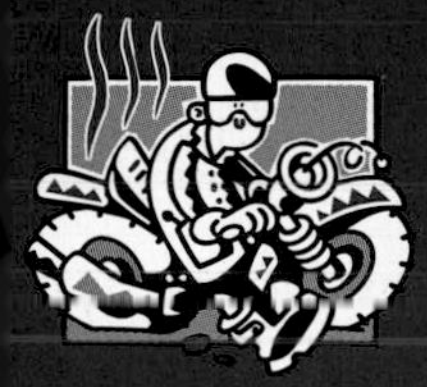

26. Genetic Disorders

Disorders with a genetic basis often manifest at birth or during the childhood years and are responsible for a major burden of both mortality and morbidity. They can be broadly divided into:

- Single gene disorders.
- Multifactorial disorders.
- Chromosomal disorders.

Clinical manifestations are of course highly variable, but it is worth remembering that many dysmorphic syndromes have a genetic basis (see Hints & Tips).

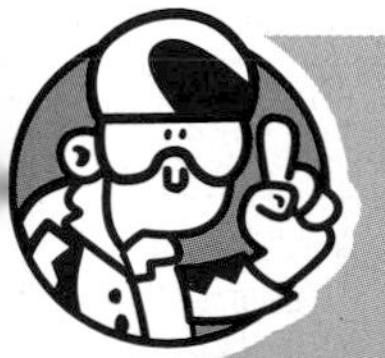

Dysmorphism and syndromes:

- **Dysmorphism is an abnormality in form or structural development, often manifested in the facial appearance and often due to an underlying genetic disorder.**
- **A syndrome is a recognizable pattern of structural and functional abnormalities or malformations known or presumed to be the result of a single cause. Dysmorphism is often a feature.**
- **Syndromes may be of unknown cause, due to teratogens, (e.g. foetal alcohol syndrome), chromosomal anomalies (e.g. Turner syndrome), or single gene disorders (e.g. Marfan syndrome).**

The revolution taking place in our understanding of genetic disease at a molecular level has led to rapid advances in diagnostic techniques and may lead to new approaches to prevention and treatment in the future.

BASIC GENETICS

Some useful definitions are shown in Fig. 26.1. The key symbols used in drawing a family tree are shown in Fig. 26.2.

Basic genetics—some definitions

Term	Definition
karyotype	A display of the set of chromosomes extracted from a eukaryotic somatic cell arrested at metaphase
genome	The totality of the DNA contained within the diploid chromosome set of a eukaryotic species and within extra-nuclear structures such as the mitochondrial genome
gene	A sequence of DNA occupying its own place (locus) on a chromosome and containing the information necessary for biosynthesis of a gene product such as a protein or ribosomal RNA molecule
allele	Any one of the variations of a gene or polymorphic DNA marker found in the members of a species. Numerous alleles may exist, but any individual usually possesses at most two alleles of the gene or polymorphic marker
genotype	The pair of alleles of a variable gene possessed by an individual, or the pairs of alleles of any number of variable genes possessed by an individual
phenotype	The entire physical, biochemical, and physiological makeup of an individual as determined by genotype and environment

Fig. 26.1 Basic genetics: some definitions.

SINGLE GENE DISORDERS

The human genome has about 80 000 genes that are packaged in the 46 chromosomes (22 pairs of autosomes and 1 pair of sex chromosomes) in the nucleus and in the mitochondrial genome (within the mitochondria in the cytoplasm). About 5000 diseases caused by mutations in single genes are known to exist. Disorders of single nuclear genes are recognizable because of their Mendelian pattern of inheritance, which may be:

- Autosomal dominant.
- Autosomal recessive.
- X-linked.

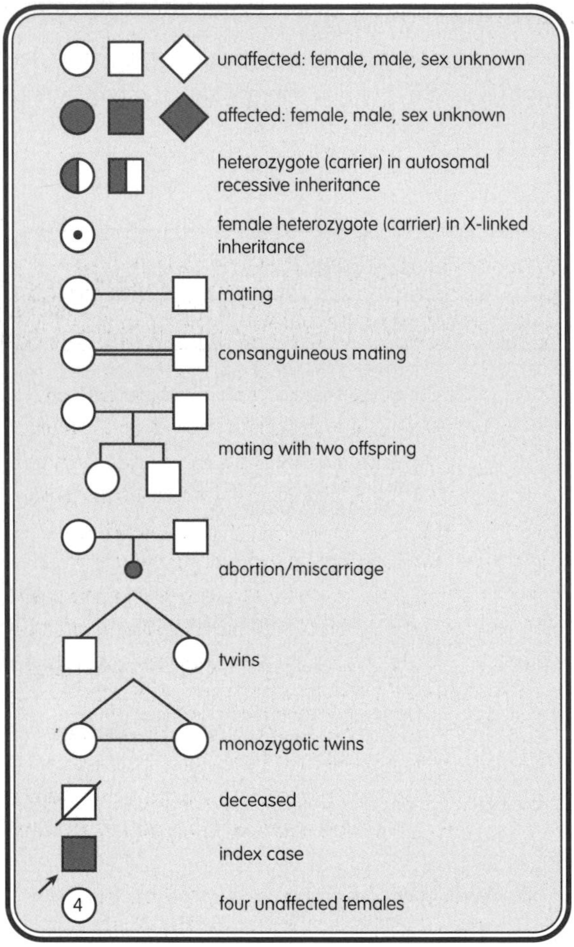

Fig. 26.2 Pedigree symbols.

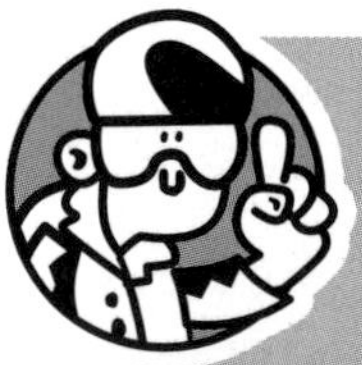

- **Autosomal dominant disorders are often caused by mutations in a gene encoding a structural protein.**
- **Autosomal recessive disorders are often caused by mutations in a gene encoding a functional protein, such as an enzyme.**

Examples of important single gene disorders are shown in Fig. 26.3.

AUTOSOMAL DOMINANT DISORDERS

An affected person has just one copy of the abnormal gene. The disease is manifested in the heterozygote. Each offspring has a 50% chance of inheriting the abnormal gene. Thus, each child of an affected individual has a 50% chance of being affected. A typical pedigree of an autosomal dominant (AD) disorder is shown in Fig. 26.4.

The features of an AD pedigree are:

- Several generations with affected individuals.

Single gene disorders: examples

Autosomal dominant (total number approximately 3000)
- myotonic dystrophy
- Marfan syndrome
- neurofibromatosis type 1
- tuberous sclerosis
- achondroplasia

Autosomal recessive (total number approximately 1500)
- cystic fibrosis
- thalassaemia
- sickle cell disease
- congenital adrenal hyperplasia
- inborn errors of metabolism (majority), e.g. phenylketonuria

X-linked recessive (total number approximately 300)
- haemophilia A and B
- Duchenne muscular dystrophy
- fragile X syndrome
- glucose-6-phosphate dehydrogenase (G6PD) deficiency
- colour blindness (red–green)

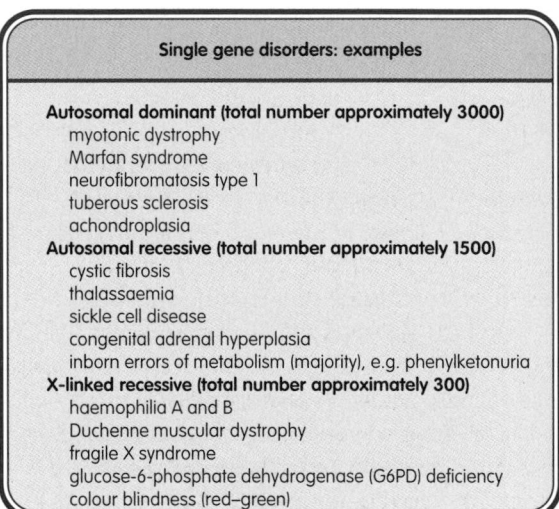

Fig. 26.3 Single gene disorders: examples.

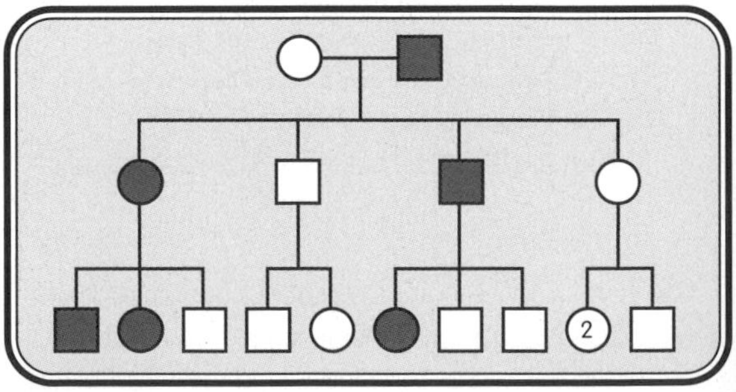

Fig. 26.4 Typical pedigree with autosomal dominant inheritance.

- Equal numbers of males and females are affected.
- Male to male transmission occurs.

Several complicating factors may occur. These include:

- Variable expression: the pattern and severity of disease varies in affected individuals within the same family.
- Non-penetrance: some individuals with the disease allele have no clinical signs or symptoms.
- Sporadic cases: a new mutation in the ovum or spermatocyte of a parent will give rise to a 'sporadic' case with no family history of the disease. The recurrence risk for new offspring from those parents is then very low.

New mutations are common in some AD disorders. For example, over 80% of individuals with achondroplasia have unaffected parents.

Marfan syndrome

This is an example of an autosomal dominant disorder that affects 1 in 10 000 newborns. It shows variable expressivity and a high new mutation rate. It is an inherited disorder of connective tissue caused by mutations in the gene encoding fibrillin located on chromosome 15. The clinical features are shown in Fig. 26.5.

The high new mutation rate and variation in severity means that up to 30% of patients do not have a parent known to be affected. If the diagnosis is suspected, further evaluation, including ophthalmological review and echocardiography to detect aortic root dilatation, is indicated. Prophylactic treatment with ß-blockers slows dilatation of the aortic root and reduces the risk of sudden death from aortic aneurysm rupture.

Major clinical features of Marfan syndrome	
skeletal	tall stature with long limbs arachnodactyly (long digits) high arched palate scoliosis
cardiac	aortic root dilatation risk of aortic aneurysm rupture
ophthalmological	lens subluxation

Fig. 26.5 Major clinical features of Marfan syndrome.

AUTOSOMAL RECESSIVE DISORDERS

An affected individual has two copies of the abnormal gene. The affected person has inherited an abnormal allele from each parent and is said to be homozygous for the disease alleles. The parents are heterozygous carriers. Many recessive disorders are caused by mutations in the genes coding for enzymes. As half of the normal enzyme activity is usually sufficient, a person with only one mutant allele will not normally be affected.

A typical pedigree of an autosomal recessive disorder is shown in Fig. 26.6.

The risk of each child being affected when both parents are carriers is 25%. Males and females are equally likely to be affected. There is usually no positive family history other than affected individuals within the sibship.

Parental consanguinity increases the risk of a recessive disease occurring in the offspring. Everyone probably carries at least one recessive disease gene allele. A couple, who are for example cousins, are more

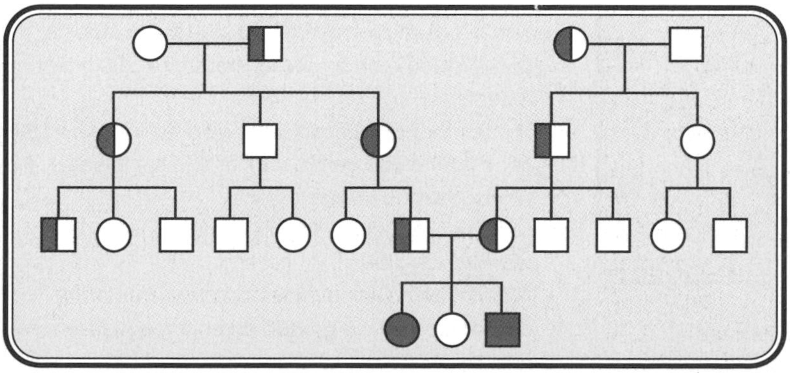

Fig. 26.6 Pedigree of an autosomal recessive disorder.

likely to have inherited the same abnormal recessive disease gene allele from their common ancestor.

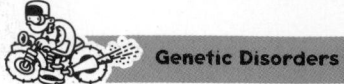

Certain recessive disorders show a founder effect. Affected individuals have inherited a founder mutation that occurred on an ancestral chromosome many generations ago. Carrier rates may be high within inbred populations (e.g. Tay–Sachs disease in Ashkenazi Jews).

Important autosomal recessive diseases are described elsewhere including cystic fibrosis (Chapter 16), thalassaemia, sickle-cell disease (Chapter 21), congenital adrenal hyperplasia (Chapter 23), and inborn errors of metabolism (Chapter 23).

X-LINKED DISORDERS

Several hundred disease genes are found on the X chromosome and give rise to the characteristic pattern of X-linked inheritance. Most X-linked disorders are recessive. In the carrier female there is a disease allele on one X chromosome, but the normal allele on her other X chromosome provides protection from the disease. The male is hemizygous for the gene because he has only a single X chromosome. The abnormal allele is not balanced by a normal allele and he manifests the disease.

A typical pedigree for X-linked recessive inheritance is shown in Fig. 26.7.

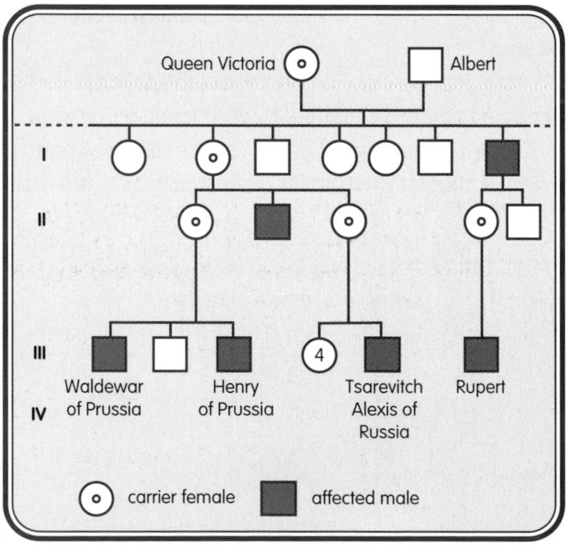

Fig. 26.7 Typical pedigree for X-linked recessive inheritance. Haemophilia in a royal family.

The characteristic features are:

- Males only are affected.
- Females are carriers and are usually healthy.
- Females may show mild signs of the disease depending on the pattern of X-chromosome inactivation (Lyon hypothesis—only one of the two X chromosomes in any cell is transcriptionally active).
- Each son of a female carrier has a 50% chance of being affected and each daughter of a female carrier has a 50% chance of being a carrier.
- Daughters of affected males are all carriers.
- Sons of affected males are never affected because a father passes his Y chromosome to his son (i.e. there is no male-to-male transmission).

New mutations are common, so there may be no family history. Several important X-linked recessive diseases including haemophilia (Chapter 21) and Duchenne muscular dystrophy (Chapter 19) are discussed elsewhere. Additional examples are fragile X syndrome and ornithine transcarbamylase deficiency.

Fragile X syndrome

After Down syndrome, this is the most common cause of severe learning impairment (mental retardation) with an incidence of 1 in 1000 men and 1 in 2000 women. It is named after a chromosomal marker, a fragile site, which can be detected on the distal end of the long arm of the X chromosome in a proportion of lymphocytes cultured in a folate-deficient medium. It is now known that this is due to expansion of a triplet repeat (CGG) in the FRAXA gene FMR1.

The clinical features of fragile X syndrome are listed in Fig. 26.8.

There are a number of unusual features accounted for in part by the triplet repeat amplification:

- The number of repeats determines status: normal individuals have less than 50 triplet repeats, carriers with a 'pre-mutation' have 50–200 triplet repeats, and affected men or women have over 200 triplet repeats.
- The number of repeats becomes amplified when the gene is inherited from a mother, but not usually when inherited from a father.
- One third of obligate female carriers have mild learning difficulties.
- 'Normal transmitting males' occur who pass the disorder on to their grandchildren through their daughters.

Clinical features of fragile X syndrome

- more common in males
- learning difficulty (IQ 20–80, mean 50)
- autistic features and hyperactivity
- physical features:
  - dysmorphic facial appearance, i.e. large forehead, long face, large prominent ears
  - macrocephaly
  - macro-orchidism—more common after puberty

Fig. 26.8 Clinical features of fragile X syndrome.

Cytogenetic analysis or direct DNA analysis confirms the diagnosis.

Ornithine transcarbamylase deficiency

This is an X-linked recessive disorder, due to mutations in the gene for a urea cycle enzyme which causes hyperammonaemia. Males are most severely affected and usually present with an overwhelming and sometimes fatal illness a few days after birth when protein-containing feeds are given.

Up to 30% of female carriers manifest symptoms, depending on the pattern of lyonization in hepatic cells (the enzyme is expressed in the liver). They may present with learning difficulties or headache and vomiting after high-protein meals.

MULTIFACTORIAL DISORDERS

These conditions are believed to be caused by a combination of genetic susceptibility, due to the interaction of several genes (polygenic), and environmental (non-genetic) factors. Multifactorial inheritance accounts for several common birth defects as well as a number of other important diseases with onset in childhood or adult life (Fig. 26.9).

A feature of the familial clustering of multifactorial diseases is that the recurrence risk is low, often in the range 3–5% (most significant for first degree relatives and decreases rapidly with more distant relatedness). Factors that increase the risk to relatives include:

- Severely affected proband (e.g. greater in bilateral cleft lip and palate than unilateral cleft lip).
- Multiple affected family members.
- The affected proband is of the less often affected sex (if there is a difference in the M:F ratio of affected individuals).

In many multifactorial disorders, the environmental factors remain obscure.

CHROMOSOMAL DISORDERS

Each human normally has 22 pairs of autosomes and 1 pair of sex chromosomes. An alteration in the amount or nature of the chromosomal material is seen in 5 in 1000 live births and is usually associated with multiple congenital anomalies and learning difficulties. A high proportion (40%) of all spontaneous abortions are caused by chromosome abnormalities.

Most chromosome defects arise *de novo*. They are classified as abnormalities of number or structure, and may involve either the autosomes or the sex chromosomes. Examples of important chromosomal disorders are shown in Fig. 26.10.

The indications for chromosome analysis are shown in Fig. 26.11. Chromosome studies are carried out on dividing cells. Most commonly, T cells from peripheral blood are used after stimulation of mitosis with phytohaemagglutinin.

Numerical autosomal abnormalities

Three autosomal trisomies are found in live born infants; others are not compatible with life and are found only in spontaneously aborted fetuses. These are:

- Down syndrome: trisomy 21 (1:700 live births).
- Edwards syndrome: trisomy 18 (1:8000 live births).
- Patau syndrome: trisomy 13 (1:15 000 live births).

Trisomy refers to the fact that three, rather than the normal two copies of a specific chromosome are

Conditions with multifactorial inheritance

Congenital malformations
- neural tube defects
- orofacial clefts (lip and palate)
- pyloric stenosis
- talipes

Common diseases
- asthma
- insulin-dependent diabetes mellitus (IDDM)
- epilepsy
- hypertension
- atherosclerosis
- psychiatric disorders, e.g. autism

Fig. 26.9 Conditions with multifactorial inheritance.

Chromosomal disorders			
Type	**Class**	**Name**	**Defect**
numerical	autosomal	Down syndrome	Trisomy 21
		Edwards syndrome	Trisomy 18
		Patau syndrome	Trisomy 13
	sex chromosomes	Klinefelter syndrome	47, XXY
		Turner syndrome	45, XO
structural	deletions	Prader–Willi syndrome	15q deletion
		Cri-du-chat syndrome	5p deletion
		Wilms tumour with aniridia	11p deletion

Fig. 26.10 Chromosomal disorders.

Indications for chromosome analysis

- phenotype consistent with known chromosomal disorder
- multiple congenital abnormalities
- dysmorphic features
- recurrent pregnancy losses
- spontaneously aborted or stillborn fetuses
- bone marrow in leukaemia, solid tumours

Fig. 26.11 Indications for chromosome analysis.

present in the cells of an individual. Trisomies occur because of a meiotic error called non-disjunction in the gamete of mother or father.

Down syndrome

Trisomy 21 is the most common autosomal trisomy compatible with life. The extra chromosomal material may result from non-disjunction, translocation, or mosaicism.

Non-disjunction

Ninety-five per cent of children with Down syndrome have trisomy 21 due to non-disjunction. The pair of chromosomes 21 fails to separate at meiosis, so one gamete has two copies of chromosome 21. Fertilization of this gamete gives rise to a zygote with trisomy 21.

Ninety per cent of non-disjunctions are maternally derived and the risk rises with maternal age, increasing steeply in mothers over 35 years (Fig. 26.12).

However, because a higher proportion of pregnancies occur in younger women, most children with trisomy 21 are born to women under 35 years of age. The recurrence risk for parents of children with trisomy 21 increases to 1–2% (unless the age-related risk is higher).

Translocation

Four per cent of Down syndrome children have 46 chromosomes with a translocation of the third number 21 chromosome to another chromosome (most commonly 14). Three-quarters of cases are *de novo* and in one-quarter, one of the parents has a balanced translocation involving one chromosome 21. If the mother is the translocation carrier, the recurrence risk may be as high as 15%. If the father is the carrier, the risk is 2.5%.

Mosaicism

In 1% of cases the non-disjunction occurs during mitosis after formation of the zygote so that some cells are normal and some show trisomy 21. The phenotype may be milder in mosaicism.

Clinical features

Down syndrome is often suspected at birth because of the characteristic facial appearance but the diagnosis may be difficult on clinical features alone. A senior paediatrician should confirm clinical suspicion. Chromosome analysis takes several days. The phenotypic features are listed in Fig. 26.13.

Risk of Down syndrome (for live births) by maternal age at deliver

Maternal age (years)	Risk
All ages	1:700
30	1:900
35	1:380
40	1:110
44	1:37

Fig. 26.12 Risk of Down syndrome (for live births) by maternal age at delivery.

Clinical features of Down syndrome	
dysmorphic facial features	round face epicanthic folds, flat nasal bridge protruding tongue small ears brushfield spots on iris
other dysmorphic features	single palmar creases flat occiput incurved little fingers gap between first and second toes (sandal toe gap) small stature
structural defects	cardiac defects in 50% duodenal atresia
neurological features	hypotonia developmental delay mean IQ = 50
late medical complications	increased risk of leukaemia respiratory infections hypothyroidism Alzheimer's disease atlantoaxial instability

Fig. 26.13 Clinical features of Down syndrome.

Management and prognosis

Parents need information about the implications of the diagnosis and the assistance available from professionals and self help groups. Feelings of disappointment, anger,and guilt are common. Genetic counselling for recurrence risks will be required. Life expectancy in Down syndrome has increased and issues relating to employment and living situations in adulthood may need to be addressed.

Sex chromosome disorders

Turner syndrome

In this condition, there is only one normal X chromosome. It affects 1 in 2500 live born females. Various underlying chromosomal defects are seen:

- In 55% of girls, the karyotype is 45, XO.
- In 25%, there is a deletion of the short arm of one X chromosome, or a so-called isochromosome with duplication of one arm and loss of the other.
- In 15%, there is mosaicism due to postzygotic mitotic non-disjunction. (45XO/46XY).

The incidence does not increase with maternal age, and the recurrence risk is the same as the general population risk.

Clinical features and diagnosis

The clinical features are shown in Fig. 26.14. Diagnosis may be made:

- Prenatally by ultrasound scan.
- At birth by presence of puffy hands and feet (lymphoedema).
- During childhood because of short stature.
- In adolescence because of primary amenorrhoea and lack of pubertal development.

Diagnosis is confirmed by a peripheral blood karyotype.

Management

Therapy with growth hormone improves final height. Ovarian hormones are not produced due to the gonadal dysgenesis (streak ovaries). Oestrogen therapy is given at the appropriate age (11 years) to produce maturation of secondary sexual characteristics including breast development. Towards the end of puberty, progestogen is added to maintain uterine health and allow monthly withdrawal bleeds (periods). Although pregnancy can occur naturally, most patients are infertile. Pregnancy can be achieved with *in vitro* fertilization.

The hallmarks of Turner syndrome are short stature and primary amenorrhoea. Intelligence is normal but there may be specific learning difficulties.

Clinical features of Turner syndrome
Dysmorphic features lymphoedema of hands and feet (at birth) neck webbing widely spaced nipples wide carrying angle (cubitus valgus) short stature **Structural and functional abnormalities** gonadal dysgenesis congenital heart disease, particularly coarctation of the aorta renal anomalies

Fig. 26.14 Clinical features of Turner syndrome.

Structural chromosomal abnormalities

These arise from chromosome breakage and include deletions, duplications, inversions, and unbalanced translocations. Deletions are the most common. Most arise *de novo*, but they may arise from inheritance of an unbalanced translocation. Examples of conditions associated with chromosomal deletions include:

- Cri-du-chat syndrome: caused by deletion of short arm of chromosome 5 (5p-). Affected children have profound mental retardation and a cat-like cry.
- Prader–Willi syndrome: caused by deletions of the paternal copy of 15q11-13 (see Hints & Tips).
- Angelman syndrome: caused by deletions of the maternal copy of 15q11-13 (see Hints & Tips).

Imprinting:

- **Some genes are 'imprinted'. The copy derived from one parent (either male or female) is active and the other is not.**
- **Deletions of chromosomal regions, which are 'imprinted' have different effects according to the parent of origin of the deleted chromosome.**
- **The most well-known example is deletion of 15q11-13. Paternal chromosome deletion causes Prader–Willi syndrome (obesity, learning difficulties). Maternal chromosome deletion causes Angelman syndrome (happy puppet syndrome: ataxia, learning difficulties, 'happy' disposition).**

GENETIC COUNSELLING

This is usually carried out as a specialist service by trained medical staff and specialist nurses. The main aim is to provide information about hereditary disorders so that parents will have greater autonomy and choice in reproductive decisions (see Hints & Tips).

The basic elements of counselling include:

- Establishing a diagnosis: this may involve physical examination of proband and family members and special investigations including DNA, cytogenetic, and biochemical analysis.
- Estimation of risk: the risk for future offspring is determined by the mode of inheritance of the disease.
- Communication: information must be conveyed in an unbiased and non-directive way,and all the possible options discussed (see Hints & Tips).

Information base in genetic counselling:

- **Magnitude of risk.**
- **Severity of disorder.**
- **Availability of treatment.**
- **Parental cultural and ethical values.**

Options in antenatal genetic counselling:

- **Not having offspring.**
- **Ignoring the risk.**
- **Antenatal diagnosis and termination of pregnancy.**
- **Pre-implantation diagnosis.**
- **Artificial insemination by donor or ovum donation.**

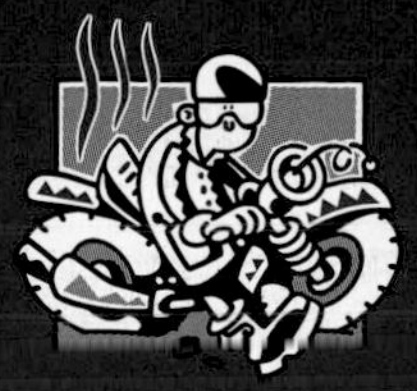

27. The Newborn

Fetal and neonatal life are best regarded as a continuum and the term 'perinatal' medicine is sometimes used to encompass the care of the pregnant mother and fetus as well as the newborn infant. Many factors from before conception to delivery influence the health of the newborn infant.

Introduction—perinatal statistics and definitions

Terms used in perinatal statistics are defined in Fig. 27.1.

Nearly half of all neonatal deaths occur in the first 24 hours. The perinatal mortality rate in developed countries has fallen steadily over the last 20 years and may be approaching an irreducible lower limit set by deaths from lethal malformations. However, disadvantaged people continue to have the highest rates of perinatal deaths and congenital malformations.

Definitions for perinatal statistics

Term	Definition
still birth	a fetus born after 24 weeks of gestation who shows no signs of life after delivery
low birth weight	a baby weighing 2500 g or less at birth
preterm	a baby born at any time before 37 weeks' gestation
term	a baby born between 37 and 42 completed weeks' gestation
post-term	a baby born after 42 weeks' gestation
neonatal period	first month of life
perinatal mortality rate	still births and deaths within the first 6 days per 1000 live and still births (i.e. total births)
neonatal mortality rate	deaths of liveborn infants during the first 28 days of age per 1000 live births

Fig. 27.1 Definitions for perinatal statistics.

MATERNAL AND FETAL HEALTH

Mother and fetus are a single physiological unit and any serious maternal disease or condition can affect the fetus. Action to optimize the chances of a healthy baby can begin even before conception. The chance of a good outcome can be enhanced by:

- Avoiding smoking, excess alcohol, and medication.
- Avoiding infections: rubella immunization before pregnancy, avoiding exposure to toxoplasmosis (via cat's litter), and avoiding exposure to listeriosis (unpasteurized dairy products).
- Folic acid supplements reduce the risk of neural tube defects.
- Optimizing treatment of maternal conditions such as hypertension and diabetes mellitus.
- Genetic counselling for couples at risk of inherited diseases.

Fetal assessment and antenatal diagnosis

Methods for assessing the growth, maturation, and wellbeing of the fetus are available. They include:

- Ultrasound: for assessing age and growth.
- Doppler blood flow studies.

Antenatal diagnosis is now available for many disorders using the methods shown in Fig. 27.2.

Antenatal diagnosis may allow the option of termination to be offered in certain disorders, therapy to be given, or neonatal management to be planned in advance. Medical treatment may be given to the fetus via the mother or directly (e.g. fetal blood transfusion for anaemia in severe rhesus isoimmunization).

Maternal conditions affecting the fetus

The fetus may be affected by:

- Maternal diseases: diabetes mellitus, thyrotoxicosis, and auto-immune disorders (e.g. systemic lupus erythematosus, myasthenia gravis, and thrombocytopenia).
- Maternal drugs, e.g. medications, alcohol and, narcotics.
- Maternal infections: congenital infections.

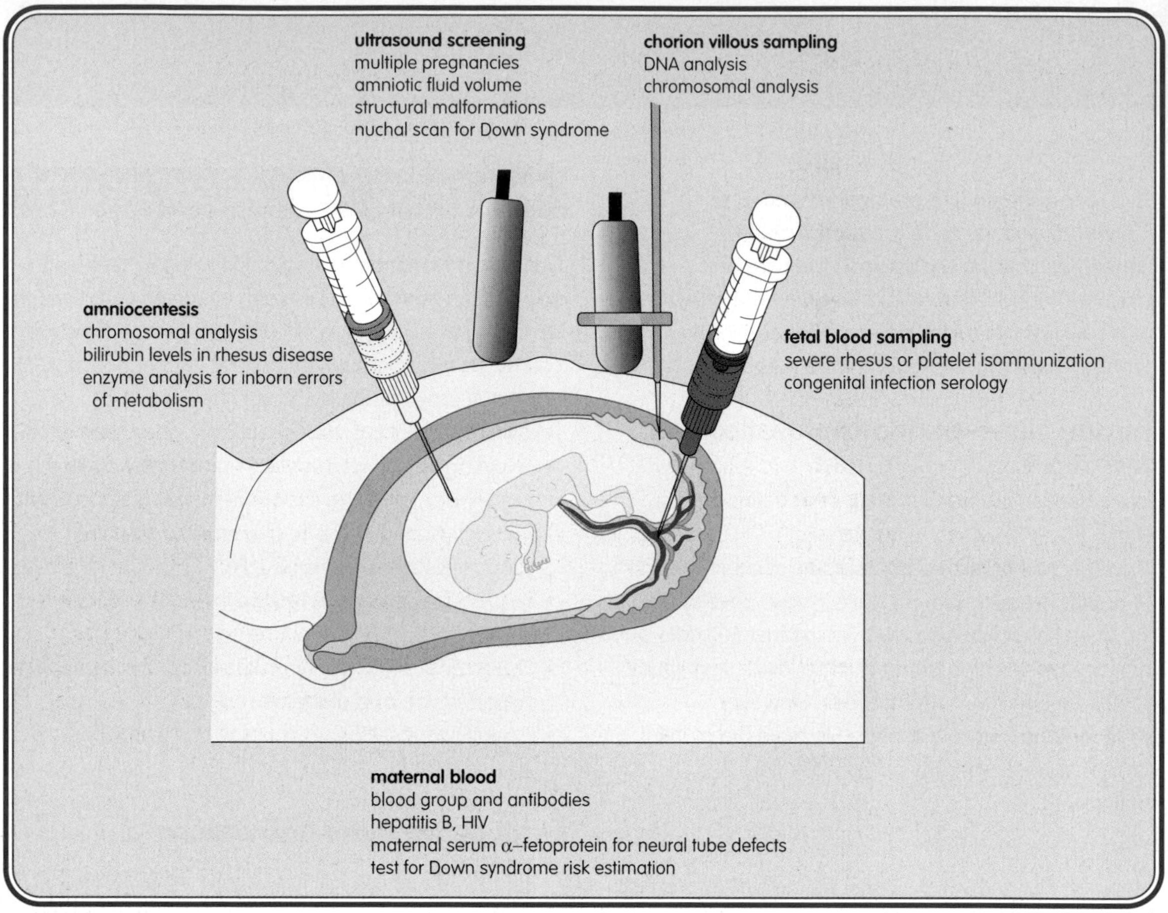

Fig. 27.2 Antenatal diagnosis: various methods and the disorders they are used to diagnose.

Maternal diseases

Diabetes mellitus

The outlook for the infant of a mother with insulin-dependent diabetes mellitus has improved greatly and is enhanced by good diabetic control during the pregnancy.

Potential fetal problems include:

- Congenital malformations: there is a three-fold increase (there is a particular increased incidence of cardiac malformations).
- Macrosomia: the fetal insulin response to hyperglycaemia promotes excessive growth, which predisposes to difficulties during delivery.

Potential neonatal problems include:

- Hypoglycaemia: transient early hypoglycaemia occurs due to fetal hyperinsulinism; early feeding can usually prevent this.
- Respiratory distress syndrome (RDS).
- Polycythaemia (haematocrit >0.65).

Maternal drugs affecting the fetus

Drugs taken by the mother may cause congenital malformations (Fig. 27.3), adverse effects by their pharmacological action on the fetus or placenta, or transient problems at birth.

Maternal infections and the fetus

A number of infections acquired by the mother may affect the fetus or newborn (Fig. 27.4). Transmission may occur *in utero*, during labour, or postpartum (Fig. 27.5).

Rubella

For rubella, see Chapter 13.

Maternal drugs and the fetus:

- **Teratogenic drugs taken during organogenesis can cause spontaneous abortions or congenital malformations.**
- **Drugs given during labour can have adverse effects, e.g. analgesics and anaesthesia (suppression of spontaneous breathing at birth), sedatives (sedation, hypotension). IV fluids: excess hypotonic fluids may cause hyponatraemia.**

Maternal medication that may harm the fetus	
Drug	**Adverse effects**
cytotoxic agents	congenital malformations
phenytoin	fetal hydantoin syndrome (growth retardation, microcephaly, hypoplastic nails)
sodium valproate	neural tube defects
carbamazepine	growth retardation, craniofacial abnormalities
warfarin	interferes with cartilage formation, risk of cerebral haemorrhage, and microcephaly
progestogens (androgenic)	masculinization of fetus
diethylstilboestrol	adenocarcinoma of vagina
thalidomide	limb shortening (phocomelia)
Drug abuse	
alcohol	fetal alcohol syndrome (characteristic facies, septal defects, mental retardation)
opiates (heroin/methadone)	growth retardation, prematurity, drug withdrawal in neonate (tremors, hyperirritability, seizures)
cocaine	spontaneous abortion, prematurity, cerebral infarction

Fig. 27.3 Maternal medication that may harm the fetus.

Varicella zoster

More than 85% of women of childbearing age have evidence of past infection with chickenpox, so a minority of pregnant women are at risk.

Infection in the first trimester does not usually cause fetal damage, but about 5% may develop the so-called 'congenital varicella syndrome' characterized by:

- Cicatricial skin lesions (scars).
- Malformed digits.
- Cataracts.
- CNS damage, chorioretinitis.

The principal problem is infection acquired late in pregnancy, particularly within 5 days before or 2 days after delivery. The fetus receives a high viral load, but little in the way of maternal antibodies. Severe infection can ensue with a mortality of up to 5%.

Exposed susceptible women can be treated with varicella zoster immune globulin (VZIG) and aciclovir. Infants exposed in the high-risk period should also be treated with VZIG. Intravenous aciclovir should be used if lesions develop in the newborn infant.

Cytomegalovirus

For cytomegalovirus, see Chapter 13.

Maternal infections transmitted to the fetus *in utero*
toxoplasmosis
rubella
cytomegalovirus
varicella zoster
HIV
Treponema pallidum (syphillis)
Listeria monocytogenes

Fig. 27.4 Maternal infections transmitted to the fetus in utero.

Infections acquired during delivery
Group B haemolytic streptococci
E. coli
HIV
hepatitis B
herpes simplex
gonococci
Chlamydia trachomatis
echoviruses

Fig. 27.5 Infections acquired during delivery.

Human immunodeficiency virus (HIV)

Vertical transmission from mother to infant may occur *in utero*, during birth, or postnatally by breastfeeding. The exact risk of infection by each of these routes is uncertain, but overall vertical transmission rates vary between 15 and 35% (see Chapter 13).

Use of zidovudine given to the mother during pregnancy and delivery, and to the neonate for the first 6 weeks of life, reduces the transmission risk.

Toxoplasmosis

Infection with the protozoan parasite *Toxoplasma gondis* occurs from the ingestion of raw or undercooked meat, or from oocytes excreted in the faeces of infected cats. Most infections are asymptomatic. Serological epidemiological studies show that in some countries (e.g. France and Austria), 80% of women of childbearing age are immune, whereas in the UK only 20% have antibodies.

About 40% of women who acquire an acute infection during pregnancy transmit the infection to the fetus. The risk of severe damage is highest following infection in the first trimester. About 10% of infected infants have clinical manifestations at birth, which may include:

- Hydrocephalus.
- Intracranial calcification.
- Chorioretinitis.
- Neurological damage.

Infants with asymptomatic infection may still develop chorioretinitis in later life.

In some countries, serological screening for infection is carried out during pregnancy. If positive (and fetal infection is confirmed by cordocentesis), termination or treatment with spiramycin can be offered. The efficacy of the latter remains uncertain. An infected newborn infant is treated with alternating courses of pyrimethamine with sulphadiazine and spiramycin until the age of 1 year.

- **Diagnosis of HIV during infancy is rendered difficult by the passage of maternal antibody which may persist for up to 18 months.**
- **Breastfeeding may increase the risk of vertical transmission by 15%.**

THE NORMAL NEWBORN—ANATOMY AND PHYSIOLOGY

There are characteristic features of newborn anatomy and physiology that are important and these are considered in turn.

Size and growth

The average term infant in the UK weighs about 3500 g. Boys weigh approximately 250 g more than girls. Infants of 2500 g or less are classified as 'low birthweight'. This important category is considered separately.

During the first 3–5 days, up to 10% of birthweight is lost. This is regained by 7–10 days. In the first month, average weight gain per week is 200 g.

Skin

The newborn skin is immature with a thin epithelial layer and incompletely developed sweat and sebaceous glands. Combined with the high surface area to body mass ratio, this renders the baby prone to heat and water losses.

Numerous benign skin lesions occur (see Chapter 10). The skin is covered with a greasy protective layer, the vernix caseosa.

Head

The average occipitofrontal head circumference is 35 cm. Significant moulding of the head may occur during birth. Two soft spots or fontanelles are present. The anterior fontanelle closes between 9 and 18 months of age and the posterior closes by 6–8 weeks.

Respiratory system

Changes occur at birth that allow the newborn to convert from dependence on the placenta to breathing air for the exchange of respiratory gases:

- *In utero*, the airways and lungs are filled with fluid that contains surfactant.
- The lung fluid is removed by the squeezing of the thorax during vaginal delivery and by reduced secretion and increased absorption mediated by fetal catecholamines during labour and after birth.

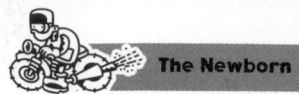

- Surfactant lines the air–fluid interface of the alveoli and reduces the surface tension thereby facilitating lung expansion. This is associated with a fall in pulmonary vascular resistance.

Newborn infants breathe mainly with the diaphragm. The rate is variable and normally ranges between 30–50 breaths per minute. Brief (up to several seconds) self-limiting apnoeic spells may occur during sleep. Small babies are obligate nose-breathers.

Cardiovascular system

Major changes in the lungs and circulation allow adaptation to extrauterine life.

In the fetal circulation, the right-sided (pulmonary) pressure exceeds the left-sided (systemic) pressure. Blood flows from right to left through the foramen ovale and ductus arteriosus (Fig. 27.6).

At birth, these relationships reverse:

- Left-sided (systemic) pressure rises with clamping of umbilical vessels.
- Right-sided (pulmonary) pressure falls as the lungs expand and the rising PO_2 triggers a prostaglandin-mediated vasodilatation.
- The foramen ovale and ductus arteriosus close functionally shortly after birth. The ductus closes due to muscular contraction in response to rising oxygen tension.

Gastrointestinal system

Most infants over 35 weeks gestation have developed the coordination necessary to 'latch on' and feed from breast or bottle. At term, the secretory and absorbing surfaces are well-developed, as are digestive enzymes with the exception of pancreatic amylase.

Meconium is usually passed within 6 hours and delay beyond 24 hours is considered abnormal.

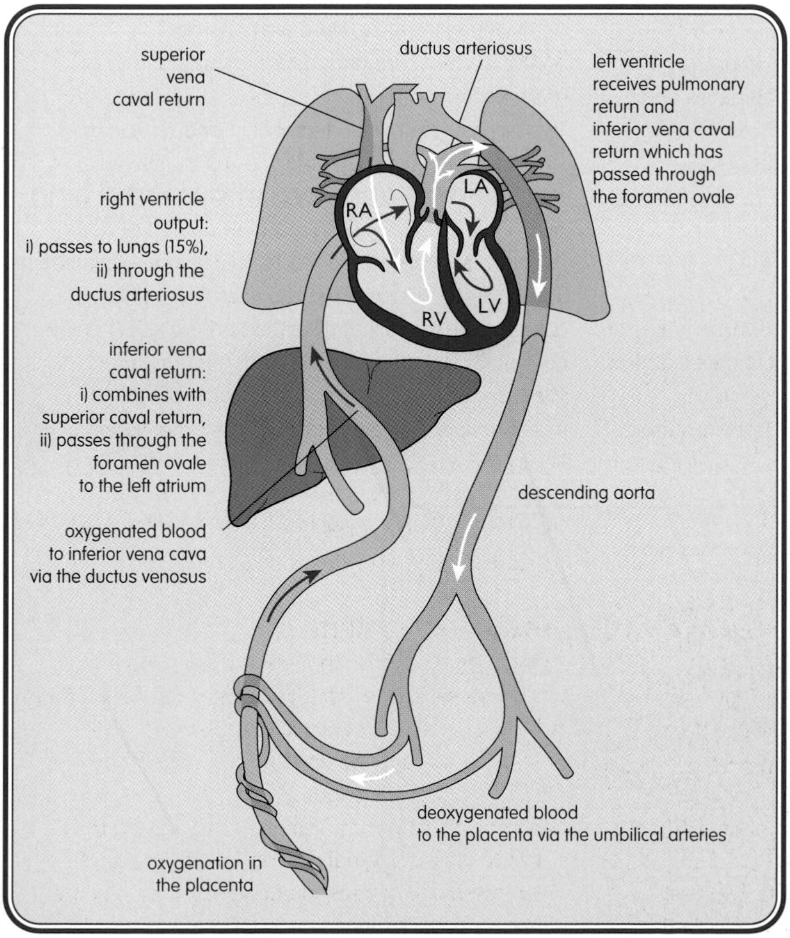

Fig. 27.6 Fetal circulation.

With normal feeding, 'changing stools' replace meconium on day 3 or 4, and thereafter the yellowish stools of the milk-fed infant develop.

Immaturity of the liver enzymes responsible for conjugation of bilirubin is responsible for the 'physiological jaundice' which may occur from the second day of life.

Genitourinary system

Urine production is occurring during the second half of gestation and accounts for much of the amniotic fluid. The infant may micturate during delivery (unnoticed) and should void within the first 12 hours of life.

Haematopoietic and immune system

The newborn's red cells contain fetal haemoglobin (HbF) which transports O_2 at lower pressures than adult haemoglobin (HbA). The haemoglobin concentration of cord blood ranges from 15–20 g/dl (mean 17 g/dl). The volume of the placental transfusion received before the cord is cut influences this value.

The neonatal immune system is also immature. Cellular immune responses such as chemotaxis and phagocytosis are reduced. The humoral response is limited and the infant depends on maternal IgG antibodies that have crossed the placenta. IgA is found in breast milk.

Central nervous system

The central nervous system (CNS) is relatively immature at birth. Myelination is incomplete and continues during the first 2 years of life.

A limited behavioural response repertoire is sufficient for survival, comprising a sleep and wake cycle, sucking and swallowing, and crying:

- Newborn infants sleep for a total of 16–20 hours each day.
- The touch of a nipple on the baby's face initiates the sequence of rooting, latching on, and the complex coordination of lip, tongue, palate, and pharynx required for sucking and swallowing.
- Crying (without tears) is the main means of communication. Usually this is in response to hunger, thirst, or pain, but some newborns cry without obvious reason and are difficult to pacify.

BIRTH

The short journey down the birth canal from the intrauterine environment to the external world is potentially hazardous. Various risk factors can be identified during labour; the most important of which is prematurity. The problems of the preterm infant are dealt with separately. Here we consider:

- The normal care and resuscitation of the term newborn.
- The problems of birth asphyxia and birth injuries.

Assessment and care at a normal birth

The infant is usually delivered after a short period of oxygen deprivation and begins to breathe within a few seconds. The Apgar score is a useful quantitative assessment of the infant's condition (Fig. 27.7) and is commonly determined at 1 and 5 minutes after birth. The Apgar score is influenced by several factors including intrapartum asphyxia, maternal sedation or

Apgar score evaluation of the newborn			
Criteria	**Score**		
	0	**1**	**2**
heart rate	absent	<100 beats/min	>100 beats/min
respiratory effort	absent/weak	irregular/gasping	regular
muscle tone	limp	some flexion	active movements
reflex response to stimulation	none	weak	cries
colour	blue or pale	extremities blue	pink

Fig. 27.7 Apgar score evaluation of the newborn.

analgesia, the gestational age, and any cardiac, pulmonary, or neurological disease in the infant.

Birth asphyxia

This refers to a condition in which the fetus is acutely deprived of oxygen and is commonly due to uteroplacental insufficiency. The incidence has fallen to 1.5–6 per 1000 live births but it remains an important cause of brain damage in newborn babies.

Asphyxia (which literally means 'absent pulse' and was a term for 'suffocation') is manifested during labour by various fetal responses (previously termed 'fetal distress'). There is fetal hypoxia, hypercapnia, and acidosis, which may be detected by:

- Abnormalities in fetal heart rate: there may be fetal bradycardia (rate under 120 beats/minute), fetal tachycardia (rate over 160 beats/minute) or an abnormal pattern of deceleration during or after uterine contractions.
- Acidosis: sampling of fetal blood from scalp or cord will demonstrate significant acidosis (pH <7.20).
- Meconium staining of the liquor: the asphyxiated infant passes meconium.

These signs are an indication for prompt delivery of the fetus.

Intrapartum asphyxia is associated with decreased oxygen supply to tissues of many organs, but the principal effect is on the brain (Fig. 27.8).

The postnatal symptoms and signs of intrapartum asphyxia vary with the degree of asphyxia, which may be classified as mild, moderate, or severe. 'hypoxic–ischaemic encephalopathy' is the term used to describe the neurological manifestations.

Complications of perinatal asphyxia (severe)

Organ	Complication
brain	hypoxic–ischaemic encephalopathy
heart	hypoxic cardiomyopathy, hypotension
lungs	persistent pulmonary hypotension
guts	ileus and necrotizing enterocolitis
kidneys	acute tubular necrosis
blood	disseminated intravascular coagulation

Fig. 27.8 Complications of perinatal asphyxia (severe).

Hypoxic–ischaemic encephalopathy

The manifestations of the effects of asphyxia on the brain vary with its severity:

- Mild: initial lethargy followed by a period of hyperalertness with irritability, staring of the eyes, and impaired feeding for 1–2 days. There are no focal signs. Prognosis is good.
- Moderate: as above with generalized seizures occurring 12–24 hours after the episode of asphyxia and resolving within a few days. Depressed conscious level. Variable prognosis.
- Severe: coma and intractable seizures worsening over 1–3 days as delayed or 'secondary' injury develops. Multiorgan failure is often present. Death is common and survival associated with poor long-term outcome.

The asphyxiated infant needs active resuscitation (Fig. 27.9). Further management may involve:

- Ventilatory support.
- Anticonvulsants for seizures.
- Fluid restriction if inappropriate antidiuretic hormone secretion develops.
- Circulatory support with inotropes.

Brain imaging and EEG may assist in predicting the outcome. Cystic lesions or cerebral atrophy will appear in the ensuing weeks.

Birth injury

Physical injury during labour and delivery is now relatively uncommon, partly because the availability of caesarean section obviates the need for heroic attempts at vaginal delivery. Predisposing factors include:

- Breech presentation.
- Cephalopelvic disproportion.
- Assisted delivery: manual or instrumental (forceps or ventouse extraction). Injuries may occur to soft tissues, nerves, or bones.

DISEASES OF THE NEWBORN

Much of neonatal care is directed towards the problems of low birthweight infants, especially those born prematurely, many of whom require intensive care. It is therefore useful to consider the disorders of low birthweight and term infants separately although there is of course significant overlap.

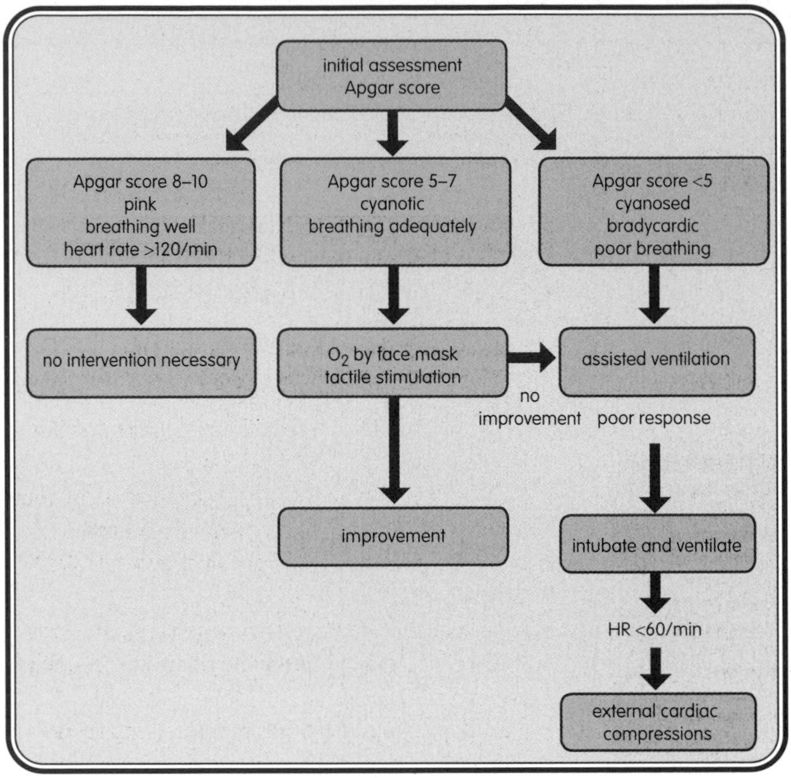

Fig. 27.9 Neonatal resuscitation.

Size and gestational age

Newborn infants may be small because they have been born preterm or because they are small in relation to their gestational age (small for dates). Some useful definitions are shown in Fig. 27.10.

Small for gestational age infants

These infants have intrauterine growth retardation (IUGR) which may be caused by:

- An intrinsic fetal problem. Poor growth is symmetrical, with head circumference proportionally reduced, e.g. chromosomal disorders, small normal fetus, and congenital infections.
- Placental insufficiency. Poor growth is asymmetrical, with brain growth relatively spared (an adaptive response), e.g. maternal pre-eclampsia, hypertension, renal disease, sickle-cell disease, and multiple pregnancy.

The fetus with IUGR is at risk from hypoxia and death and is closely monitored using cardiotocography and Doppler ultrasound to profile blood flow velocity in the uterine and umbilical arteries.

Postnatal problems encountered by the fetus with IUGR include:

- Hypothermia.
- Hypoglycaemia from low fat and glycogen stores.
- Hypocalcaemia.
- Polycythaemia (haematocrit >0.65).

Large for gestational age infants

The most common cause of macrosomia is maternal diabetes mellitus. Potential associated problems include birth asphyxia from a difficult delivery and birth trauma especially from shoulder dystocia.

The preterm infant

About 3 in every 100 babies are born prematurely (before 37 weeks gestation) and are classified as 'preterm'. Most weigh less than 2500 g and are therefore 'low birthweight' babies. These infants provide much of the work in neonatal units and account for 60% of neonatal deaths.

The major problems encountered by preterm infants are determined by the immaturity of their organ systems particularly the lungs (Fig. 27.11). The limits of

Definitions for size and gestational age	
Term	**Definition**
preterm	gestation <37 completed weeks
post-term	gestation >42 completed weeks
low birth weight	<2500 g
very low birth weight	<1500 g
extremely low birth weight	<1000 g
small for gestational age	birthweight <10th centile for gestational age
large for gestational age	birthweight >90th centile for gestational age

Fig. 27.10 Definitions for size and gestational age.

viability are currently in the region of 23–24 weeks of gestation.

Characteristics of the preterm infant

A typical infant of 28 weeks gestation would have the following features:

- Large head in relation to chest which is small and narrow.
- Shiny, smooth skin.
- Skull soft, ears floppy and lacking cartilage
- Eyes closed
- Extended posture, jerky frog-like movements.
- Weak cry.

The physiology of the major organ systems and bodily functions are immature as shown by:

- Temperature control: heat production is low (no brown fat, limited muscle activity). Heat loss is high (high surface area to volume, lack of fat insulation).
- Blood and circulation: hypotension, easy bruising and bleeding.
- Respiratory system: narrow nasal airways, soft thoracic cage, poor cough reflex, unstable respiratory drive with irregular breathing and apnoea. Alveolar collapse due to surfactant deficiency.
- Gastrointestinal tract: uncoordinated suck or swallow (before 32–34 weeks). Regurgitation common. Increased severity and incidence of 'physiological' jaundice.
- Renal function: tendency to lose sodium but unable to excrete fluid load. Oedema and hyponatraemia may occur.
- Immune system: active and passive immunity are both limited.

General care of the preterm infant

Some basic principles apply to the care of all preterm infants. These are considered separately from the

Major problems in preterm infants	
System	**Problems**
respiratory system	surfactant deficiency (hyaline membrane disease) apnoeic attacks
cardiovascular system	hypotension patent ductus arteriosus
temperature control	hypothermia
gastrointestinal tract	nutrition reflux jaundice necrotizing enterocolitis
nervous system	intracranial haemorrhage/ischaemia retinopathy of prematurity sensorineural hearing loss
immune system	infection
metabolism	hypoglycaemia osteopenia of prematurity

Fig. 27.11 Major problems in preterm infants.

specific problems that arise in different systems. Attention must be paid to:

- Prevention and predelivery care.
- Resuscitation at birth.
- Maintaining body temperature.
- Avoiding infection.
- Nutrition and fluids.
- Physiological monitoring.

Prevention and predelivery care

Preterm labour may be avoided in the presence of risk factors by bed rest and ß-mimetic drugs, e.g. ritodrine. Once labour has started it may be delayed by using the same group of drugs. This may give time for the administration of a corticosteroid to reduce the risk of respiratory distress syndrome (hyaline membrane disease).

Resuscitation at birth

Delivery should ideally take place in a location with full paediatric backup including a neonatal special care unit. At birth the baby should be handled gently, dried, and placed under a source of radiant heat.

Many preterm infants of 32 weeks gestation or less will not achieve adequate spontaneous ventilation and intermittent positive pressure ventilation or nasal continuous positive airways pressure is advisable and lessens severity of subsequent respiratory disease.

Body temperature

Preterm infants rapidly lose heat through evaporation, radiation, and convection (see Hint & Tips), and have limited heat-production mechanisms. Strategies for maintaining body temperature have to take into account the need for observation and access. They include:

- Ambient temperature: incubators provide a controlled microenvironment.
- Insulation with clothing: monitoring equipment can be attached to a clothed infant so most do not need to be kept naked. A bonnet prevents excessive loss from the relatively large head.
- Radiant heat: this is useful in the resuscitation area as access is optimized, but it causes excessive fluid loss over prolonged periods.

Avoiding infection

Meticulous attention to hand-washing before and after handling is the most important safeguard against transmitting infection. Obviously, staff with skin or bowel infections should not be at work until clear. Infected babies require barrier nursing.

Body temperature in the preterm infant:

- **Heat loss is excessive due to high surface area to volume ratio, poor insulation, and transepidermal water loss.**
- **Heat generation is limited by reduced muscular activity, lack of brown fat, and inability to shiver.**

Nutrition and fluids

Infants of 35 weeks gestation or more are usually able to take oral feeds of milk from breast or bottle without difficulty. Although preterm infants can digest and absorb enteral feeds, their sucking and swallowing reflexes may be ineffective and some or all of the feeds must be delivered through a small bore polyethylene tube passed via the nose or mouth into the stomach. The approach to giving nutrition and fluids therefore depends on the size and maturity of the individual baby.

The majority of small preterm infants (under 1500 g) require their fluid and calorie requirements intravenously during the first 24–48 hours. This is usually given as 10% dextrose. The volume required increases during the first week, but is variable.

If enteral feeds by mouth or nasogastric tube are not tolerated, more prolonged maintenance of nutrition is achieved by total parenteral nutrition. A mixture of amino acids, dextrose, lipids, and electrolytes is given intravenously via a long line, the lumen of which is placed centrally in the vena cava or right atrium.

Which milk for preterm infants?

Breast milk is not designed to meet the specific needs of the preterm infant. Early breast milk is rather variable in quality and may be too low in electrolytes and calories to be ideal. Artificial feeds have now been designed that are adapted for the nutritional needs of very low birthweight infants and appear to enhance both growth and development. They have higher calorific and electrolyte contents.

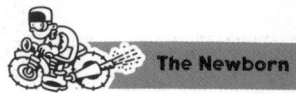

Supplements
Breastfed preterm infants need supplements of phosphate and vitamin D to ensure adequate bone mineralization. A multivitamin preparation is usually given from the third week and an iron supplement from 4–6 weeks of age onwards.

DISORDERS OF THE PRETERM INFANT

Respiratory disorders

Surfactant deficiency (hyaline membrane disease, respiratory distress syndrome)

This syndrome is caused by a deficiency of surfactant associated with immaturity of the Type II alveolar cells. Surfactant is a lipoprotein that lowers surface tension in the alveoli and prevents collapse of the alveoli during expiration. At postmortem, an exudate of proteinaceous hyaline material is seen in the alveoli and terminal bronchioles (hence, the alternative term 'hyaline membrane disease' used for this disorder).

Surfactant deficiency is uncommon in term infants but will occur in the majority born before 28 weeks' gestation. It tends to be worse in boys, and hypoxia, acidosis, or hypothermia exacerbates surfactant deficiency.

Clinical features
Respiratory distress is the major feature. This may be present from birth or develop within the first 4 hours. The signs include:

- Tachypnoea.
- Cyanosis.
- Subcostal and intercostal recession.
- Expiratory grunting.

The disease displays a spectrum of severity from mild, to severe, and life-threatening. A chest X-ray (CXR) will show a diffuse granular or 'ground glass' appearance of the lungs, and an air bronchogram outlining the larger airways.

Management
Glucocorticoids given antenatally for 48 hours stimulate fetal surfactant production, but, of course, many preterm births occur without this period of warning. Effective resuscitation, at birth, of infants at risk reduces the severity of the disease.

The mainstays of management include:

- Surfactant therapy.
- Oxygen.
- Assisted ventilation.

Exogenous surfactant therapy represents a significant advance. A suspension is instilled into the lungs via the endotracheal tube. It reduces mortality and morbidity from respiratory distress syndrome (RDS) in babies between 26 and 34 weeks gestation.

An increased concentration of inspired oxygen is required and in more severe disease this needs to be supplemented with continuous positive airways pressure via the nasal airways or intermittent positive pressure ventilation via an endotracheal tube. Ventilation is guided by monitoring of the arterial blood gas tensions (PaO_2 and $PaCO_2$). High frequency oscillatory ventilation is a new and effective approach for treating very immature infants.

Complications of RDS are shown in Fig. 27.12.

Mild to moderate RDS resolves spontaneously in a few days. Extremely preterm, very low birthweight infants, have lungs that are both anatomically immature as well as surfactant deficient. Ventilatory support may be required for weeks or months and chronic lung disease may ensue.

Apnoeic attacks

Many small, preterm infants display 'periodic respiration' with some spells of very shallow breathing or complete cessation of breathing for up to 10 seconds. This reflects immaturity of the respiratory centre.

Apnoeic attacks are more serious. Breathing stops suddenly for 20 seconds or more and there is associated bradycardia or cyanosis. Predisposing factors include:

- Respiratory distress syndrome.
- Hypoxia.
- Infection.
- Anaemia or hypoglycaemia.

The differential diagnosis includes seizures, which may mimic apnoeic attacks.

Apnoea alarms set to respond at an appropriate interval are useful for alerting staff to the need for action. Breathing will usually start again with physical stimulation. If frequent, and in the absence of an underlying cause, they may be prevented by oral theophylline or caffeine, or continuous positive airways pressure.

Complications of respiratory distress syndrome

- pneumothorax, pulmonary interstitial emphysema. Air leaks from alveoli into the pleural space or interstitium, a tension pneumothorax causes rapid deterioration and requires rapid relief by insertion of a chest drain
- patent ductus arteriosus
- intraventricular haemorrhage

Fig. 27.12 Complications of respiratory distress syndrome.

Cardiovascular problems

Patent ductus arteriosus

A patent ductus arteriosus (PDA) is a common problem in preterm infants and is often associated with RDS. Failure of closure occurs because of gestational immaturity and hypoxia.

As the pulmonary vascular resistance falls blood is shunted across the ductus from left to right. The clinical features are a widened pulse pressure with prominent peripheral pulses, tachycardia, and the classic 'machinery' murmur loudest in the second left intercostal space. A large shunt causes congestive heart failure. CXR shows an enlarged heart with pulmonary plethora.

Treatment

Fluid restriction and diuretics may be sufficient until spontaneous closure occurs. If these measures fail, a prostaglandin inhibitor, such as indomethacin, may be used to facilitate closure. (The local action of prostaglandin maintains an open ductus.) Surgical closure may occasionally be required.

Intracranial lesions

Preterm infants are at risk of:

- Intracranial haemorrhage: into the germinal matrix or ventricles.
- Ischaemia: of the periventricular white matter.

Risk factors for both include asphyxia, hypovolaemia, hypotension, and hypoxia in association with RDS.

Gastrointestinal problems

Necrotizing enterocolitis

This is a necrosis of the intestine involving usually the distal ileum or proximal colon. The aetiology is uncertain but established predisposing factors include:

- Preterm birth.
- Hypotension.
- Umbilical vessel catheters.
- Early oral feeding.

Clinical features include abdominal distension, vomiting, and bloody stools. Abdominal X-rays may show intramural gas, a pathognomonic finding. Bowel perforation may occur.

Treatment

This comprises:

- Gastric aspiration and IV fluids.
- Antibiotics—broad spectrum.
- In severe cases, surgical resection of the necrosed segment may be required.

Long-term sequelae and prognosis

Although the majority of preterm infants survive intact without sequelae, a number of significant problems may persist especially in the very low birthweight group. These include:

- Retinopathy of prematurity (retrolental fibroplasia).
- Chronic lung disease of prematurity (bronchopulmonary dysplasia).
- Neurodevelopmental problems.

Retinopathy of prematurity

This comprises a spectrum of vascular abnormalities of the retina which occur in preterm infants in response to various injurious factors especially hyperoxia (PaO_2 >12 kPa). There is abnormal vascular proliferation which may progress to fibrosis, retinal detachment, and blindness.

All infants weighing less than 1500 g should have their eyes screened 6–8 weeks after birth by indirect ophthalmoscopy. Most cases resolve spontaneously but cryosurgery or laser therapy may be indicated for severe disease.

Chronic lung disease of prematurity

Chronic lung disease of prematurity or bronchopulmonary dysplasia occurs in newborns who for any reason require prolonged assisted ventilation with high pressures and high concentrations of oxygen. It is particularly common in very low birthweight infants and positive pressure ventilation (barotrauma) is believed to be the main causative factor. The CXR shows widespread opacities with patchy translucent areas.

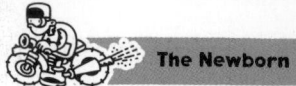

Treatment

- Initially there may be a continued requirement for assisted ventilation or continuous positive airways pressure and supplemental O_2.
- Dexamethasone may allow weaning from the ventilator and a reduction in O_2 requirement.
- Bronchodilators and diuretics may be required.

Complete recovery of lung function can occur over several months, but severely affected babies may die from cor pulmonale.

Neurodevelopmental problems

The prospects for normal survival in preterm infants are good, especially for those weighing more than 1500 g at birth.

However, very low birthweight infants and those with a gestation period of under 28 weeks are at risk of a range of neurodevelopmental problems including:

- Cerebral palsy.
- Cognitive delay.
- Visual impairment.
- Hearing loss.
- Seizures.
- Behavioural problems.
- Educational difficulties.

About 20% of these infants will have a measurable and lasting disability, and their developmental progress should be closely monitored to allow early detection and treatment of neurodevelopmental problems.

DISORDERS OF THE TERM INFANT

Respiratory disorders

Respiratory distress in term infants is characterized by:

- Tachypnoea.
- Cyanosis.
- Nasal flaring and recession.
- Expiratory grunting.

The causes are considered in Chapter 9 and are listed again in Fig. 27.13.

The pulmonary causes are considered in turn.

Respiratory distress in full-term infants

Pulmonary
- transient tachypnoea of the newborn
- pneumonia
- pneumothorax
- meconium aspiration
- persistent fetal circulation
- milk aspiration
- diaphragmatic hernia

Non-pulmonary
- congenital heart disease
- severe anaemia
- metabolic acidosis

Fig. 27.13 Respiratory distress in term infants.

Transient tachypnoea of the newborn

This is caused by delay in reabsorption of fetal lung fluid and is more common after birth by caesarean section. There is early onset of mild to moderate respiratory distress and the CXR shows prominent pulmonary vasculature and fluid in the horizontal fissure. Treatment with increased ambient O_2 may be required. The condition usually settles within a day or two.

Pneumonia

Early onset, congenital pneumonia is acquired prenatally especially when the membranes have been ruptured for more than 24 hours before the onset of labour. It is most commonly due to the group B-haemolytic streptococcus. Respiratory distress is the chief sign and the condition may mimic surfactant deficiency in preterm infants. Preterm infants with respiratory distress are therefore given antibiotics. Pneumonia of later onset is more likely to be due to Gram-negative bacilli and rarely, *Staphylococcus aureus*.

Treatment

This comprises:

- Physiotherapy to prevent local accumulation of secretions.
- Humidified O_2.
- Nasogastric feeds.
- Intravenous antibiotics.

Pneumothorax

A pneumothorax may occur spontaneously but is most commonly seen as a complication of positive pressure ventilation. Tension pneumothorax results in partial collapse of the lung with a sudden deterioration in the infant's condition manifested by cyanosis and hypotension. Diagnosis is confirmed by transillumination with a fibre-optic cold light source, or CXR. Urgent treatment by insertion of a chest drain is indicated.

Meconium aspiration

Passage of meconium into the amniotic fluid is triggered by fetal distress in term or post-term infants. The infant is at risk of inhaling meconium and developing meconium aspiration syndrome. This severe condition causes respiratory distress and cyanosis and has a high mortality rate. This condition can be ameliorated by suctioning thick meconium from the upper airway as soon as the head is delivered and by suctioning any meconium from the trachea under direct vision after delivery. However, most severe cases are probably due to antenatal aspiration *in utero* and cannot be prevented by suction at delivery.

Persistent fetal circulation

This condition is characterized by high pulmonary vascular resistance and is usually found in term or post-term infants. There is right-to-left shunting of blood at atrial and ductal levels with severe cyanosis. Persistent fetal circulation may be primary or secondary to birth asphyxia, meconium aspiration, or respiratory distress syndrome.

A CXR shows a normal cardiac shadow and pulmonary oligaemia, and an echocardiogram may be necessary to exclude cyanotic congenital heart disease.

Treatment

This includes:

- Assisted ventilation.
- Prostacyclin, or inhaled nitric oxide for pulmonary vasodilatation.
- Extracorporeal membrane oxygenation for severe cases.

Milk aspiration

Aspiration of milk or stomach contents into the lungs may occur especially in:

- Preterm infants with RDS or neurological problems.
- Infants with chronic lung disease of prematurity.
- Infants with cleft palate.
- Infants with tracheo–oesophageal fistula.

Diaphragmatic hernia

See Chapter 9. This congenital malformation:

- Occurs in 1 in 4000 live births.
- Is usually left-sided.
- Can be diagnosed on antenatal ultrasound.
- Is repaired surgically.
- Has a high mortality due to coexisting pulmonary hypoplasia.

Gastrointestinal and hepatic disorders

Congenital anomalies of the gastrointestinal tract including cleft lip and palate, tracheo–oesophageal fistula, duodenal stenosis or atresia, and exomphalos or gastroschisis are considered in Chapter 9.

Small bowel obstruction

This presents with:

- Persistent, bile-stained vomiting.
- Delayed or absent passage of meconium.
- Abdominal distension.

Important causes are listed in Fig. 27.14.

Diagnosis is made on clinical features and abdominal X-ray. Treatment depends on the cause and is often surgical. Administering gastrograffin contrast medium may relieve meconium ileus.

Large bowel obstruction

Hirschsprung's disease or rectal atresia may cause this.

Hirschsprung's disease

Congenital aganglionic megacolon or Hirschsprung's disease is a genetic disorder in which there is absence of ganglion cells from the myenteric and submyenteric plexuses of a segment of the large bowel. (See Chapter 17.)

Clinical features

Presentation is usually in the neonatal period with failure to pass meconium in the first 24 hours followed by abdominal distension and bile-stained vomiting. Diarrhoea may occur and alternate with periods of constipation.

Causes of small bowel obstruction
duodenal stenosis or atresia—30% have Down syndrome
malrotation with volvulus
meconium ileus—occurs in cystic fibrosis

Fig. 27.14 Causes of small bowel obstruction.

Diagnosis
This is made by demonstration of the absence of ganglion cells on a suction rectal biopsy.

Management
Treatment is surgical. A preliminary colostomy is usually performed in the neonatal period followed later by an operation to anastomose normally innervated bowel to anus.

Jaundice
Clinical jaundice appears in newborns when the serum bilirubin exceeds 80–120 μmol/L. The causes are considered in Chapter 9.

Jaundice is important as it may be indicative of underlying problems such as infection, and because unconjugated bilirubin can be deposited in the brain and cause kernicterus. Causative conditions are most usefully considered by age of onset of the jaundice.

Jaundice in the first 24 hours
The most common cause is haemolysis, which may be due to:

- Haemolytic disease of the newborn: rhesus or ABO incompatibility.
- Intrinsic red cell defects: spherocytosis, G6PD deficiency or pyruvate kinase deficiency.

Congenital infections may also cause early onset jaundice.

Haemolytic disorders

Isoimmune haemolysis is caused by the destruction of fetal and neonatal red blood cells by maternal IgG antibodies that cross the placenta during pregnancy. Maternal sensitization is caused by fetal-maternal transfusion during current or previous pregnancies, or from mismatched blood transfusions.

The incidence of rhesus (Rh) haemolytic disease has fallen since the introduction of prevention by the use of anti-D immune globulin given to the Rh-negative mother immediately after birth of a Rh-positive infant. Affected infants are usually diagnosed antenatally and given fetal therapy as necessary. Severe haemolysis causes anaemia and hydrops fetalis, which is treated by intrauterine blood transfusion.

ABO incompatibility is more common than Rh haemolytic disease. The usual combination is a group O mother with a group A, or less commonly group B infant. The anti-A or anti-B haemolysins are comparatively weak. There is mild anaemia, no organomegaly, a weakly positive Coombs' test, and mild jaundice peaking in the first few days.

G6PD deficiency may cause neonatal jaundice as may congenital spherocytosis.

Jaundice at 2 days to 2 weeks of age
The most common cause is physiological jaundice, due to the combination of liver enzyme immaturity and an increased load of bilirubin from red cell breakdown. Prematurity, bruising, or polycythaemia (haematocrit >0.65) may exacerbate it. Physiological jaundice usually peaks on the third day of life.

Infection, particularly of the urinary tract, also causes unconjugated hyperbilirubinaemia at this time.

Jaundice at more than 2 weeks of age
Persistent (prolonged, protracted) jaundice is usually an unconjugated hyperbilirubinaemia, which may be due to:

- 'Breast milk' jaundice: affects 15% of healthy breastfed infants. The cause is unknown. It usually resolves by 3–4 weeks of age.
- Infection, particularly of urinary tract.
- Congenital hypothyroidism should have been detected on neonatal screening.

Prolonged conjugated hyperbilirubinaemia is usually associated with dark urine and pale stools. Causes include neonatal hepatitis syndrome and biliary atresia. Early diagnosis of biliary atresia is important as delay in surgical treatment beyond 6 weeks of age compromises outcome.

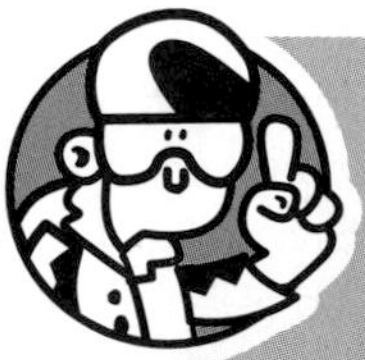

- **Physiological jaundice is the most common cause of jaundice in the newborn. It is associated with unconjugated hyperbilirubinaemia.**
- **Conjugated hyperbilirubinaemia, in excess of 15% of total serum bilirubin, suggests cholestasis due to hepatobiliary disease.**

Management of neonatal jaundice
Investigations are directed towards establishing the cause (see Chapter 9). Clinical estimation of the severity is unreliable and a plasma bilirubin must be measured in any significantly jaundiced infant. The main concern is to prevent kernicterus.

Kernicterus occurs when unconjugated bilirubin is deposited in the brain, especially in the basal ganglia and cerebellum. Bilirubin encephalopathy occurs initially with lethargy, rigidity, eye-rolling, and seizures. The long-term sequelae include choreo-athetoid cerebral palsy, sensorineural deafness, and learning difficulties.

Many factors in addition to the bilirubin level influence the risk of kernicterus. These include:

- The infant's gestational age—risk increases for preterm infants.
- The postnatal age—risk decreases with increasing postnatal age.
- Serum albumin level—risk increases with hypoalbuminaemia.
- Coexistent asphyxia, acidosis, or hypoglycaemia.

Charts exist indicating levels at which treatment should be initiated, bearing those factors in mind.

Treatment options are:

- Phototherapy.
- Exchange transfusion.

Phototherapy
Blue light (not ultraviolet) of wavelength 450 nm converts the bilirubin in the skin and superficial capillaries into harmless water-soluble metabolites, which are excreted in urine and through the bowel. The eyes are covered to prevent discomfort and additional fluids are given to counteract increased losses from skin.

Exchange transfusion
This is required if the bilirubin rises to levels considered dangerous despite phototherapy. It rapidly reduces the level of circulating bilirubin, and in isoimmune haemolytic disease also removes circulating antibodies and corrects anaemia. Techniques vary, but conventionally the exchange is done via umbilical artery and vein catheters. Aliquots of baby's blood (10–20 ml) are withdrawn, alternating with infusions of donor blood of the same volumes. Twice the infant's blood volume (i.e. 2 x 80 ml/kg) is exchanged over about 2 hours. The procedure may need to be repeated.

Haematological disorders
Haemolytic diseases of the newborn are considered with jaundice.

Haemorrhagic disease of the newborn
This is caused by a deficiency of the vitamin K-dependent coagulation factors II, VII, IX, and X. It characteristically affects the fully breastfed infant between the third and sixth day of life. Mothers taking anticonvulsant drugs, which interfere with vitamin K metabolism, such as phenytoin, are at increased risk.

Bleeding usually occurs from the gastrointestinal tract but may rarely be intracranial or from the umbilical stump.

This disease is prevented by intramuscular injection of 1 mg of vitamin K at birth, or repeated oral administration after birth. In the UK, it is recommended that all newborn infants receive this prophylaxis.

Infections
The newborn infant is vulnerable to infection by bacteria, viruses, and fungi. *In utero,* infection may take place across the placenta or by ascending the birth canal.

After birth, the skin and umbilicus are colonised by staphylococci, the gut by *Escherichia coli* and the upper respiratory tract by streptococci. Important bacterial pathogens in the neonate include:

- Group B β-haemolytic streptococci.
- *Escherichia coli.*
- *Staphylococcus aureus.*
- *Staphylococcus epidermidis.*

The range of acquired infections in the newborn is shown in Fig. 27.15.

Minor infections
Skin pustules and paronychia
These are caused by staphylococcal infection and typically occur in moist areas such as groins and axillae. Inflammation of the skin in the area of a nail fold may evolve into a pustular lesion. Treatment with oral flucloxacillin is indicated.

Acute mastitis
This is an inflamed swelling under the nipple in a febrile infant. It is usually caused by *Staphylococcus aureus* infection in an engorged neonatal breast. Flucloxacillin is the antibiotic of choice.

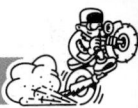

Conjunctivitis

A 'sticky eye' in the first day or two of life is often due to chemical irritation and clears spontaneously.

Conjunctivitis with a purulent discharge may be due to:

- Staphylococci, streptococci, *Escherichia coli*.
- Gonococcus—ophthalmia neonatorum (see below)
- *Chlamydia trachomatis*.

Swabs for culture should be taken and treatment initiated with chloramphenicol 1% eye ointment. If infection is persistent and does not respond, *Chlamydia trachomatis* should be suspected. The organism is difficult to culture but an antigen detection test is available. Treatment is with tetracycline eye ointment together with oral erythromycin in severe cases.

Thrush (moniliasis)

Infection with *Candida albicans* may affect the mouth or nappy area. Oral thrush appears as white plaques on the tongue and inside of the mouth. Nystatin suspension 1 ml (100 000 units) after feeds for 7–10 days is usually effective. Topical preparations include miconazole and clotrimazole are used for perineal thrush.

Major infections

Septicaemia

Infection with potential pathogens may occur before, during, or after birth. The major problem is infection with group B β-haemolytic streptococci, but other organisms often responsible include *Escherichia coli, Pseudomonas aeruginosa, Listeria monocytogenes,* and *Staphylococcus epidermidis* (especially in very preterm infants).

Acquired infections in the newborn

Minor infections
- skin pustules
- paronychia
- acute mastitis
- conjunctivitis
- thrush

Major infections
- septicaemia
- meningitis
- pneumonia
- urinary tract infection
- ophthalmia neonatorum

Fig. 27.15 Acquired infections in the newborn.

The incidence of serious acute infections in the newborn period is about 3 per 1000 live births in the UK.

Initial presentation is often non-specific with:

- Lethargy and drowsiness.
- Poor feeding, vomiting.
- Temperature instability.
- Pallor.
- Irritability.

Specific signs relating to a site of infection may then emerge. These include:

- Tense fontanelle, seizures: meningitis.
- Respiratory distress: pneumonia.

Group B streptococcal infection

Early onset disease presents on day 1–3 of life with pneumonia, septicaemia, and occasionally meningitis. Mortality is up to 20%. Late-onset disease presents between 1 week and 3 months of age and usually causes meningitis.

Diagnosis

If systemic infection is suspected, prompt investigation is essential. The following investigations are performed to confirm the diagnosis and identify a causative organism.

- 'Septic' screen: blood culture, urine culture, lumbar puncture, and cerebrospinal fluid culture. Swabs from the throat, nose, and ear.
- Full blood count.
- CXR.

Treatment

Antibiotics are started immediately without waiting for culture results, which may not be available for 24–72 hours. Intravenous broad-spectrum antibiotics are given, e.g. benzylpenicillin combined with an aminoglycoside (gentamicin) or third-generation cephalosporin (cefuroxime or cefotaxime). Treatment can be changed according to the sensitivity of any organism recovered on culture. All the supportive measures of intensive care may be required in severe infections.

Meningitis

Neonatal meningitis is usually due to a different range of pathogens from that in the older infant or child. In infants, the infective organisms include:

- *Escherichia coli*.
- Group B β-haemolytic streptococci.
- *Listeria monocytogenes*.

Meningeal infection usually follows a septicaemic stage. Clinical features include poor feeding, pallor, and temperature instability. Fullness of the anterior fontanelle and fits are late signs.

Diagnosis

Lumbar puncture is required to confirm the diagnosis.

Treatment and outcome

Intravenous antibiotics are given. Good penetration into cerebrospinal fluid is important and is a feature of cephalosporins, such as cefotaxime. Mortality and morbidity remains high despite effective treatment.

Pneumonia

This is most commonly due to the group B β-haemolytic streptococcus. Respiratory distress is the chief presenting sign together with features of septicaemia.

Urinary tract infection

The most common pathogen is *Escherichia coli,* although other Gram-negative organisms are occasionally responsible. There is a relatively high incidence of underlying congenital anomalies or vesicoureteric reflux.

Symptoms and signs are usually non-specific. Urine must be cultured in all infants with poor feeding, lethargy, vomiting, failure to thrive, and jaundice.

The diagnostic problem is obtaining an uncontaminated specimen of urine. Options include a 'clean catch', a 'bag' urine, or suprapubic aspiration of the bladder. Any growth in urine obtained by the latter method is indicative of infection.

Antibiotic treatment with IV gentamicin is indicated initially, with a change to oral antibiotics later if the clinical state and sensitivity tests allow. Subsequent imaging of the renal tracts is essential to identify underlying congenital anomalies or renal scarring.

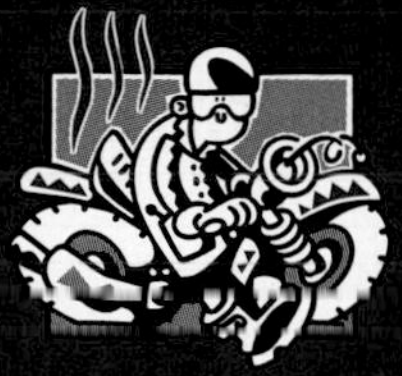

28. Accidents and Emergencies

ACCIDENTS

Accidents in children are extremely common and are the leading cause of death between the ages of 1 and 14 years. The pattern of accidents varies with age (Fig. 28.1). Road traffic accidents account for the majority of fatal accidents (Fig. 28.2).

Trauma

Physical trauma causing multiple serious injuries is an important cause of death and early, correct management of the multiply injured child is vital to reduce mortality and long-term morbidity. Injuries to the head are the most important class of local injury.

Major trauma

Initial assessment and management is described in Fig. 28.3. Events during the first 'golden hour' determine the outcome.

Once the initial steps of immediate resuscitation have been carried out, a careful secondary survey of the complete child must be undertaken to detect and treat all injuries (Fig. 28.4).

Head injury

Minor head injuries in children are very common and most children recover without ill effect. A small minority, about 1 in 800 of those admitted, develops serious complications such as intracranial haemorrhage. Causes of head injury include:

- Road traffic accidents (RTAs): the most common cause of severe and fatal head injuries.
- Falls from trees, walls, bicycles, etc.
- Child abuse: especially 'shaking' injuries in infants.

Damage to the brain may be primary or secondary (Fig. 28.5).

The history should establish:

- When and how the injury occurred?
- Was consciousness lost?
- Subsequent symptoms—vomiting, drowsiness, seizures, bleeding from nose or ears.

Clinical features

Clinical examination should look for the following signs:

- Head: external injury including haematoma, laceration, depressed fracture. In babies, the anterior fontanelle tension provides a useful indicator of intracranial pressure, as does the head circumference. Look for blood or cerebrospinal fluid leak from the ears or nose.
- Central nervous system: assess Glasgow coma scale, fundi and pupillary reflexes. Examine for focal neurological signs.
- General: full examination to exclude other injuries.

Diagnosis

Investigations may include:

- Skull X-ray: for all but most minor.
- Cranial computed tomography (CT): if severe with signs of raised intracranial pressure or intracranial haemorrhage or severe fracture (i.e. compound or depressed).

Accidents in childhood

Toddlers are prone to:
falls
scalds
drowning
accidental ingestion
choking
School-age children are prone to:
falls while climbing
road traffic accidents

Fig. 28.1 Accidents in childhood.

Causes of fatal accidents	
road traffic accidents	50%
home accidents: fire, falls, choking, suffocation	30%
drowning	10%

Fig. 28.2 Causes of fatal accidents.

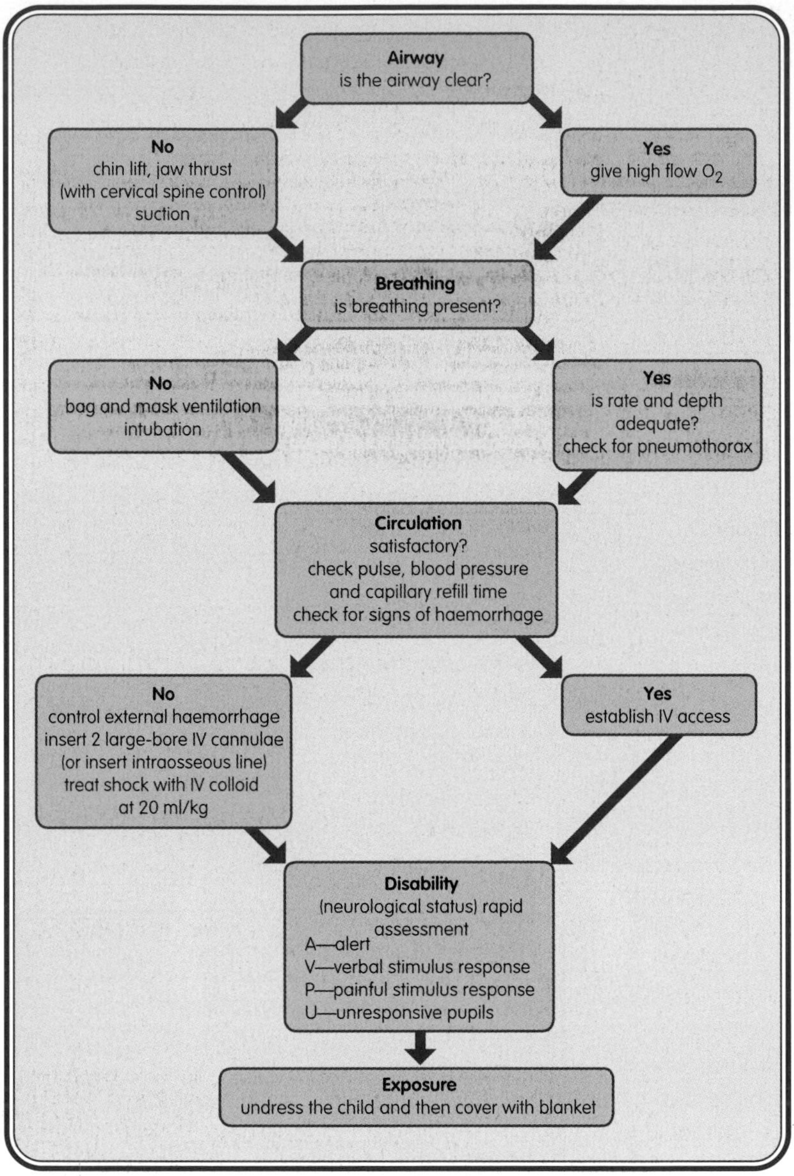

Fig. 28.3 Major trauma. Initial assessment and management—A, B, C, D, E.

Secondary survey and treatment—multiple trauma		
detailed history of accident	previous medical history, allergies	
complete examination	chest:	open chest wound, tension pneumothorax, flail chest, cardiac tamponade
	abdomen:	ruptured organs—spleen, liver, kidney, bowel
	head:	most common cause of death in injured children
	spine:	assume patient has a spinal injury until proved otherwise
	limbs:	check for fractures
investigations include:	X-rays:	lateral cervical spine, CXR, pelvis
	blood tests:	FBC, cross-match, glucose, U&Es, arterial blood gas

Fig. 28.4 Secondary survey and treatment—multiple trauma.

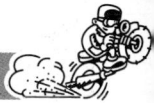

Brain damage in head injury	
Primary	cerebral contusion dural tears
Secondary	intracranial haemorrhage reduced cerebral perfusion due to hypotension and raised intracranial pressure hypoxia—hypoventilation infection—from penetrating injury or CSF leak

Fig. 28.5 Brain damage in head injury.

Management

Minor and moderate injuries

These are the majority. Admit to hospital for observation if:

- History of seizure or loss of consciousness.
- Declining level of consciousness.
- Severe headache or persistent vomiting.
- Skull fracture.
- Suspected non-accidental injury.
- Child has a bleeding tendency.
- Supervision at home is inadequate.

If the child is not admitted, the parents should be given written instructions to bring the child back if there is severe headache, recurrent vomiting, or a declining level of consciousness.

Neurological observations should be made at intervals dictated by clinical state.

Severe injuries

These usually occur in the context of multiple major trauma requiring intensive care.

Additional measures in severe head injury are directed towards the management of complications such as raised intracranial pressure, intracranial bleeding, seizures, and risk of infection.

Urgent referral to a neurosurgeon is indicated if there is any evidence of an expanding haematoma, such as:

- Declining level of consciousness.
- Focal neurological signs.
- Signs of rising intracranial pressure—bradycardia, rise in systolic blood pressure.

Burns and scalds

Scalds from contact with hot liquids are the most common form of thermal trauma in childhood (most of the fatalities are from house fires, but those are due to gas and smoke inhalation rather than burns). Burns and scalds may be non-accidental. Toddlers are most at risk of accidental scalds.

Assessment

The extent, depth, and distribution of the injury should be estimated (Figs 28.6 and 28.7 and see Hints & Tips).

Diagnosis

Investigations should include:

- Full blood count: packed cell volume is increased with significant hypovolaemia.
- Urea and electrolytes.
- Group and save (if burns are greater than 15–20%).
- Serum albumin.

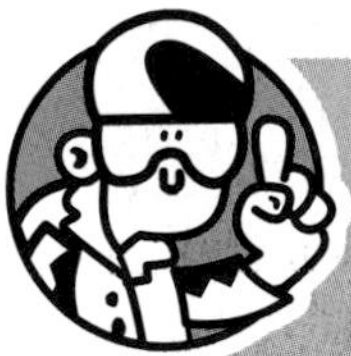

Electrical burns are usually full thickness. Most scalds are deep, partial thickness.

Assessment of the depth of burn		
Thickness	**Depth**	**Characterisitics**
partial	superficial	pink, sensitive, blanches epithelium intact (e.g. mild sunburn)
	deep	pink or red, sensitive, blanches blistered
full	-	white or charred leathery, dry to touch insensitive

Fig. 28.6 Assessment of the depth of burn.

Location of the burn is important, as well as extent:

- **Face—potential airway involvement, scarring.**
- **Hands—contractures and functional loss.**
- **Genitalia—difficult to nurse, risk of infection.**

Management

Recommended first aid is:

- Run cold water over the affected part for 5 minutes.
- Cover the burn with a clean, non-fluffy dressing, e.g. a tea towel.

Admit to hospital if:

- Extent is over 5% full thickness or deep partial thickness.
- A difficult area is involved,e.g. face, hands and feet, perineum, or genitalia.
- There is any possibility of child abuse.

The important aspects of management are shown in Fig. 28.8.

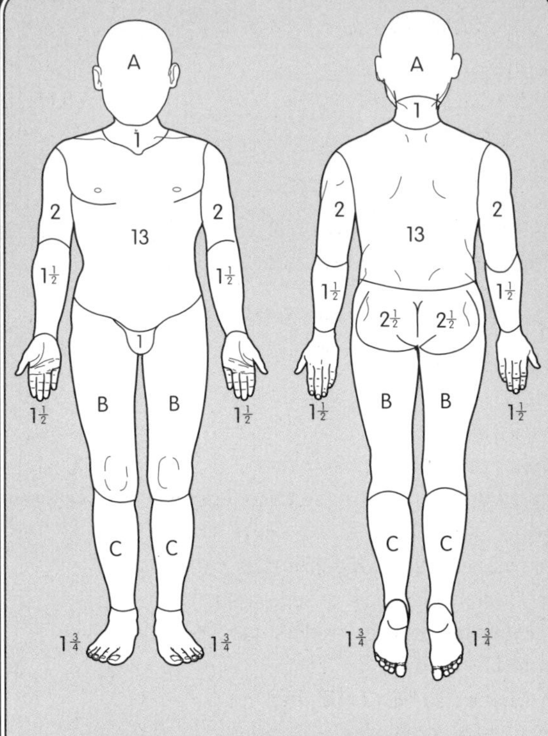

area indicated	surface area at 1 year	5 years	10 years	15 years
A	8.5	6.5	5.5	4.5
B	3.25	4.0	4.5	4.5
C	2.5	2.75	3.0	3.25

Fig. 28.7 Assessment of the extent of a burn. The percentage body surface area affected is calculated from this standard body diagram. Note that the area corresponding to head and lower limbs (A, B, C) changes with age. The small child has a relatively big head and short legs.

Management of burns

Analgesia
pain relief is a priority—patients with major burns will need intravenous morphine
IV fluids
essential if extent >10%, as fluid and protein loss causes severe hypovolaemia
formula for initial regimen:
n ml of 4.5% albumin over 4 hours where
[n = weight (kg) × % burn] ÷ 2
full thickness burns require a blood transfusion
Wound toilet and dressing
Tetanus toxoid if not vaccinated
Monitor urine output

Fig. 28.8 Management of burns.

Near drowning

Drowning is more common in boys than girls. It is the third most common cause of childhood accidental death in the UK. In the UK, drowning incidents are more common in freshwater canals and lakes, swimming pools, and domestic baths than in the sea.

The two principal problems in near drowning are:

- Hypoxia—due to laryngospasm (15% dry drowning) or water in the lungs (85%) which causes alveolar damage and pulmonary oedema.
- Hypothermia—this leads to bradycardia and asystole (extreme hypothermia can be protective).

Haemolysis or electrolyte problems caused by the ingestion or inhalation of large amounts of fresh water are unusual.

Management

Skilled on-site treatment with mouth to mouth resuscitation and warming is vital. All children should

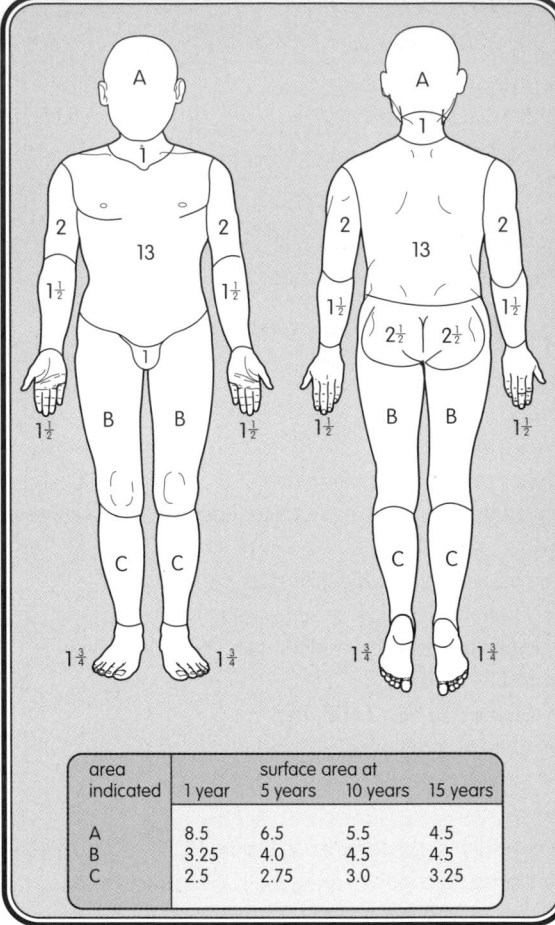

be hospitalized for at least 24 hours. Patients admitted in asystole or respiratory arrest should undergo cardiopulmonary resuscitation in the normal way. In hypothermic patients, resuscitation must be continued until the core temperature has been at or near normal for 15 minutes.

Late respiratory sequelae may occur in the 72-hour period after near drowning. These include pneumonia and pulmonary oedema.

Poisoning

Most cases of poisoning in young children follow accidental ingestion by an inquisitive, fearless toddler. In adolescents most poisoning is deliberate self-harm. Children may also be poisoned deliberately by their parents (or inadvertently by their doctors). Although many thousands of children attend hospital each year, very few die as a result of accidental ingestion.

The history should establish:

- What was ingested—identify from carton or bottle.
- Amount ingested—usually an approximation.
- Time ingested—important in relation to management.

The toxicity of the ingested substance can then be assessed (Fig. 28.9) or the Regional Poisons Information Centre contacted if there is any doubt concerning the agent's identity or toxicity.

Clinical features

Examination should include the following:

- Inspect oropharynx and any vomitus.
- Assess level of consciousness.
- Look for features specific to various poisons (e.g. small pupils—opiates or barbiturates, tachypnoea—salicylate poisoning, cardiac arrhythmias—tricyclic antidepressants or digoxin).

Diagnosis

Relevant investigations include:

- Blood levels (at optimum time after ingestion) can be measured for salicylates, paracetamol, digoxin, iron, lithium, and tricyclic antidepressants.
- Keep specimens of vomitus and urine for analysis.

Management

If the agent ingested was relatively innocuous the patient may be allowed home or briefly observed in hospital. Efforts should be made to remove the poison if there has been a large ingestion of a highly toxic substance. These may include:

- Ipecacuanha: still used but unpleasant and may cause persistent vomiting. Contraindicated if the patient is drowsy and following ingestion of paraffin, caustics, or acids.
- Activated charcoal: give 1 g/kg, if necessary by nasogastric tube. It binds a wide range of toxic drugs, with the exception of iron and lithium.

Specific treatment is indicated for certain drugs and toxins (see Fig. 28.9).

Deliberate self-poisoning in older children

This is a serious occurrence which may reflect a significant underlying psychiatric disorder such as depression. In most cases, there is no serious suicidal

Poison-specific adverse effects and treatments

Poison	Adverse effect	Treatment
iron	gastric ulceration liver failure	IV and enteral desferrioxamine
opiates	respiratory depression	naloxone (IV and IM)
paracetamol	liver toxicity	oral methionine or IV N-acetylcysteine
digoxin	arrhythmias	antibodies for life-threatening toxicity
salicylates	metabolic acidosis	alkalinization with sodium bicarbonate
alcohol	hypoglycaemia	monitor blood glucose IV dextrose

Fig. 28.9 Poison specific adverse effects and treatments.

intent. Alcohol intoxication is often a predisposing element. All children who deliberately poison themselves should be admitted to hospital and assessed by a child and adolescent psychiatrist.

EMERGENCIES

Children are not little adults. They differ in important ways that are relevant to emergency care (Fig. 28.10).

The seriously ill child

A seriously ill child is on one of the pathways leading to cardiopulmonary arrest (Fig. 28.11). Such arrests in children are rarely unheralded, but are preceded by a period of progressive circulatory, respiratory, or central neurological failure. It is vital to recognize such a critically ill child and intervene to prevent the progression to cardiac arrest.

Rapid assessment

An initial ABCD assessment should be carried out to identify features of:

- Airway and breathing—respiratory failure.
- Circulation—circulatory failure.
- Disability—central neurological failure.

Airway and Breathing

A critical state is indicated either by:

- An increase in the work of breathing (respiratory distress).
- Absent or decreased respiratory effort (exhaustion or respiratory depression).

Key signs include:

- Respiratory rate—increased or decreased.

Anatomical and physiological characteristics of young children

Anatomical
large body surface area to weight ratio
increased fluid needs and heat loss
airways are small and easily obstructed

Physiological
respiratory:
- compliant chest wall
- infants rely on diaphragmatic breathing
- relatively small alveolar surface area
- high O_2 consumption

cardiovascular:
- circulating volume is higher per kilogram body weight (70–80 mL/kg), but absolute volume is small
- cardiac stroke volume small, so heart rate is higher

Fig. 28.10 Anatomical and physiological characteristics of young children.

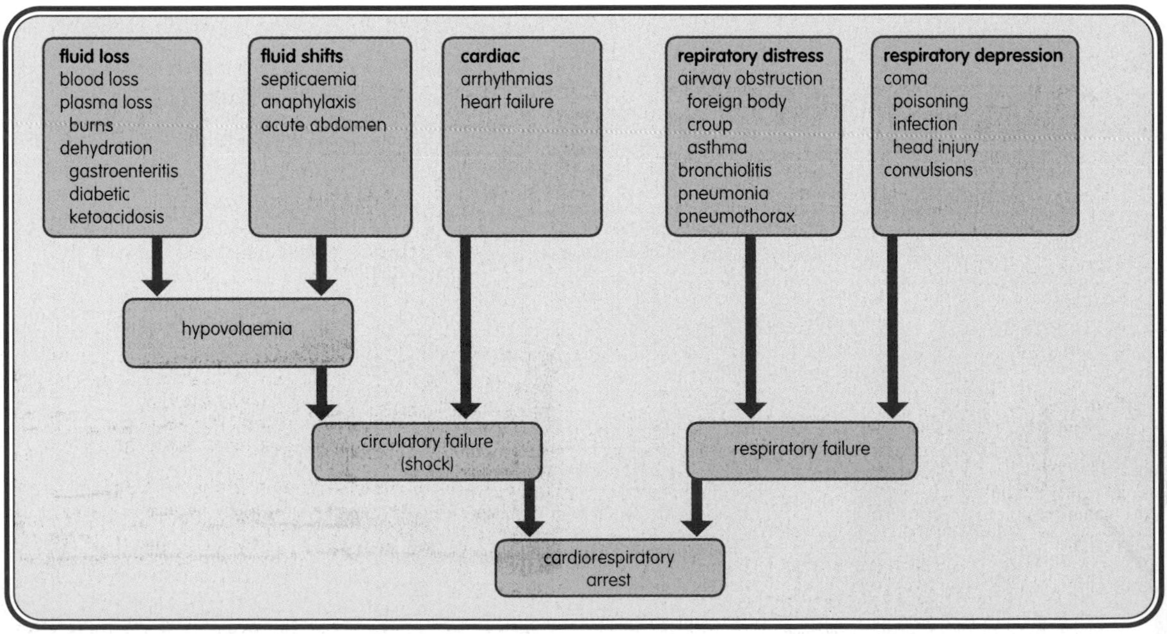

Fig. 28.11 The critically ill child: pathways to cardiorespiratory arrest.

- Recession—intercostal, subcostal, or sternal.
- Accessory muscle use.
- Stridor, wheezing, or grunting.
- Flaring of alae nasi.
- Auscultation.

Signs of hypoxia include:
- Skin pallor due to vasoconstriction (via catecholamine release).
- Cyanosis—a late and preterminal sign.
- Tachycardia.
- Altered mental state—agitation or drowsiness.

Circulation

Signs of potential circulatory failure (shock) include:
- Tachycardia
- Pulse volume reduction: absent peripheral pulses and weak central pulses are serious signs of advanced shock.
- Capillary refill time of over 2 seconds.
- Blood pressure: hypotension is a late and preterminal sign of circulatory failure.

The effects of circulatory failure encompass:
- Metabolic acidosis with increased respiratory rate.
- Skin—mottled, cold, pale skin peripherally.
- Mental state—agitation followed by drowsiness due to reduced cerebral perfusion.
- Urine output—oliguria due to renal hypoperfusion.

Disability

Signs of potential central neurological failure are:
- Level of consciousness—reduced (see Hints & Tips).
- Posture—most are hypotonic; stiff posture is a sign of serious brain dysfunction.
- Pupils—most sinister signs are dilatation, unreactivity, and inequality.

Circulatory and respiratory failure have central neurological effects.
Central neurological failure has respiratory and circulatory consequences.

Central neurological failure has important effects on both respiration and circulation:
- Respiratory depression.
- Abnormal respiratory patterns.
- Systemic hypertension with sinus bradycardia (Cushing's response) indicates herniation of the cerebellar tonsils through the foramen magnum.

Cardiorespiratory arrest

A standard procedure exists for applying basic life support in the event of a cardiorespiratory arrest (Figs 28.12–14).

Following basic life support procedures, it may be necessary to proceed to:
- Intubation and ventilation.
- Circulatory access—venous or intra-osseous.
- ECG monitoring—to identify the rhythm, asystole is most common. Protocol for drug use in asystole is shown in Fig. 28.14.

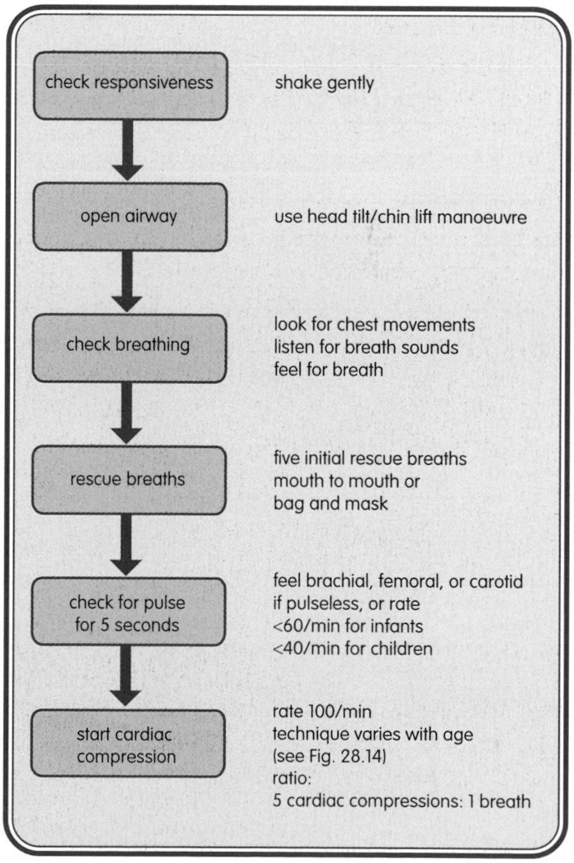
check responsiveness
shake gently
open airway
use head tilt/chin lift manoeuvre
check breathing
look for chest movements
listen for breath sounds
feel for breath
rescue breaths
five initial rescue breaths
mouth to mouth or
bag and mask
check for pulse
for 5 seconds
feel brachial, femoral, or carotid
if pulseless, or rate
<60/min for infants
<40/min for children
start cardiac
compression
rate 100/min
technique varies with age
(see Fig. 28.14)
ratio:
5 cardiac compressions: 1 breath

Fig. 28.12 Basic life support.

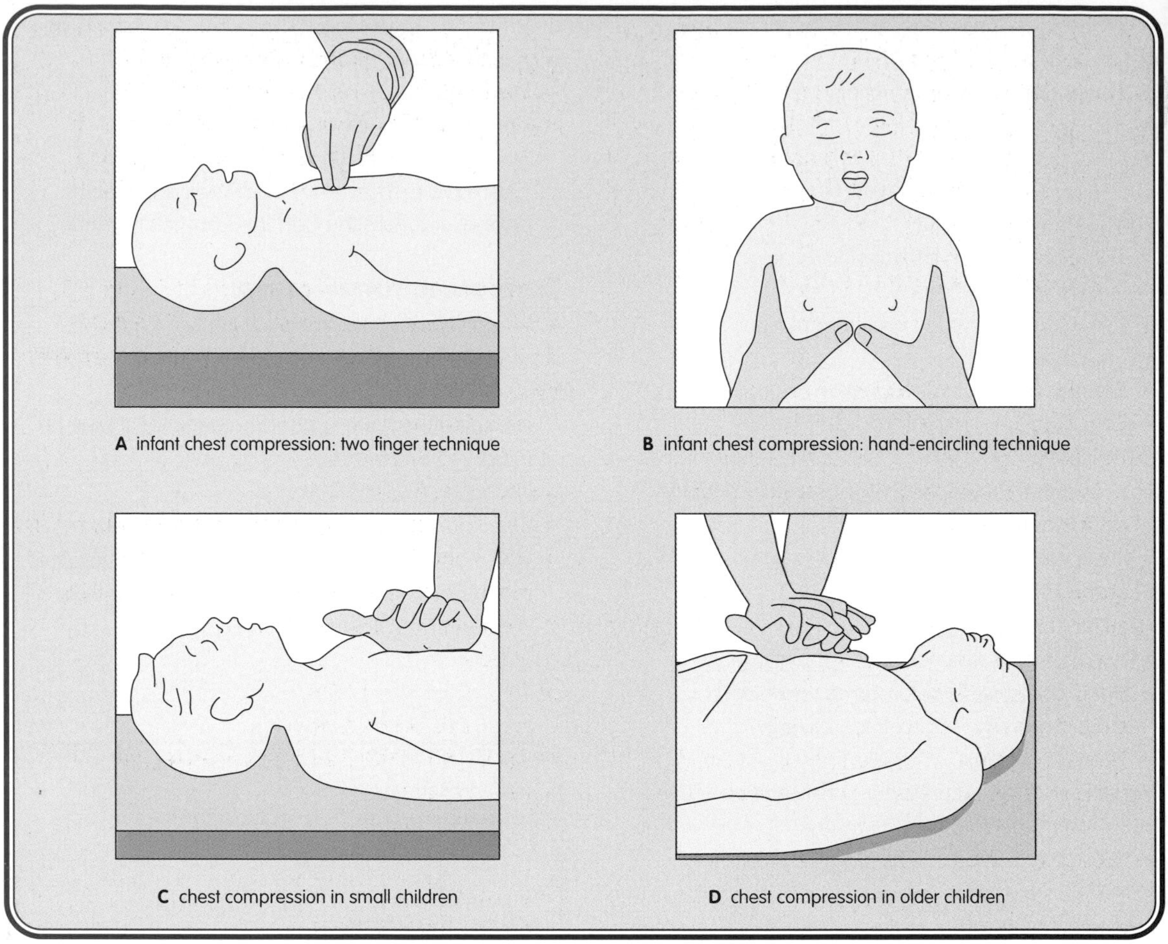

A infant chest compression: two finger technique
B infant chest compression: hand-encircling technique
C chest compression in small children
D chest compression in older children

Fig. 28.13 Cardiac compression techniques.

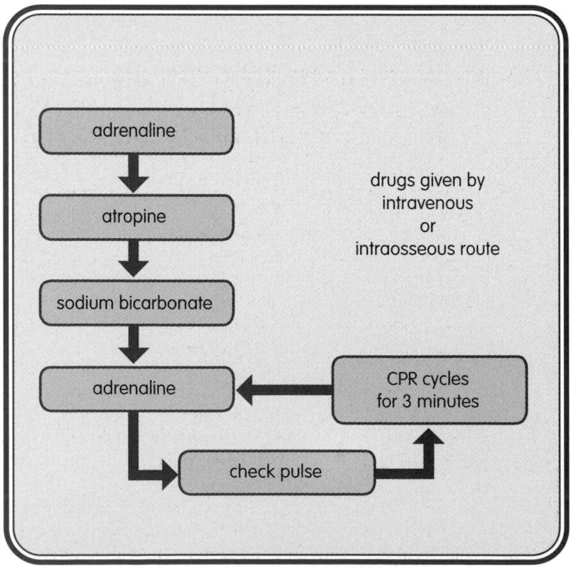

Fig. 28.14 Protocol for drug use in asystole.

Neurological emergencies

Coma

This is a reduced level of consciousness in which the child is unrousable. There are many causes (see Fig. 5.4). Some are self-evident but others may only be identified after careful clinical evaluation and special investigations.

Assessment

A rapid history should include information about:

- Chronic medical conditions such as epilepsy and diabetes mellitus.
- Any recent injury.
- Access to poisons including drugs.
- Clinical state in the 24 hours before onset of coma.

Clinical examination should pay attention to:

- External signs of trauma.
- Fever or rash—especially a purpuric rash.

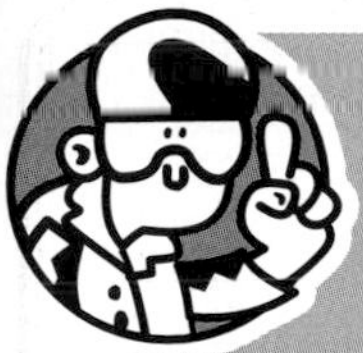

Hypoglycaemia is an important cause of both coma and seizures in children. Recognition and treatment is simple. If missed, brain damage may result.

- Blood pressure and respiratory pattern.
- CNS: Glasgow coma score (see Fig. 5.5), signs of meningism (nuchal rigidity), focal neurological signs, pupil size and reaction to light, fundi—papilloedema or haemorrhages.

Diagnosis

Investigations are determined by the clinical evaluation and may include:

- Blood analysis for glucose, electrolytes.
- Urine for toxins.
- Lumbar puncture for suspected meningitis.
- Brain imaging—cranial CT or magnetic resonance imaging.
- EEG for seizures, metabolic encephalopathy.

Management

Initial management should be directed towards maintaining airway, breathing, and circulation. Further specific treatment depends on aetiology, e.g.

- IV dextrose for hypoglycaemia.
- IV antibiotics for bacterial meningitis.
- IV naloxone for opiate poisoning.

A raised intracranial pressure is treated (e.g. mannitol, steroids, hyperventilation) to prevent secondary brain damage.

Convulsions

A 'convulsion' is a generalized tonic–clonic seizure. The causes of a convulsion vary with age (Fig. 28.15). The most common cause in young children is a 'febrile convulsion' (see Chapter 19).

A continuous convulsion lasting more than 30 minutes, or repeated convulsions without recovery of consciousness lasting more than 30 minutes is called 'convulsive status epilepticus' (CSE).

Prolonged convulsions may result in brain damage or death from hypoxia. Cerebral blood flow and O_2 consumption increase five-fold to meet the extra metabolic demand. Oxygen delivery to the brain will be impaired if there is inadequate ventilation or hypotension.

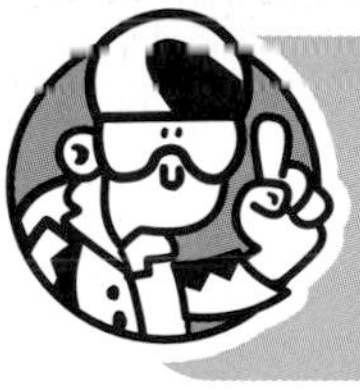

Check blood sugar in a comatose or convulsing child to identify treatable hypoglycaemia.

Management

An algorithm for management of the convulsing child is shown in Fig. 28.16.

While initiating emergency management, establish the history and examine the child:

History:

- Duration of convulsion.
- History of recent trauma.
- Known epileptic? If so, medication regime.
- Known diabetic?
- Preceding illness.

Examination:

- Cardiorespiratory status.
- Signs of head trauma.
- Fever, petechial rash, meningism.
- Nature of convulsion: generalized or focal.

Causes of convulsions	
Age	**Causes**
all ages	hypoglycaemia head injury poisoning meningitis epilepsy
birth to 6 months	hypoglycaemia hypocalcaemia inborn errors of metabolism meningitis
6 months to 5 years	febrile convulsion meningitis
>5 years	epilepsy (most common cause)

Fig. 28.15 Causes of convulsions.

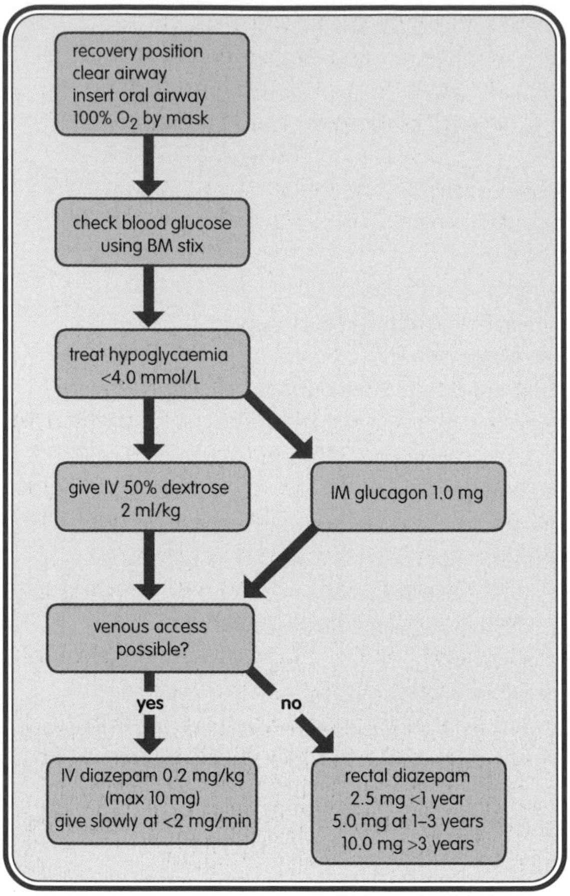

Fig. 28.16 The convulsing child.

If diazepam in maximum dosage fails to stop the seizure, further options include, in order:

- Paraldehyde: rectal administration as 10% solution 1 ml/year of age. Safe and usually effective within 5 minutes.
- Summon senior anaesthetic help.
- IV Phenytoin—15 mg/kg over 15 minutes followed by an infusion under ECG and blood pressure monitoring.

Status epilepticus (convulsive)

Protracted convulsions (of over 30 minutes) may occur in:

- Epilepsy.
- Febrile convulsion.
- Head injury.
- Intracranial infection: meningitis or encephalitis.
- Metabolic seizures: hypoglycaemia, or poisoning.

Diazepam, paraldehyde, and phenytoin are used in order as indicated above. If convulsions persist, the child should be paralysed, ventilated, and managed on an Intensive Care Unit where a thiopentone or benzodiazepine infusion can be safely instituted.

Cardiac emergencies

Serious illness arising from a primary cardiac problem is uncommon outside the newborn period. The causes and management of heart failure are considered elsewhere (see chapter 2), as is the management of circulatory failure (shock) and cardiac arrest. Cardiac arrhythmias, uncommon but treatable conditions in childhood, are considered in Chapter 15.

Respiratory emergencies

The pattern of severe respiratory illness in children is determined by features of the anatomy and physiology of their respiratory system, including:

- Small airways: easily obstructed with rapid increase in airways resistance.
- Compliant thoracic cage: reduced breathing efficiency.
- Inefficient respiratory muscles: rapid development of fatigue.
- Susceptibility to infection.

The illnesses most commonly presenting as emergencies are:

- Upper airway obstruction: croup, acute epiglottitis.
- Lower airway obstruction: asthma, bronchiolitis.
- Pneumonia.

Upper airways obstruction

The cardinal sign of upper airway obstruction is stridor. This is a noise associated with breathing and due to obstruction of the extra thoracic airway. It tends to be worse on inspiration.

The important common causes of acute stridor are:

- Croup—acute laryngotracheobronchitis.

Not all respiratory distress has a respiratory cause:

- **Metabolic acidosis causes deep, rapid breathing.**
- **Heart failure is associated with tachypnoea.**

- Inhaled foreign body.
- Epiglottitis.

Features distinguishing croup from epiglottitis are shown in Fig. 28.17. Epiglottitis has become uncommon since the introduction of Hib vaccination.

Croup

This is a clinical diagnosis. Investigations are not usually required. Management depends on the severity of upper airways obstruction. Children requiring hospital admission are given supportive care:

- Gentle, confident handling.
- Monitoring of transcutaneous O_2 saturation, heart rate.
- O_2 therapy.
- Nebulized budesonide—reduces severity.
- Nebulized adrenaline—gives transient relief of severe obstruction.

Up to 5% of children admitted to hospital with croup require endotracheal intubation. The differential diagnosis of severe croup includes bacterial tracheitis. (See Chapter 16.)

Acute epiglottitis

The diagnosis is clinical. Any disturbance of the child, such as lying down, examining the throat, or venepuncture must be avoided as total airway obstruction and death may be precipitated. The procedure is:

- Call for help: paediatric team, senior anaesthetist, ear, nose, and throat surgeon.
- Arrange examination under anaesthesia.
- If the diagnosis is confirmed, secure an airway by endotracheal intubation. Take blood cultures and start IV antibiotics (e.g. cefuroxime).

Most children can be extubated within a day or two and will have recovered fully within a week. (See Chapter 16.)

Distinguishing croup from epiglottitis

Feature	Croup	Epiglottitis
appearance	unwell	toxic ill
onset	over days	over hours
initial coryza	yes	no
cough	severe, barking	absent or minimal
able to drink	yes	no
drooling	no	yes
stridor	harsh, rasping	soft

Fig. 28.17 Distinguishing croup from epiglottitis.

Lower airways obstruction

Acute asthma

An algorithm for the management of acute severe asthma is shown in Fig. 28.18. Features of severe or life-threatening asthma are shown in Fig. 28.19.

Nebulized β_2-bronchodilators, steroids and oxygen are the mainstays of treatment of acute asthma:

- The nebulizer should be driven by oxygen.
- Steroids take several hours to exert their effect so should be given early.
- Intravenous aminophylline has a role in children who do not respond adequately to nebulizers.
- Nebulized therapy can be given continuously, but it is important to monitor for sinus tachycardia and hypokalaemia. IV fluids should be two-thirds the normal requirement as there is often inappropriate antidiuretic hormone (ADH) secretion.

Antibiotics are unnecessary unless there are clear signs of infection. Mechanical ventilation is rarely required. (See Chapter 16.)

Bronchiolitis

This is the most common, serious respiratory infection of childhood (see Chapter 16). It is predominantly a disease of infants aged 1–9 months and occurs as an annual winter epidemic. Respiratory syncytial virus is the pathogen in 75% of cases.

Infants at high risk of developing severe disease complicated by apnoeic episodes or respiratory failure include:

- Preterm infants.
- Infants under 6 weeks of age.
- Infants with chronic lung disease (e.g. cystic fibrosis, bronchopulmonary dysplasia).
- Infants with congenital heart disease.

Clinical features

Features of severe disease include:

- Irregular breathing or recurrent apnoea.

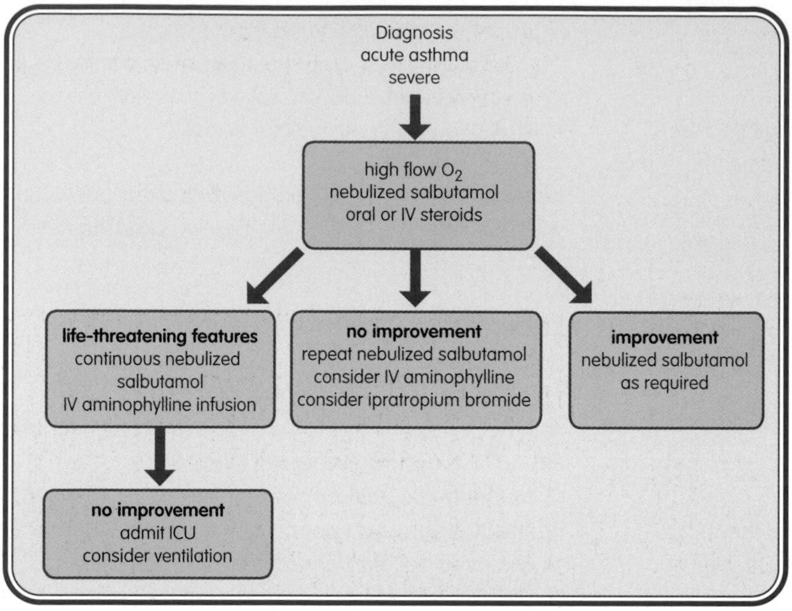

Fig. 28.18 Management of acute severe asthma.

Clinical features of severe and life-threatening asthma		
Feature	**Severe**	**Life-threatening**
altered consciousness	±	yes
cyanosis	±	yes
O_2 saturation in air	>92%	<92%
accessory muscles	±	yes
wheeze	+	silent chest
peak flow (predicted)	<50%	<33%

Fig. 28.19 Clinical features of severe and life-threatening asthma.

- Tachypnoea: respiratory rate >60/min.
- Hypoxia: O_2 saturation <85% in O_2 concentrations over 60%.

Management

Management is supportive and includes:

- Monitoring O_2 saturation by pulse oximetry: apnoea alarm.
- Humidified O_2 by head box or nasal cannulae to maintain O_2 saturation above 94%.
- Fluids: nasogastric feeds or IV fluids.

Antibiotics, bronchodilators, and steroids have not been shown to be of value, and the role of the nebulized antiviral agent ribavirin remains unclear.

Shock (circulatory failure)

Shock is a clinical syndrome resulting from acute failure of circulatory function and is commonly present in the critically ill child. It tends to progress through three phases (Fig. 28.20):

- Compensated.
- Uncompensated.
- Irreversible.

Causes of shock are shown in Fig. 28.21 and in Fig. 28.11. The two most common mechanisms are hypovolaemia or pump failure (cardiogenic).

Clinical features

A brief history may identify the cause. The early physical signs of shock include:

- Pallor—due to vasoconstriction.
- Tachycardia with reduced pulse volume.
- Poor skin perfusion—capillary refill time >2 seconds, core/toe temperature difference >2°C.
- Hypotension.

The late physical signs of shock include:

- Rapid, deep breathing—response to metabolic acidosis.

- Agitation, confusion—due to brain hypoperfusion.
- Oliguria—urine flow less than 2 ml/kg/h in infants, 1 ml/kg/h in children.

Management of shock—general

An algorithm for the general management of circulatory failure is shown in Fig. 28.22. If there is not rapid improvement, or there is evidence of organ failure, transfer to an Intensive Care Unit will be required for assisted ventilation, intensive monitoring, and inotropic support.

Three phases of shock

Phase	Clinicopathological features
compensated shock	vital organ function (brain, heart) is preserved by sympathetic response. Pallor, tachycardia, cold periphery, poor capillary return but systolic blood pressure is maintained
decompensated shock	inadequate perfusion leads to anaerobic metabolism, metabolic acidosis, and, on occasion, a bleeding diathesis. Blood pressure falls, acidotic breathing, very slow capillary return, altered consciousness, anuria
irreversible shock	a retrospective diagnosis. Damage to heart and brain irreversible, with no improvement even if circulation is restored

Fig. 28.20 Three phases of shock.

Causes of shock

Mechanism	Causes
hypovolaemia	fluid loss • haemorrhage • burns • diarrhoea and vomiting • diabetic ketoacidosis fluid shifts • septicaemia • anaphylaxis • peritonitis
cardiogenic	arrhythmias heart failure

Fig. 28.21 Causes of shock.

Specific shock syndromes

The three important specific syndromes in which shock occurs are:

- Anaphylactic shock.
- Septicaemic shock.
- Diabetic ketoacidosis.

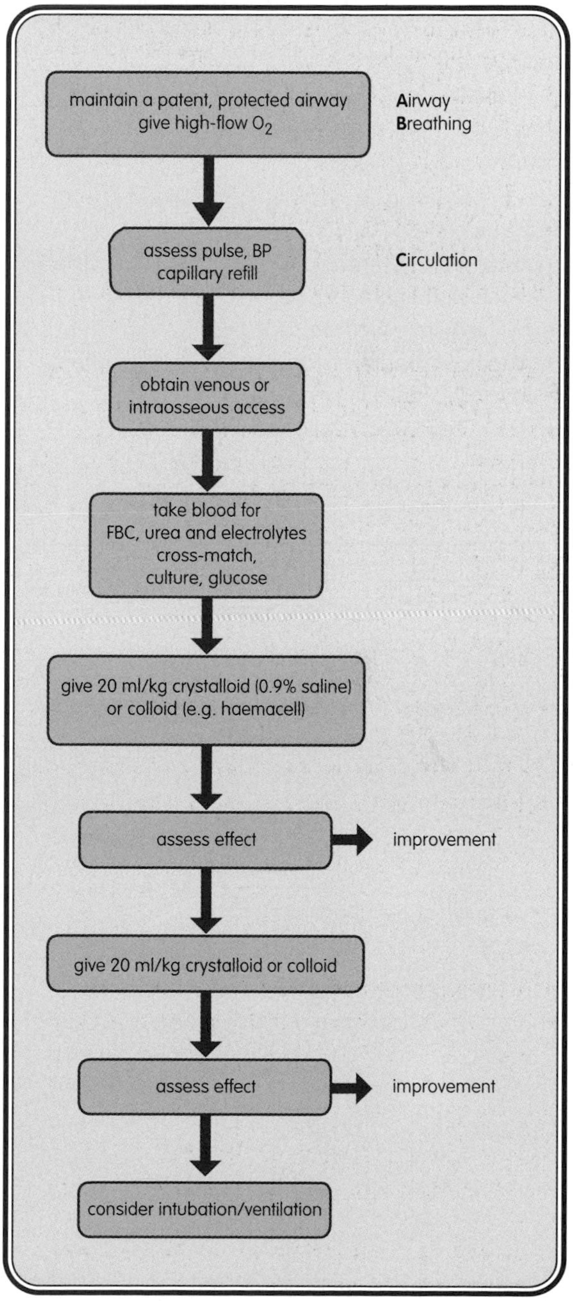

Fig. 28.22 Management of shock (ABC).

Anaphylactic shock

The most common causes are allergy to:

- Drugs, e.g. penicillin.
- Radiographic contrast media.
- Food, especially nuts.

Prodromal symptoms of itching, abdominal pain, and diarrhoea with flushing, facial swelling and urticaria may progress to stridor, wheeze, and circulatory failure. The shock is hypovolaemic due to vasodilatation and capillary leakage.

A protocol for management is shown in Fig. 28.23. If repeated boluses of adrenaline are not effective an infusion may be given.

Septicaemic shock

Septicaemia is an important cause of shock in children. The main pathogens include:

- *Neisseria meningitidis.*
- *Haemophilus influenzae* (unless Hib immunized).
- Staphylococci, pneumococci, streptococci.
- Gram-negative bacteria.

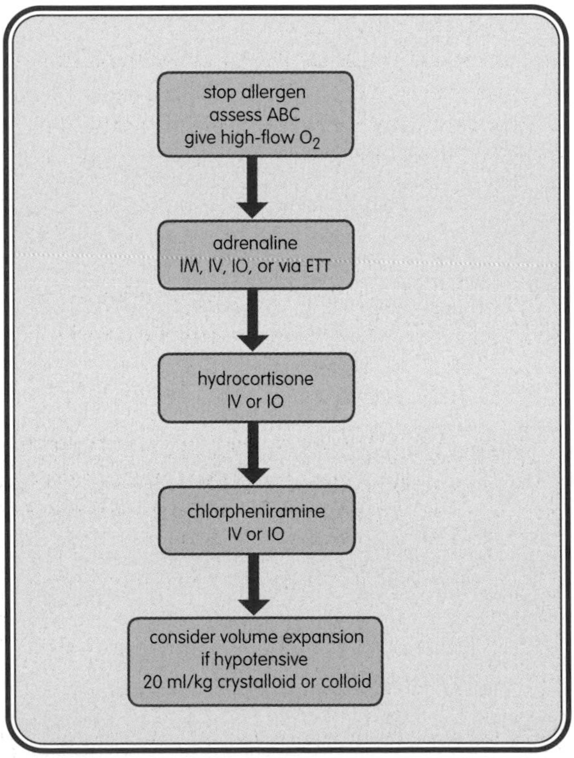

Fig. 28.23 Management of anaphylactic shock.

Meningococcal septicaemia is the most fulminant variety. Death can occur within 12 hours of the first symptom; early diagnosis is vital.

Bacterial toxins trigger the release of various mediators and activators, which may:

- Cause vasodilatation or vasoconstriction.
- Depress cardiac function.
- Disturb cellular oxygen consumption.
- Cause 'capillary leak' with hypovolaemia.
- Promote disseminated intravascular coagulation.

Clinical features

The clinical features progress from early (compensated) to late (decompensated) shock:

- 'Early' shock: increased cardiac output, decreased systemic resistance, warm extremities, high fever, and mental confusion.
- 'Late' shock: reduced cardiac output, hypotension, cool peripheries, and metabolic acidosis.

The cardinal sign of meningococcal septicaemia is a petechial or purpuric rash. In the early stages, this may be subtle, and a careful search for petechiae is required. (In 10% of cases a blanching erythematous rash may occur first.) An injection of benzylpenicillin should be given immediately if a diagnosis of meningococcal septicaemia or meningitis is suspected.

Management

Key points in initial management include:

- Oxygen: 100% O_2 by face mask.
- Fluids: 20 ml/kg of colloid given as a bolus (up to 60 ml/kg may be required if there is substantial capillary leakage).
- Antibiotics: IV benzylpenicillin and a third-generation cephalosporin (e.g. cefotaxime).
- Investigations (Fig. 28.24).

In severe illness, intensive care facilities are required to allow continuous monitoring of circulatory parameters (including central venous pressure), urine output and pulse oximetry. Assisted ventilation and inotropic agents may be required.

Diabetic ketoacidosis

This is an important and life-threatening complication of insulin-dependent diabetes mellitus. It is now relatively uncommon for new cases of diabetes to present in a ketoacidotic state. The majority of episodes are seen in

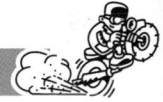

Investigations in septic shock
full blood count and differential blood glucose urea and electrolytes coagulation screen blood culture urine culture blood gases CXR consider lumbar puncture

Fig. 28.24 Investigations in septic shock.

patients known to have type 1 diabetes mellitus.

Diabetic ketoacidosis represents the endstage of insulin deficiency. Deficiency of insulin blocks use of glucose leading to hyperglycaemia. As glucose levels exceed the renal threshold, an osmotic diuresis ensues with severe dehydration and electrolytes losses (sodium and potassium). Without insulin, fat is used as a source of energy leading to the generation of ketones and metabolic acidosis.

Clinical features

The clinical features evolve as the severity of dehydration and acidosis worsens.

- The new diabetic has a history of polyuria, polydipsia, and weight loss. This is followed by the rapid development of vomiting, lethargy, and abdominal pain.
- The known diabetic may have an intercurrent illness with vomiting, poor control, and documented hyperglycaemia and ketonuria.

Characteristic physical signs are listed in Fig. 28.25.

Diagnosis

Essential initial investigations include:

- Blood glucose.
- Urea and electrolytes.
- Arterial blood gas analysis.
- Urine glucose and ketones.

The typical metabolic abnormalities in diabetic ketoacidosis, which will be revealed by these investigations include:

- Hyperglycaemia: blood glucose over 15 mmol/L and glycosuria.
- Ketoacidosis: ketonuria, metabolic acidosis on arterial blood gas analysis (ABG) (pH—low, $[HCO_3]$—reduced, $PaCO_2$—low, respiratory compensation with hypocapnia).
- Dehydration: raised urea.
- Sodium and potassium depletion. Serum sodium concentration is often slightly reduced. Serum potassium concentration may be low, normal, or high depending on renal function and the degree of acidosis.

Management

The mainstays of management are the restoration of fluid and electrolyte status, and insulin (Fig. 28.26).

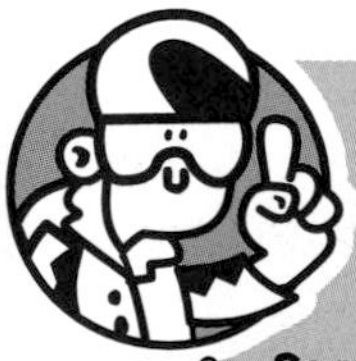

In diabetic ketoacidosis:

- **Total body potassium depletion is always present.**
- **Serum potassium concentration may be high initially if there is severe acidosis (bringing potassium out of cells) and impaired renal perfusion (reducing excretion).**
- **Serum potassium concentration falls with treatment as potassium is driven into cells (with insulin action and correction of acidosis) and renal function improves.**
- **IV fluids need to include potassium to avoid hypokalaemia as treatment proceeds.**

Physical signs in diabetic ketoacidosis	
dehydration	dry mucous membranes loss of skin turgor if severe, circulatory failure (shock) develops
acidosis	smell of ketones on breath Kussmaul breathing: rapid, deep, sighing respiration
altered consciousness	confusion and coma are late signs

Fig. 28.25 Physical signs in diabetic ketoacidosis.

The acidosis will usually correct with correction of fluid balance and insulin therapy. Administration of bicarbonate is rarely required. A nasogastric tube should be passed if there is vomiting or evidence of gastric dilatation.

Careful monitoring is required of:

- Fluid status: weight, input and output.
- Electrolytes: check urea and electrolytes 2–4 hourly initially.
- Acid–base status: check ABG 2–4 hourly initially.
- Blood glucose: monitor hourly.
- ECG monitoring allows early identification of hyperkalaemia or hypokalaemia.
- Vital signs and neurological observations.

Complications

Major complications include:

- Cerebral oedema: manifested by reduced conscious level, headache, irritability, and fits. Prevent this by avoiding *rapid* falls in blood glucose or serum sodium concentrations.
- Cardiac dysrhythmias: usually secondary to electrolyte (potassium) disturbances. Acute renal failure is uncommon.

After the initial 24–48 hours, it is usually possible to switch to oral fluids and 4-hourly subcutaneous soluble insulin on a sliding scale determined by the blood glucose concentration.

Management of diabetic ketoacidosis

Fluids
- if there is severe dehydration (>10%), initial resuscitation is given with 20 mL/kg, 0.9% saline (or colloid)
- ongoing IV fluid requirement is calculated from the deficit and maintenance fluids used, initially, 0.9% or 0.45% NaCl—potassium is added unless anuria present
- when blood glucose falls to <12 mmol/L change to dextrose-containing fluid, e.g. 4% dextrose/0.18% saline

Insulin
- continuous infusion of soluble insulin is given IV
- initial dose is 0.1 IU/kg/h
- aim to reduce blood glucose by about 5 mmol/L/h

Fig. 28.26 Management of diabetic ketoacidosis.

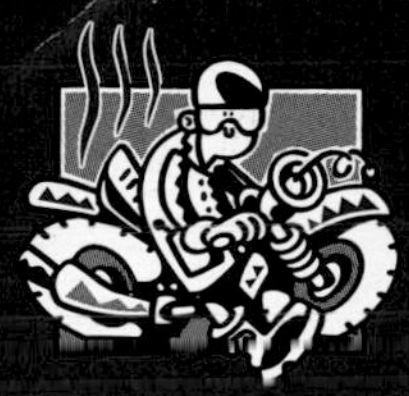

29. Nutrition, Fluids, and Prescribing

Infants and children are more vulnerable than adults to inadequate nutrition or the derangement of fluid and electrolyte balance. Their high surface area to volume ratio is associated with a high metabolic rate, large calorific requirements, and corresponding rapid fluid turnover.

Globally, malnutrition is probably directly or indirectly responsible for half of all deaths of children under 5 years of age. In the developed world, nutrition is a vital consideration in the management of many diseases (such as cystic fibrosis) and special diets are indicated for some disorders (such as coeliac disease, phenylketonuria, and food allergy).

Dehydration associated with diarrhoeal diseases is a major killer worldwide and its treatment with oral rehydration solution represented a major advance. However, attention to fluid and electrolyte status is an important aspect of a wide spectrum of disorders including diabetes mellitus, pyloric stenosis, and postoperative care.

Prescribing for infants and children involves many considerations unique to this age group. The route and frequency of administration must be adapted to the age, and dosage must take into account bodyweight, surface area, and age-dependant changes in drug metabolism and excretion.

NUTRITION

Normal nutritional requirements

A satisfactory dietary intake should meet the normal requirements for energy and protein, together with providing an adequate supply of vitamins and trace elements. Reference values for energy and protein requirements are shown in Fig. 29.1.

Infants and children are vulnerable to undernutrition because of:

- Low nutritional stores of fat and protein.
- Growth creating high nutritional demands (at 4 months of age, 30% of an infant's energy intake is used for growth, but at 3 years of age this has fallen to 2%).

Reference values for energy and protein requirements		
Age	Energy (kcal/kg/day)	Protein (g/kg/day)
0–6 months	115	2.2
6–12 months	95	2.0
1–3 years	95	1.8
4–6 years	90	1.5
7–10 years	75	1.2
11–14 years	60	1.0
15–18 years	50	0.8

Fig. 29.1 Reference values for energy and protein requirements.

- Brain growth: the brain is proportionally larger in infants and is growing rapidly during the last trimester and first 2 years of life. It is vulnerable to energy deprivation during this period.

Infant feeding

An infant's primary source of nutrition is milk, either human breast milk or so-called 'formula' milk based on modified cow's milk. Weaning, the introduction of solid foods is usually initiated between the ages of 3 and 6 months.

Breastfeeding

This is the preferred method for most infants. In general, there is no doubt that 'breast is best'. The many advantages, and few disadvantages, of breastfeeding are listed in Fig. 29.2.

The composition of breast milk, cow's milk, and infant formula does differ significantly (Fig. 29.3).

Breastfeeding in early infancy may be life-saving in developing countries. The popularity of breastfeeding in developed countries is subject to fashion and custom.

Advantages and disadvantages of breast-feeding
Advantages quality: • breast milk has anti-infective properties including secretory IgA, lysozyme, phagocytic cells, lactoferrin (iron-binding agent), a factor that promotes growth of non-pathogenic flora • breast milk has better nutritional qualities, including easily digested protein, low renal solute load, and a favourable calcium to phosphate ratio emotional—if successful, promotes maternal–infant bonding reduction in risk of maternal breast cancer **Disadvantages** volume of intake uncertain transmission of drugs, e.g. laxatives, anticoagulants, antineoplastics nutrient deficiencies: • insufficient vitamin K to prevent haemorrhagic disease of the newborn • vitamin D deficiency (rickets) may occur if there is prolonged breast-feeding and delayed weaning emotional—failure to establish breast-feeding may be a cause of emotional upset

Fig. 29.2 Advantages and disadvantages of breastfeeding.

Unmodified, whole, pasteurized cow's milk is unsuitable as a main diet for infants under the age of 1 year because:

- It contains too much protein and sodium.
- It is deficient in iron and vitamins.

Modified cow's milk formulas have a modified casein to whey ratio, reduced mineral content, and are fortified with iron and vitamins.

Soya formulas

Milks based on soya bean protein have been widely used on the basis that they may prevent the development of atopic features provoked by exposure to cow's milk proteins. They do appear to help infants with genuine cow's milk protein intolerance, but should not be indiscriminately prescribed for vague symptoms of uncertain origin. Disadvantages include a higher aluminium content.

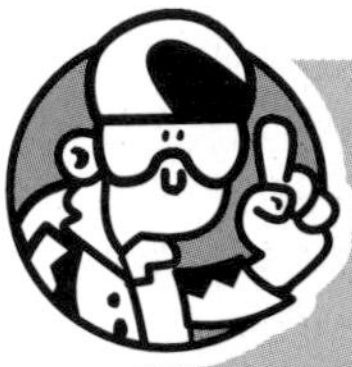

Establishing breastfeeding:

- **The baby should be put to the breast as soon as possible after birth.**
- **Thereafter the baby should be fed on demand (indicated by crying).**
- **Frequent suckling promotes lactation.**
- **The baby's mouth needs to be well applied round the areola, with the nipple drawn into the back of the baby's mouth.**
- **Colostrum (high content of protein and immunoglobulin) rather than milk is produced in first few days.**
- **The interval between feeds gradually lengthens from 2–3 hours to approximately a 4-hourly schedule.**

Composition of different milks (per 100 mL)

	Breast milk	Cow's milk	Infant formula
protein (g)	1.3	3.3	1.5
casein:whey	40:60	60:40	variable
carbohydrate (g)	7.0	4.5	7.0–8.0
fat (g)	4.2	3.6	2.6–3.8
energy (kcal)	70	65	65
sodium (mmol)	0.65	2.3	0.65–1.1
calcium (mmol)	0.87	3.0	1.4
iron (μmol)	1.36	0.9	10
vitamin D (μg)	0.6	0.03	1.0

Fig. 29.3 Composition of different milks (per 100 ml).

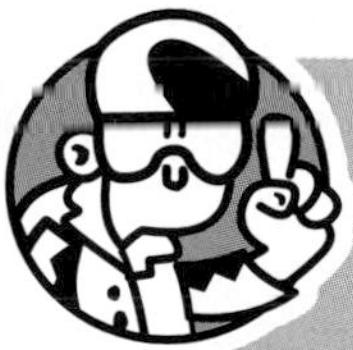

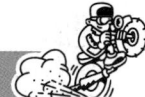

Bottle feeding:

- Is less restrictive for mothers as others can do the feeding.
- Available as a dry powder requiring reconstitution or as ready made liquid feeds.
- Changing 'brands' in response to feeding difficulties is usually a futile gesture.

Weaning

The introduction of solid foods (weaning) is usually undertaken between 3 and 4 months of age. At this age the infant can coordinate swallowing and has reasonable head control. After 6 months of age, breast milk alone becomes nutritionally inadequate and continued breastfeeding without introduction of solids will lead to energy, vitamin, and iron deficiency.

A typical scheme for the introduction of solids is shown in Fig. 29.4.

Introduction of solids	
Age	**Feeding**
3–4 months	cereals, e.g. baby rice
4–5 months	pureed fruit and vegetables, meat (e.g. chicken)
6–7 months	able to chew, e.g. rusks introduce lumpy foods and variety of tastes and textures
8–9 months	bread and butter, fruit
12 months	'real' food in small bits

Fig. 29.4 Introduction of solids.

Special milks

A variety of specialized milks exist that are used in infants who are intolerant of specific constituents. Examples include:

- Low phenylalanine milk: phenylketonuria.
- Low lactose milk: lactose intolerance.
- Soya milk: cow's milk protein intolerance.

Malnutrition

Worldwide, malnutrition due to inadequate intake (starvation) is responsible for millions of childhood deaths. However, malnutrition may also complicate many childhood diseases (Fig. 29.5) and specific nutritional deficiencies such as iron deficiency are not uncommon in the developed world.

Severe malnutrition affects many systems (Fig. 29.6).

Malnutrition in childhood—causes

Inadequate intake
- starvation due to famine
- poverty
- restrictive diets—parental, iatrogenic, self-inflicted
- anorexia nervosa
- anorexia due to chronic illness

Malabsorption
- pancreatic disease, e.g. cystic fibrosis
- coeliac disease
- short gut (postoperative)

Increased energy requirements
- cystic fibrosis
- malignant disease
- burns
- trauma

Fig. 29.5 Malnutrition in childhood—causes.

Consequences of severe malnutrition

- impaired immunity
- delayed wound healing
- apathy and inactivity
- impaired intellectual development

Fig. 29.6 Consequences of severe malnutrition.

The most common dietary deficiencies in the UK are iron and vitamin D.

Assessment of nutritional status

Evaluation involves:

- Dietary history.
- Anthropometry and clinical examination.
- Laboratory investigations.

Dietary history

The food intake, as recalled by the parents or recorded in a diary, is determined over a period of several days.

Anthropometry

This involves measurement of:

- Height—height for age is reduced (stunted growth) in chronic malnutrition.
- Weight—reduced weight with normal height (wasting) is an index of acute malnutrition.
- Midarm circumference—an indication of skeletal muscle mass.
- Skinfold thickness—triceps skinfold thickness is a measure of subcutaneous fat stores.

Clinical syndromes of protein-energy malnutrition include:

- Marasmus—wasted (weight less than 60% of mean for age) wizened appearance, withdrawn, and apathetic.
- Kwashiorkor—occurs in children weaned late from the breast and fed on a relatively high-starch diet. May be precipitated by an acute intercurrent infection. Features include wasting, oedema, sparse hair and depigmented skin, angular stomatitis, and hepatomegaly.

Laboratory investigations

Useful laboratory tests include:

- Serum albumin—reduced in severe malnutrition.
- FBC—low Hb and lymphocyte count.
- Blood glucose.
- Calcium, Phosphate, and vitamin D levels.
- Serum potassium and magnesium levels.

Management

Nutrition may be supplied:

- Enterally, via the gastrointestinal tract: this route is preferred wherever possible.
- Parenterally, directly into the circulation.

In many cases, malnutrition is due to inadequate intake and can be managed by the provision of supplementary enteral feeds given via a nasogastric or gastrostomy tube.

Examples of chronic diseases requiring such supplemental feeding include:

- Cystic fibrosis.
- Congenital heart disease.
- Cerebral palsy.
- Chronic renal failure.
- Malignancy.
- Inflammatory bowel disease.
- Anorexia nervosa.

Vitamin deficiencies

Several important vitamin deficiency diseases still occur in childhood. These include in particular:

- Vitamin D deficiency: rickets.
- Vitamin A deficiency: blindness.
- Vitamin K deficiency: haemorrhagic disease of the newborn.

Scurvy due to vitamin C deficiency is now extremely rare in developed countries.

Vitamin D deficiency—rickets

The effects of vitamin D deficiency on growing bone cause rickets. The bone matrix (osteoid) of the growing bone is inadequately mineralized, giving rise to the clinical features described in Fig. 29.7. The undermineralized bone is less rigid and bends and twists in an abnormal way.

The normal pathways of vitamin D absorption and metabolism are shown in Fig. 29.8.

The most common cause is nutritional deficiency. The minimum daily requirement of vitamin D is 400 IU and may not be attained in infants who are breast fed for a protracted period. An additional important factor is decreased exposure to the sun as vitamin D is synthesized from precursors in the skin under the effect of ultraviolet light. This may occur especially in:

- Infants with dark skin pigmentation.
- Urban living conditions.
- Winter.

Less common causes of rickets include:

- Inherited abnormalities of vitamin D metabolism or of the vitamin D receptor.
- Mineral deficiency, e.g. X-linked hypophosphataemia.

Clinical features of rickets

General
misery
hypotonia
developmental delay
growth failure

Skeletal
craniotabes (thin, soft, skull bones)
enlarged metaphyses (especially wrists and knees)
rickety rosary (enlarged costochondral junctions)
bowing of legs (caused by weight bearing)

Fig. 29.7 Clinical features of rickets.

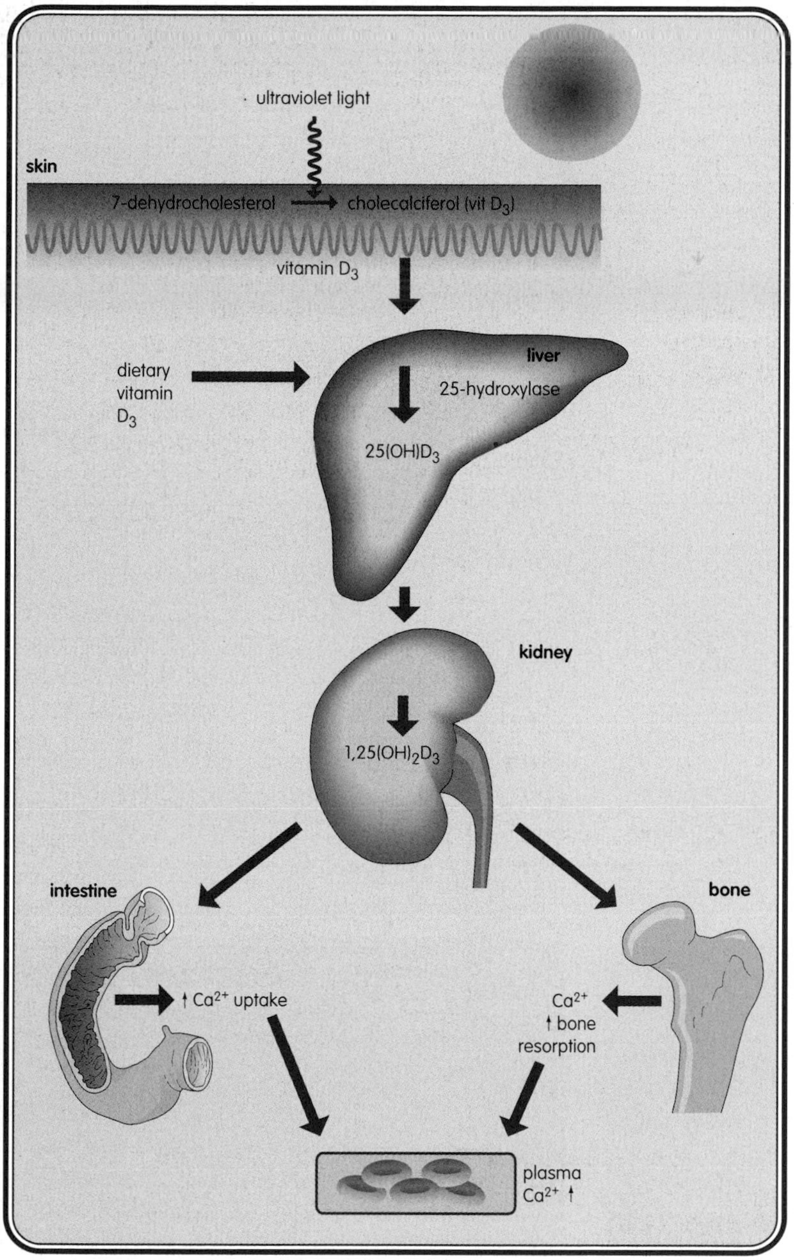

Fig. 29.8 Normal pathways of vitamin D metabolism and action.

- Chronic renal disease.
- Decreased activity of 1α-hydroxylase in the kidneys leads to rickets as one component of renal osteodystrophy.
- Rickets of prematurity. Metabolic bone disease in the premature infant occurs if the milk used contains inadequate calcium and phosphate (1,25-dihydroxycholecalciferol levels are elevated because of the hypophosphataemic stimulus, but there is osteopenia and inadequate mineralization of growing bone).

Diagnosis

This is confirmed by X-ray imaging and blood biochemistry. X-ray of the wrist shows cupping and fraying of the metaphysis and a widened metaphyseal plate (Fig. 29.9).

The biochemical changes in classic nutritional rickets include:

- Serum calcium: low or normal (may be normalized by secondary hyperparathyroidism).
- Serum phosphate: low.
- Serum alkaline phosphatase: elevated.
- Serum parathormone (PTH): elevated.
- Serum 1,25-dihydroxycholecalciferol: low.

Treatment

Prevention is obviously preferred and this is achieved by health education, exposure to sunlight, and supplementation of the diet with minerals and vitamin D when indicated.

Treatment of nutritional rickets is with vitamin D_3 (1,25-dihydroxycholecalciferol) 5000–10 000 IU/day initially for several weeks, followed by provision of 400 IU/day in the diet.

Higher doses may be required in the inherited forms. Biochemistry and radiography monitor the effect of therapy.

Vitamin A (retinol) deficiency

Vitamin A is necessary for membrane stability and it plays a role in vision, keratinization, cornification, and placental development. The body's need for vitamin A can be met by milk, butter, eggs, liver, and dark green or orange-coloured (e.g. carrots) vegetables.

Worldwide about 150 million children are at risk of vitamin A deficiency and it has been calculated that up to a third of a million children go blind each year from vitamin A deficiency. In addition, vitamin A deficiency carries increased mortality from infection and poor growth.

The eye disease develops insidiously with impaired dark adaptation followed by drying of the conjunctiva and cornea (xerophthalmia).

Obesity

If obesity is defined as a weight more than 20% greater than ideal weight for height, then up to 5% of UK school children are obese.

Aetiological factors include:

- Genetic factors.
- Excess carbohydrate intake.
- Reduced activity.

Rarely, an endocrine or chromosomal cause is present such as Cushing syndrome, hypothyroidism, or Prader–Willi syndrome.

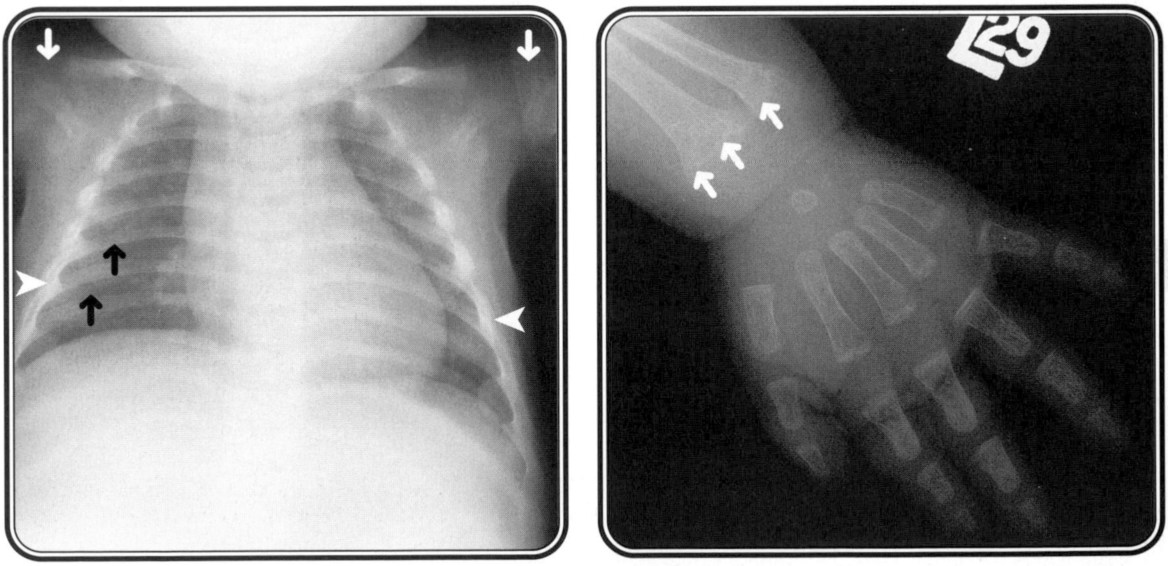

Fig. 29.9 X-ray appearance of rickets. (A) CXR of a young child with partially treated rickets. Note (i) changes at the metaphyses (white arrows), (ii) periosteal reaction on several ribs (white arrowheads), and (iii) bulging of anterior rib ends, the rickety rosary (black arrows). (B) Left wrist X-ray. note the irregular 'cupped' metaphyses with loss of bone density (white arrows).

Obesity has several deleterious consequences including:

- Emotional disturbance—weight gain may lead to low self-esteem and trigger a vicious circle of 'comfort' eating and increased weight.
- Hypoventilation—if severe, Pickwickian syndrome of hypoventilation and hypercapnia with somnolence may occur.
- Long-term complications—75% of obese school children remain obese in adult life, with increased risk of cardiovascular disease, hypertension, and maturity onset diabetes.

Management

This is often difficult, especially as obesity in a child is often accompanied by parental obesity and inappropriate eating habits.

The aim is a reduced-energy diet together with a programme of increased exercise (e.g. swimming and bicycling). All the family should follow the same dietary pattern. The target should be either to keep weight steady or to lose up to 1 kg per week. Sustained compliance is unusual.

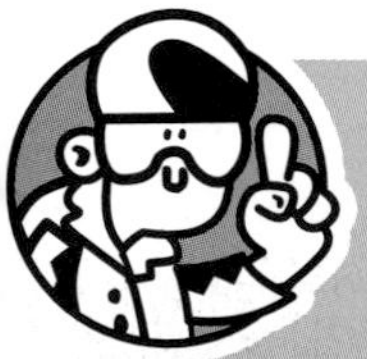

- **Most obese children are tall and above the 50th centile for height.**
- **In Cushing syndrome or hypothyroidism, obesity is associated with low growth velocity and short stature.**

FLUIDS AND ELECTROLYTES

Important physiological factors render children more vulnerable than adults to disturbances of fluid and electrolyte balance (Fig. 29.10). Such disturbances are common in paediatric practice and occur in a number of important clinical contexts (Fig. 29.11).

Basic physiology

It is useful to know how fluid is distributed between the different compartments of the body and what the normal requirements for fluid and electrolytes are. Important changes occur with age as the ratio of surface area to volume alters.

Fluid compartments

These are shown in Fig. 29.12. Infants are more 'watery' and have a higher proportion of fluid in the extracellular space. The percentages can be expressed as volumes: e.g., 70% is equivalent to 700 ml/kg bodyweight (see Hints & Tips).

Blood volume is about 100ml/kg at birth and falls to about 80 ml/kg at 1 year.

Fluid and electrolyte balance in children
Children have a larger surface area to volume ratio than adults
Total body water is a higher percentage of body weight in children
The rate of turnover of fluids and electrolytes is higher in children

Fig. 29.10 Fluid and electrolyte balance in children.

Clinical conditions associated with fluid and electrolyte disturbance
gastroenteritis
burns
diabetic ketoacidosis
renal disease
surgery: preoperative and postoperative care

Fig. 29.11 Clinical conditions associated with fluid and electrolyte disturbance.

Body fluid compartments (as a percentage of body weight)			
Age	**Total body water**	**Extracellular fluid**	**Intracellular fluid**
newborn	70	35	35
12 months	65	25	40
adult	60	20	40

Fig. 29.12 Body fluid compartments (as a percentage of body weight).

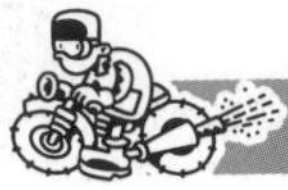

Normal requirements

Fluid requirement is that needed to make up for normal fluid losses, which include essential urine output and 'insensible' losses through sweat, respiration and the GI tract.

Of course, in pathological states there will be additional abnormal losses such as those associated with diarrhoea or vomiting.

A simple formula for calculating normal fluid requirements according to bodyweight is shown in Fig. 29.13.

There are obligatory electrolyte losses in the stools, urine, and sweat, and these require replacement. The electrolyte composition of various body fluids, which may be lost in excessive amounts, is shown in Fig. 29.14. The maintenance requirement for sodium is about 3 mmol/kg/day.

Normal fluid requirements

Body weight	Fluid requirement per 24 hours
first 10 kg	100 ml/kg
second 10 kg	50 ml/kg
further kg	20 ml/kg
example: 24-hour requirement for child weighing 25 kg	
10 kg at 100 ml/kg	= 1000 ml
10 kg at 50 ml/kg	= 500 ml
5 kg at 20 ml/kg	= 100 ml
total	= 1600 ml

Fig. 29.13 Normal fluid requirements.

- **As body density is close to that of water, and 1 litre of water weighs close to 1 kilogram, weights and volumes are freely interchangeable. For example 1000 ml=1000 g (1 litre=1 kg).**
- **Changes in bodyweight are the best guide to short-term changes in fluid balance (e.g. a weight loss of 500 g indicates a fluid deficit of 500 ml).**

Intravenous fluids

These can be divided into colloids, which include large molecules such as proteins, and crystalloids, which usually contain dextrose (glucose) and electrolytes. Colloids are used for plasma volume expansion and crystalloids are used for the management of most fluid and electrolyte disturbances.

The compositions of commonly available crystalloid fluids for intravenous use are shown in Fig. 29.15.

The important features of these solutions are that:

- They are isotonic—their osmolality is close to that of plasma. Clearly, a hypotonic (dilute solution) would lyse red cells and a very hypertonic solution would draw fluid into the circulation.
- Normal saline—is useful for replacing deficits and for rapid volume expansion. However, it is *not* a maintenance fluid, as it contains too much sodium chloride: five times the maintenance requirement.
- 4% dextrose and 0.18% sodium chloride—this is the usual maintenance fluid, but may require addition of potassium chloride.
- Potassium chloride can be added to give a concentration between 5–40 mmol/L.

Electrolyte content of body fluids

Fluid	Na^+ (mmol/L)	K^+ (mmol/L)	Cl^- (mmol/L)
plasma	135–141	3.5–5.5	100–105
gastric	20–80	5–20	100–150
intestinal	100–140	5–15	90–130
diarrhoea	10–90	10–30	10–110

Fig. 29.14 Electrolyte content of body fluids.

Isotonic crystalloid fluids: composition

Fluid	Na^+ (mmol/L)	K^+ (mmol/L)	Cl^- (mmol/L)	Energy (kcal/L)
0.9% saline (normal saline)	150	0	150	0
4% dextrose/ 0.18% saline	30	0	30	160

Fig. 29.15 Isotonic crystalloid fluids: composition.

Specific fluid and electrolyte problems

These are mostly considered elsewhere:

- Dehydration (see Chapter 17).
- Diabetic ketoacidosis (see Chapter 28).
- Burns (see Chapter 28).

Important features concerning certain electrolyte disturbances are considered here.

Sodium

Hypernatraemia is usually a reflection of water loss with a high-solute intake. Correction must be undertaken gradually, to avoid osmotic disequilibrium between the plasma and the brain, with water passing from a rapidly diluted plasma into the brain causing brain swelling.

Hyponatraemia is usually due to water overload, which is reflected in a gain of bodyweight. Management is by fluid restriction.

Potassium

Hypokalaemia is usually seen in combination with alkalosis, such as occurs in pyloric stenosis and hyperaldosteronism.

Hyperkalaemia is potentially dangerous, but it is rare in children for arrhythmias to occur until the level exceeds 7.5 mmol/L. The most common cause is renal failure, but it also occurs in:

- Severe acidosis.
- Hypoaldosteronism.
- Iatrogenic potassium overload.

Immediate management involves:

- Promotion of cellular potassium uptake by β_2 stimulants (nebulized salbutamol).
- Treatment of acidosis (if present) with intravenous sodium bicarbonate.
- Administration of insulin and dextrose.

PAEDIATRIC PRESCRIBING

Prescribing for babies and children is different in several important ways. Firstly, the dose must be adjusted to the body size of the patient. Secondly, the route and frequency of administration of any drug must take into account factors peculiar to childhood. Infants and children do not take kindly to painful intramuscular injections and the administration of medication during school hours generates its own problems.

Prescribing rules

It is essential to

- Write legibly.
- Write in ink, not erasable pencil.
- Date all prescriptions.
- Sign all prescriptions.
- Prescribe the dose correctly (see Hints & Tips).

Calculating the dose

This can be done according to:

- Age.
- Bodyweight.
- Body surface area.

For drugs with a wide therapeutic range, doses are often quoted according to age ranges.

Bodyweight is the most frequently used guide to dose calculation. Body surface area is a more precise physiological guide to dosage, but requires calculation from a nomogram that includes height and weight measurements and is only required for very exact dosage calculations.

A formulary may quote the dose as:

- The total daily dose, with an indication of how it is to be divided.
- The individual dose, with an indication of frequency (e.g. 6-hourly).

Mean bodyweight and body surface area values at various ages are shown in Fig. 29.16.

Route of administration

A variety of routes are available (Fig. 29.17):

- Oral administration is usually most acceptable but some drugs, such as insulin, cannot be given by this route.

Body weight and body surface area by age

Age	Weight (kg)	BSA (m^2)
newborn	3.5	0.25
6 months	7.7	0.40
1 year	10	0.50
5 years	18	0.75
12 years	36	1.25
adult	70	1.80

Fig. 29.16 Body weight and body surface area (BSA) by age.

- Elixirs rather than capsules or tablets are required for infants and often preferred by older children.
- Liquid medicines can be given to young babies using a syringe.
- Intramuscular injections can usually be avoided.
- Ease of IV access makes this the route of choice for most drugs requiring systemic administration.

Insulin is routinely given subcutaneously, the antimitotic agent methotrexate may be given intrathecally, and diazepam is the drug most commonly given per rectum.

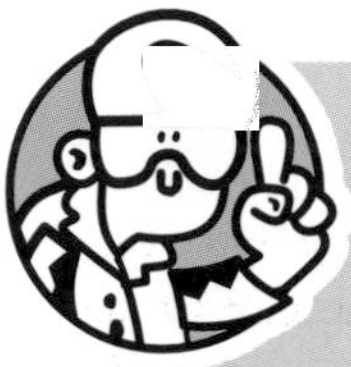

Prescribing the dose:

- **Avoid decimal points, e.g. prescribe 500 mg, *not* 0.5 g.**
- **If the decimal point is unavoidable, use a zero before the point, e.g. 0.5 ml, *not* .5 ml.**
- **Avoid prescribing by volume, unless the medicine is a complex mixture, e.g. Abidec vitamin drops.**
- **Never abbreviate 'micrograms'. The scribbled Greek 'μ' is easily mistaken for 'm'.**

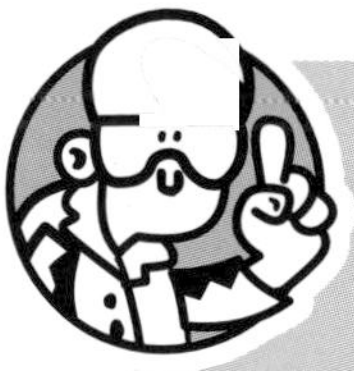

The metric system:

- **Remember that each unit differs by a factor of 1 000, so wrong units are incorrect by a massive amount.**
- **1000 nanograms = 1 microgram *(do not abbreviate).***
- **1000 micrograms = 1 milligram (mg).**
- **1000 milligrams = 1 gram (g).**
- **1000 grams = 1 kilogram (kg).**
- **Most drug dosages are in milligrams, but there are important exceptions.**

Routes of administration

Route	Abbreviation
oral	p.o.
intravenous	i.v.
intramuscular	i.m.
subcutaneous	s.c.
intrathecal	i.t.
rectal	p.r.
inhaled	inh
topical	top

Fig. 29.17 Routes of administration.

PAEDIATRIC FORMULARY

There are a small number of commonly used drugs for which it is important to know the indications, mode of action, and side effects. These are considered here. Dosages are given for some, but do not need to be memorized.

Drugs of major importance in paediatric practice are listed in Fig. 29.18.

Antibiotics

A reasonable first-line choice of antibiotic in some common clinical contexts are listed in Fig. 29.19.

Analgesics/antipyretics

Paracetamol

This is the preferred drug for the prophylaxis and management of fever and for general pain relief. It should be given every 4 hours. Adverse effects are uncommon, but of course, an overdose may cause hepatic toxicity. It is not an anti-inflammatory drug.

Ibuprofen is a useful alternative and does have an anti-inflammatory action. Aspirin is not used in children under 12 years because of the danger of Reye's syndrome.

Bronchodilators

The β_2 agonists salbutamol and terbutaline are very similar in their properties. Inhalation is the most effective mode of delivery. They are very safe, but in excessive dosage may cause tremor, tachycardia, and hypokalaemia.

Ipratropium bromide is an anticholinergic drug that causes bronchodilation. It is believed to be more useful than β_2 agonists for the treatment of wheezing in infants (under 1 year old).

Aminophylline is used intravenously in acute severe asthma. There is a danger of cardiac arrhythmias in overdose especially in the presence of hypoxia.

Steroids

Prednisolone is the most commonly used oral preparation and is available in an enteric-coated form. It is used in acute asthma, the nephrotic syndrome, and for induction of remission in acute leukaemia. The most important side effects in protracted usage are growth suppression and the vulnerability to viral infections such as chickenpox.

Hydrocortisone is used on occasion when rapid systemic treatment is required (such as in acute asthma or anaphylactic shock). It is also the usual first-line topical steroid (as a 1% ointment or cream) for eczema.

Important drugs in childhood

Category	Class	Drug
antibiotics	penicillins	penicillin V and G amoxycillin flucloxacillin co-amoxiclav
	cephalosporins	cefuroxime cefotaxime
	macrolides	erythromycin clarithromycin
	aminoglycosides	gentamicin
	folate inhibitor	trimethoprim
analgesics/ antipyretics		paracetamol ibuprofen
antiasthma drugs	bronchodilators	salbutamol terbutaline ipratropium bromide aminophylline
	inhaled steroids	budesonide beclomethasone
hormones	steroids	prednisolone hydrocortisone
	insulins	soluble insulin
antiepilepsy drugs		sodium valproate carbamazepine diazepam
laxatives		senokot lactulose
nutritional supplements	vitamins	abidec iron

Fig. 29.18 Important drugs in childhood.

Antiepilepsy drugs

Sodium valproate is the first choice for oral monotherapy in most generalized epilepsies, including those characterized by generalized tonic–clonic seizures, absence seizures, and myoclonic seizures. Side effects are uncommon, but include increased appetite (weight gain) and transient hair loss. Rare cases of fatal hepatic failure have been reported.

Carbamazepine is first-line oral monotherapy for most partial epilepsies. It should be introduced gradually to avoid excessive drowsiness.

Diazepam is used for the treatment of protracted generalized seizures and may be given rectally or intravenously. The most important side effect is respiratory depression.

Laxatives

The two most useful laxatives are senna, which acts by increasing intestinal mobility, and lactulose, which is a semisynthetic disaccharide and acts as a stool softener. Senna is given as syrup. Both are very safe and the most common mistake is to use too low a dose. Senna can cause cramping abdominal pain.

Nutritional supplements

Abidec, as the name implies, is a multivitamin preparation that contains vitamins A, B, D, and C.

Iron preparations may contain any of the various iron salts, most commonly ferrous sulphate or sodium iron edetate. When estimating the dosage, the relative ratio of iron salt to elemental iron should be taken into account. Iron is highly toxic in overdose.

Antibiotics usage in common infections

Condition	Antibiotic
acute tonsillitis	amoxycillin
otitis media	amoxycillin
pneumonia—lobar	cefuroxime
pneumonia—'atypical'	erythromycin
bacterial meningitis	cefotaxime
osteomyelitis	flucloxacillin
septic skin spots, boils	flucloxacillin
urinary tract infection	trimethoprim

Fig. 29.19 Antibiotics usage in common infections.

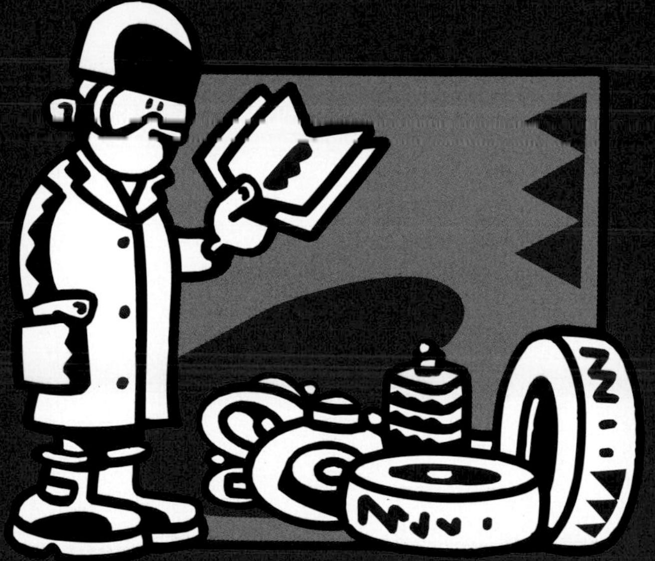

SELF-ASSESSMENT

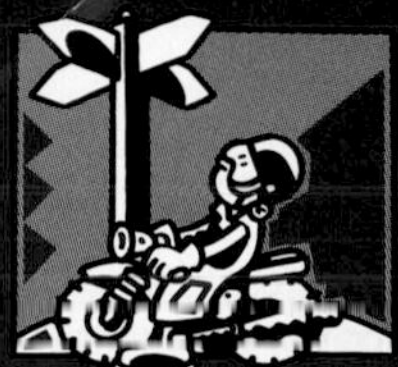

Multiple-choice Questions

Indicate whether each answer is true or false.

1. An 'innocent' cardiac murmur:

a) Is usually heard in diastole.
b) Is associated with a thrill.
c) May vary with posture.
d) Is always asymptomatic.
e) Does not require antibiotic prophylaxis for dental procedures.

---

2. The following are examples of cyanotic heart disease:

a) Coarctation of the aorta.
b) Ventricular septal defect.
c) Fallot's tetralogy.
d) Pulmonary stenosis.
e) Transposition of the great arteries.

---

3. Thrombocytopenia (low platelet count) is a recognized feature of:

a) Henoch–Schönlein purpura.
b) Acute lymphoblastic leukaemia.
c) Kawasaki disease.
d) Disseminated intravascular coagulation.
e) Haemolytic disease of the newborn.

---

4. Sickle-cell disease:

a) Is inherited as an autosomal recessive disorder.
b) Can be diagnosed antenatally.
c) Presents with severe anaemia at birth.
d) Is associated with hyposplenism.
e) Is caused by a single amino acid change in the α-globin chain

---

5. Wilms tumour (nephroblastoma):

a) May be associated with aniridia.
b) May present with painless haematuria.
c) May be associated with raised levels of urinary catecholamines
d) Occurs most commonly under the age of 3 years.
e) Is never treated surgically.

---

6. Recognized features of Kawasaki disease (mucocutaneous lymph node syndrome) include:

a) Protracted fever.
b) Preceding streptococcal infection.
c) Bilateral conjunctivitis.
d) A cardiac murmur.
e) Sudden death from myocardial infarction.

7. Intussusception in childhood:

a) Is most commonly ileocaecal.
b) Is usually painless.
c) Most commonly occurs under 2 years of age.
d) Characteristically is associated with a mass in the right hypochondrium.
e) Always requires surgical treatment.

---

8. The following conditions are inherited as autosomal recessive traits:

a) Duchenne muscular dystrophy.
b) Cystic fibrosis.
c) Haemophilia.
d) Marfan syndrome.
e) Phenylketonuria.

---

9. In meningococcal septicaemia:

a) There is characteristically a rash which blanches.
b) Meningitis is always present.
c) Antibiotic therapy should be withheld until blood cultures have been taken.
d) Mortality is high if treatment is delayed.
e) Household contacts should receive antibiotic prophylaxis.

---

10. Respiratory distress syndrome due to surfactant deficiency in the newborn:

a) Can be treated with exogenous surfactant.
b) Has an increased incidence in infants of mothers with diabetes mellitus.
c) Is strongly correlated with preterm birth.
d) Shares no clinical features with neonatal pneumonia.
e) Responds to antibiotic treatment.

---

11. Turner syndrome is characterized by:

a) Short stature.
b) Karyotype 45, XO.
c) Precocious puberty.
d) Ambiguous genitalia.
e) Associated congenital heart disease.

---

12. The following are characteristic features of rickets:

a) Normal or low serum alkaline phosphatase.
b) Hypercalcaemia.
c) Widening and 'fraying' of epiphyses on X-ray.
d) Association with protracted breastfeeding in dark-skinned patients.
e) Secondary hypoparathyroidism.

13. With regard to fluid and electrolyte balance in children:

a) Normal saline is an ideal fluid for intravenous maintenance requirements.
b) For initial resuscitation of hypovolaemia a volume of 20ml/kg body weight is suitable.
c) Pyloric stenosis is often associated with hyperchloraemic acidosis.
d) Hypernatraemia (serum sodium >150 mmol/L) should be corrected as rapidly as possible.
e) Oral rehydration solutions contain dextrose to enhance palatability.

---

14. Chickenpox (varicella zoster) is characterized by:

a) Low infectivity.
b) Sequential appearance of different 'crops' of vesicles.
c) Initial appearance of the rash on the extremities.
d) An unusually mild course in immunosuppressed children.
e) Cerebellitis as an occasional postinfectious complication.

---

15. The following are features of Duchenne muscular dystrophy:

a) Increased incidence in girls.
b) An increased incidence of mild learning impairment.
c) Raised serum creatine phosphokinase.
d) Usually presents in the first year of life.
e) Pseudohypertrophy of calf muscles.

---

16. Febrile convulsions:

a) Are very common under 6 months of age.
b) Have an average duration of 30 minutes.
c) Are best prevented by long-term prophylaxis using carbamazepine.
d) Are not classified as a form of epilepsy.
e) May show a familial occurrence.

---

17. In congenital adrenal hyperplasia:

a) Inheritance is X-linked recessive.
b) 21-hydroxylase is the enzyme most commonly deficient.
c) Presentation with a salt-losing crisis may occur in the first few weeks of life.
d) Male infants usually have ambiguous genitalia (intersex).
e) ACTH is the treatment of choice.

---

18. Infantile hypertrophic pyloric stenosis:

a) Characteristically presents at birth.
b) Is more common in female than male infants.
c) Has a familial occurrence.
d) Is associated with a hypokalaemic alkalosis.
e) Is not treated surgically.

19. In the management of a 3-year-old child admitted with bruising and suspected non-accidental injury:

a) A skeletal survey is indicated.
b) Normal coagulation studies exclude any underlying bleeding diathesis.
c) Parental visiting should not be allowed until a case conference has been held.
d) History taken directly from the child at this age is unreliable.
e) The law can allow the child to be kept in hospital against the parents' wishes.

---

20. Brain tumours in children:

a) Are most commonly in the posterior fossa.
b) Rarely present with seizures.
c) Commonly present with symptoms and signs of raised intracranial pressure.
d) Never show calcification on skull X-ray.
e) Are usually primary rather than metastatic.

---

21. In the management of diabetic ketoacidosis:

a) All patients with diabetic ketoacidosis are depleted of total body potassium.
b) The severe metabolic acidosis causes a shift of potassium from extracellular fluid into cells.
c) Rehydration is more important than insulin treatment in the early phase.
d) Sodium bicarbonate should be given for metabolic acidosis.
e) A long-acting insulin preparation should be used.

---

22. In the assessment and investigation of a child with suspected idiopathic epilepsy:

a) Cranial imaging by MR is mandatory.
b) An abnormal interictal EEG is an absolute indication for treatment.
c) Rapid recovery of consciousness after an episode favours a 'faint' rather than a fit.
d) A family history of epilepsy would be highly exceptional.
e) Sodium valproate is first line monotherapy for generalized epilepsy in a 10-year-old.

---

23. In childhood asthma:

a) Nebulized salbutamol is used in an acute attack.
b) There is an association with atopic eczema.
c) Regular oral steroid therapy is indicated for prophylaxis of moderate to severe asthma.
d) Swimming should be discouraged.
e) Most 2-year-olds can use a metered dose (aerosol) inhaler without a spacer.

---

24. The following vaccines are live, attenuated vaccines:

a) Mumps, measles, and rubella (MMR).
b) BCG.
c) Diphtheria.

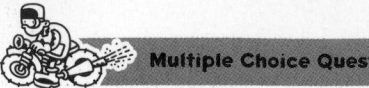

d) Pertussis.
e) Oral (Sabin) poliomyelitis vaccine.

25. Haemorrhagic disease of the newborn:

a) Usually occurs in breastfed infants.
b) Is associated with thrombocytopenia.
c) Can be prevented by vitamin K.
d) Is an inherited condition.
e) Usually presents within 24 hours of birth.

26. Systemic oral steroids have an established role in the management of:

a) Classical 'minimal-change' nephrotic syndrome.
b) Transient synovitis (irritable hip).
c) Status asthmaticus.
d) Idiopathic thrombocytopenia purpura.
e) Septic arthritis.

27. Haemophilia:

a) Is inherited as an X-linked recessive disorder.
b) Rarely presents in the newborn.
c) Is characterized by bleeding into skin and mucous membranes.
d) May be complicated by chronic arthropathy.
e) Is due to factor IX deficiency.

28. Urticaria in childhood:

a) Is usually benign.
b) May be caused by food allergy.
c) Requires treatment with oral steroids.
d) Antihistamines are contraindicated.
e) Usually involves the mucous membranes.

29. Napkin dermatitis (nappy rash):

a) Is an indication of neglect.
b) Spares skin creases if due to candida (thrush) infection.
c) Should be treated with topical hydrocortisone.
d) May be caused by staphylococcal exotoxins.
e) Is more common in bottle-fed infants.

30. The cerebrospinal fluid:

a) Has a normal glucose concentration two thirds that in blood.
b) Is normally slightly opalescent.
c) Has a high white cell count in encephalitis.
d) Shows increased protein concentration in bacterial meningitis.
e) Never contains microorganisms visible on microscopy in health.

31. With regard to viral infections in childhood:

a) Sixth disease (roseola infantum) is due to infection with human herpes virus type 6.
b) Measles may be complicated by encephalitis.
c) Viral gingivostomatitis is most commonly caused by coxsackie virus infection.
d) Acute infection with hepatitis B virus (HBV) is associated with IgM antibodies to HBc antigen.
e) The average incubation period for chickenpox is 4 weeks.

32. Signs of heart failure in a baby include:

a) Swollen ankles.
b) Bradycardia.
c) Hepatomegaly.
d) Tachypnoea.
e) Poor weight gain.

33. Whooping cough (pertussis) in children:

a) Is spread by droplet infection.
b) Has an incubation period of 3 weeks.
c) Is characterized by a paroxysmal cough which may persist for up to 100 days.
d) Is often associated with lymphopenia.
e) Is less dangerous in very young infants.

34. Cystic fibrosis is:

a) Due to mutations in a gene encoding an ATP-binding cassette transporter.
b) Associated with a carrier rate of 1:25 in White people.
c) Not possible to diagnose antenatally.
d) Associated with low concentrations of sodium and chloride in sweat.
e) Associated with high levels of fertility in surviving adult males.

35. With regard to tuberculosis in childhood:

a) Affected children are highly infectious.
b) BCG immunization provides close to 100% protection.
c) A positive response to tuberculin testing is an indication of previous or present infection with mycobacterium.
d) Isoniazid and rifampicin are commonly used for treatment of childhood TB.
e) Cultures of the bacillus will be positive within 10 days.

36. Gastrooesophageal reflux is:

a) More common in preterm infants.
b) Can cause recurrent aspiration pneumonia.
c) Characterized by projectile vomiting.
d) Often helped by thickening feeds.
e) Not helped by early introduction of solid feeds.

37. Recurrent abdominal pain in childhood:

a) Usually has an organic cause.
b) May be caused by thread worms.
c) Should be intensively investigated in most cases.
d) Is more likely to be organic if periumbilical.
e) Responds well to drug therapy with non-steroidal anti-inflammatory agents.

38. Urinary tract infections in childhood:

a) Are more common in boys up to age 3 months.
b) *Proteus* or *Klebsiella spp.* are the usual pathogens.
c) Can be diagnosed without resort to urine culture.
d) Oral trimethoprim is a suitable antibiotic for initial treatment of an uncomplicated UTI in an older child.
e) Ultrasound is the imaging method used to identify vesicoureteric reflux.

---

39. Acute nephritis:

a) Is associated with very heavy proteinuria.
b) May complicate Henoch–Schönlein purpura.
c) Is usually postinfectious following a streptococcal throat or skin infection.
d) Is rarely associated with macroscopic haematuria.
e) Is characterized by hypovolaemia and low blood pressure.

---

40. The nephrotic syndrome:

a) Is usually associated with macroscopic haematuria.
b) Causes oedema restricted to the face and eyes.
c) Is associated with 'minimal change' histology on light microscopy in 90% of childhood cases.
d) Requires renal biopsy for confirmation of diagnosis in all cases.
e) Most commonly responds to oral steroid therapy.

---

41. Hydrocephalus in infants:

a) Is the most common cause of significant macrocephaly.
b) Can be diagnosed using cranial ultrasound.
c) May occur as a complication of intraventricular haemorrhage.
d) Is usually treated with a ventriculoatrial shunt.
e) May be associated with upward deviation of the eyes (sun-rising sign).

---

42. Infantile spasms (West syndrome) is:

a) A benign form of childhood epilepsy.
b) Rarely occurs under 1 year of age.
c) Is associated characteristically with a 3Hz spike-wave pattern on EEG.
d) May be misdiagnosed as infantile colic.
e) Associated with tuberous sclerosis.

---

43. Developmental dysplasia of the hip:

a) Is more common in boys.
b) Is less common after breech delivery.
c) Can be diagnosed by ultrasound scan.
d) Is a cause of delayed walking.
e) Is associated with limited abduction of the flexed hip.

---

44. Bacterial infections of the bones or joints:

a) Are most comonly caused by *Staph. aureus.*
b) Can be diagnosed by X-ray changes found early in the course of the illness.
c) Commonly involve the hip or knee.
d) Are rarely associated with a fever.
e) Can be treated initially with oral antibiotics.

---

45. Juvenile chronic arthritis:

a) May present with a systemic illness without evidence of arthritis.
b) The polyarticular subtype is more common in boys.
c) Rheumatoid factor is positive in the majority of patients.
d) Uveitis is an important cause of morbidity in the pauciarticular subtype.
e) Systemic steroids may be indicated for severe disease.

---

46. Attention-deficit hyperactivity disorder:

a) Is more common in boys than girls.
b) Is characterized by impulsive behaviour.
c) Responds well to sedative drugs.
d) Usually reflects an underlying brain disorder.
e) Is partly caused by genetic factors.

---

47. In anorexia nervosa:

a) There is a disturbed body image.
b) The peak age of onset is 14 years.
c) Girls outnumber boys by 3 to 1.
d) The mortality rate is less than 5%.
e) Fine lanugo hair over the trunk and limbs is a characteristic feature.

---

48. The Children Act (England and Wales 1989, Scotland 1995):

a) Defines parental responsibilities rather than rights.
b) Places the welfare of the child paramount.
c) Requires local authorities to keep a register of children with disabilities.
d) Includes new laws on adoption.
e) Lays down court orders related to child protection.

---

49. Fragile X syndrome:

a) Is due to expansion of a triplet repeat (CGG) in the FRAXA gene.
b) Is the second most common cause of severe learning impairment.
c) Does not occur in females.
d) Is associated with small testes in males.
e) Is associated with macrocephaly.

---

50. Protracted jaundice in the newborn:

a) Is present if jaundice persists beyond 2 weeks of age.
b) Is usually a conjugated hyperbilirubinaemia.
c) Affects 1% of healthy breastfed infants.
d) May be a sign of urinary tract infection.
e) May be caused by biliary atresia.

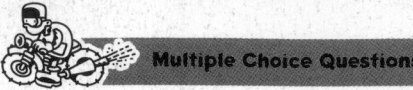

Short-answer Questions

1. Discuss the clinical manifestations of infection with *Staphylococcus aureus* in infants and children.

2. How would you manage moderately severe atopic eczema in a 9-month-old infant?

3. Describe the presentation and management of ventricular septal defect.

4. Write short notes on acute viral bronchiolitis.

5. Discuss the clinical features, diagnosis, and management of viral gastroenteritis in a 1-year-old infant.

6. Discuss the management of nocturnal enuresis ('bed-wetting') in childhood.

7. Write brief notes on cerebral palsy.

8. Discuss the differential diagnosis of acute onset of a limp in a 3-year-old child.

9. Give an account of the causes of iron deficiency anaemia in infancy and childhood.

10. Write brief notes on acute leukaemia in childhood.

11. Describe the aetiology and pathophysiology of insulin-dependent (type 1) diabetes mellitus of childhood.

12. Write brief notes on attention-deficit hyperactivity disorder.

13. Give an account of the current UK schedule for primary immunization.

14. Describe the clinical features and diagnosis of Down syndrome.

15. Give an overview of the common clinical problems encountered by a newborn infant born at 28 weeks gestation and weighing 1000 g.

16. Describe the aetiology and management of jaundice in the newborn.

17. Write brief notes on head injuries in children.

18. Discuss the diagnosis and management of acute convulsions in a child aged 18 months.

19. What are the advantages and disadvantages of breast feeding?

20. Discuss the diagnosis and management of short stature.

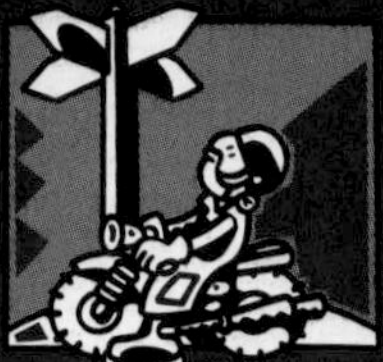

Case-based Questions

1. A 3-year-old Malaysian boy presents with a history of fever and extreme irritability which has lasted for 5 days. On examination he has bilateral conjunctivitis, marked cervical lymphadenopathy, and swollen, erythematous palms, and soles. His lips are red and cracked. Cardiovascular examination is normal except for a tachycardia of 110 beats/min. His temperature is 38.7°C.

a. What is the most likely diagnosis?
b. What investigations are indicated?

---

2. A 6-week-old White female is brought to A&E with a history of becoming pale, breathless, and unresponsive over the preceding hour. On examination she appears severely ill with pallor and cool extremities. On examination the heart rate is 220 beats/min with a blood pressure of 60/40 mmHg. No murmur is audible. She is tachypnoiec, respiratory rate is 55 beats/min, and there is an enlarged liver (4 cm).

a. What is the most likely diagnosis?
b. What investigation is indicated and what management manoeuvre is indicated if the suspected diagnosis is confirmed?

---

3. An 8-month-old male infant presents with a 10- hour history of recurrent vomiting, episodic screaming, and pallor, and recent passage of a stool which his parents describe as looking like 'redcurrant jelly'. On examination he appears well and afebrile. Abdominal examination is recorded as normal by the junior resident, but the specialist registrar suspects a palpable mass in the right hypochondrium.

a. What is the most likely diagnosis?
b. What investigation is indicated?

---

4. A 4-year-old Asian boy presents with a history of swelling around the eyes, most noticeable in the mornings, for the preceding 5 days. The parents have noted that his urine appears 'frothy' and is reduced in volume. On examination he has generalized oedema involving the periorbital region, the abdominal wall, and the lower limbs. The BP is 95/60 mmHg. There is dullness to percussion and reduced breath sounds at the right base. Abdominal examination reveals generalized tenderness.

a. What is the most likely diagnosis?
b. What investigations are indicated to confirm or exclude this diagnosis?

5. A 4-year-old boy presents with difficulty in climbing stairs. Birth and neonatal history were normal but he has delayed motor milestones. He sat at 1 year, stood at 15 months, and walked at 19 months. Two siblings are both well. On examination he has lordosis and a waddling gait. The calf muscles appear hypertrophied and the tendon reflexes are slow.

a. What is the most likely diagnosis?
b. List three useful investigations.

---

6. A 7-year-old girl presents with a 3-day history of recurrent, colicky abdominal pain and arthralgia affecting one wrist and both ankles. On examination she is afebrile and has minimal, generalized abdominal tenderness. Her BP is elevated at 150/95mmHg. There is a petechial rash over her buttocks and lower limbs bilaterally, and oedema over the dorsal surface of both feet. Urine testing is positive for protein and blood.

a. What is the most likely diagnosis?
b. Which systems are affected by the disease process?

---

7. A 15-month-old girl wakes in the night with difficulty breathing. She has been unwell for the preceding 3 days with a coryzal illness. On examination she is mildly pyrexial with a loud, predominantly inspiratory stridor and an intermittent 'barking' cough. There is a marked tracheal tug and tachypnoea, respiratory rate is 45 breaths/min. Auscultation of the chest is normal.

a. What is the most likely diagnosis?
b. Describe the initial management.

---

8. A 6 -year-old girl has generated concern at school on account of excessive 'day dreaming'. A history from the mother indicates that she has frequent episodes lasting 10–15 seconds during which she appears to be unaware of her surroundings. There is no loss of posture or abnormal movements. If an attack occurs when she is talking she will stop midsentence. Her previous history and neurodevelopmental progress is normal and neurological examination reveals no abnormality. An EEG shows generalized 3Hz spike–wave activity which is provoked by hyperventilation.

a. What is the most likely diagnosis?
b. What is the treatment of choice?

9. A 7-year-old Nigerian boy presents with a high fever. He was born in the UK and returned 2 weeks previously from a visit to his uncle in the Gambia. On examination he has a temperature of 40°C. There is mild clinical anaemia and the spleen is just palpable. His mother is known to have sickle-cell disease but his father's sickle status is unknown. Investigation reveals Hb 8.5g/dl, WBC 15 x 10^9/L and platelet count 40 x 10^9/L.

a. What disease must now be excluded and how?
b. What treatment is he likely to require?

10. A 12 year-old girl presents with frequency of micturition. She has been treated 10 days previously for a presumed urinary tract infection by her GP. Further enquiry reveals excessive thirst and a history of significant weight loss over the preceding 2 months. She has vomited once that morning. On examination she is moderately dehydrated with sweet-smelling breath and a respiratory rate of 35 breaths/min.

a. What investigations are required to confirm the most likely diagnosis?
b. Outline the initial management.

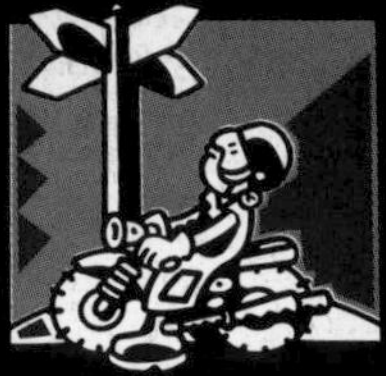

MCQ Answers

1. a) F, b) F, c) T, d) T, e) T

2. a) F, b) F, c) T, d) F, e) T

3. a) F, b) T, c) F, d) T, e) F

4. a) T, b) T, c) F, d) T, e) F

5. a) T, b) T, c) F, d) T, e) F

6. a) T, b) F, c) T, d) F, e) T

7. a) T, b) F, c) T, d) T, e) F

8. a) F, b) T, c) F, d) F, e) T

9. a) T, b) F, c) F, d) T, e) T

10. a) T, b) T, c) T, d) F, e) F

11. a) T, b) T, c) F, d) F, e) T

12. a) F, b) F, c) T, d) T, e) F

13. a) F, b) T, c) F, d) F, e) F

14. a) F, b) T, c) F, d) F, e) T

15. a) F, b) T, c) T, d) F, e) T

16. a) F, b) F, c) F, d) T, e) T

17. a) F, b) T, c) T, d) F, e) F

18. a)F, b) F, c) T, d) T, e) F

19. a) T, b) F, c) F, d) F, e) T

20. a) T b) T, c) T, d) F, e) T

21. a) T, b) F, c) T, d) F, e) F

22. a) F, b) F, c) T, d) F, e) T

23. a) T, b) T, c) F, d) F, e) F

24. a) T, b) T, c) F, d) F, e) T

25. a) T, b) F, c) T, d) F, e) F

26. a) T, b) F, c) T, d) T, e) F

27. a) T, b) T, c) F, d) T, e) F

28. a) T, b) T, c) F, d) F, e) F

29. a) F, b) F, c) F, d) F, e) T

30. a) T, b) F, c) F, d) T, e) T

31. a) T, b) T, c) F, d) T, e) F

32. a) F, b) F, c) T, d) T, e) T

33. a) T, b) F, c) T, d) F, e) F

34. a) T, b) T, c) F, d) F, e) F

35. a) F, b) F, c) F, d) T, e) F

36. a) T, b) T, c) F, d) T, e) F

37. a) F, b) F, c) F, d) F, e) F

38. a) T, b) F, c) F, d) T, e) F

39. a) F, b) T, c) T, d) F, e) F

40. a) F, b) T, c) T, d) F, e) T

41. a) T, b) T, c) T, d) T, e) F

42. a) F, b) F, c) F, d) T, e) T

43. a) F, b) F, c) T, d) T, e) T

44. a) T, b) F, c) T, d) F, e) F

45. a) T, b) F, c) F, d) T, e) T

46. a) T, b) T, c) F, d) F, e) T

47. a) T, b) T, c) F, d) T, e) T

48. a) T, b) T, c) T, d) T, e) T

49. a) T, b) T, c) F, d) F, e) T

50. a) T, b) F, c) F, d) T, e) T

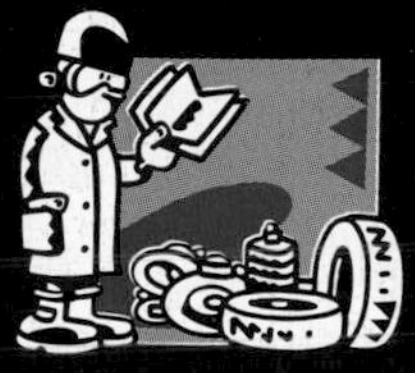

SAQ Answers

1. *Staphylococcus aureus* is carried in the nares and skin in up to 50% of children and infections occur when local defences are compromised. It most commonly causes superficial infections such as impetigo, septic skin spots, and boils. However, haematogenous spread may lead to deep infections of the bones, joints, or lungs. Abscesses may form.

   Impetigo is a highly contagious skin infection occurring on the face in young infants and children. A boil (or furuncle) is an infection of a hair follicle or sweat gland. Osteomyelitis most commonly occurs in the long bones and septic arthritis in the hip or knee.

   Certain types of *S. aureus* cause disease by producing exotoxins. Clinical syndromes produced by toxin-producing organisms include staphylococcal scalded skin syndrome and toxic shock syndrome.

   The antibiotic of choice for treating infection with S. *aureus* is flucloxacillin.

2. Management of moderate atopic eczema in a 9-month-old infant would include

   a) Avoidance of aggravating factors such as:
      - Synthetic or woollen fabrics (cotton clothing is best).
      - Allergens such as dander from furry pets.
      - Excessive heat.

   b) Emollients (e.g. aqueous cream) to moisturize and soften the skin.
   c) Mild topical steroids, e.g. 1% hydrocortisone to affected areas twice daily.
   d) Oral antihistamines at night to reduce itching and help sleep.
   e) Treatment of complications such as secondary bacterial infection with oral antibiotics.

3. The presentation, prognosis, and management depend on the size and position of the ventricular septal defect (VSD).

   a) Small VSD (maladie de Roger). The child is asymptomatic and the murmur is usually picked up on routine examination. Antibiotic prophylaxis is required for dental extractions, but no other treatment is required. Spontaneous closure often occurs.

   b) Medium VSD. These present with symptoms during infancy including failure to thrive, poor feeding, and recurrent chest infections. On examination there may be a thrill and a harsh pansystolic murmur loudest at the third and fourth left intercostal spaces.

      If cardiac failure develops, it should be treated with diuretics. If there is still a significant left-to-right shunt at 4 years of age, closure should be undertaken before the child starts school.

   c) Large VSD. Heart failure develops early. The systolic murmur may be soft in a large defect. Banding of the pulmonary artery (to reduce the left-to-right shunt) may be necessary and medical treatment of any cardiac failure until the child is big enough for definitive surgical correction.

4. Bronchiolitis is most commonly caused by respiratory syncytial virus (RSV). It occurs in annual winter epidemics, predominantly affecting infants aged 1–9 months. Coryzal symptoms are followed by a cough and increasing difficulty in breathing. Clinical signs include tachypnoea, intercostal recession, chest hyperinflation, bilateral fine crackles, and high pitched rhonchi. CXR shows hyperinflation and patchy collapse and oxygen saturation monitoring may reveal hypoxia. A nasopharyngeal aspirate is examined by a fluorescent antibody test to detect RSV. Management is supportive and depends on severity. Most infants require supplemental oxygen and more severely affected infants may require IV fluids. A minority become severely ill (young infants, ex preterm infants with chronic lung disease, and babies with congenital heart disease are at high risk) and require assisted ventilation for respiratory failure or recurrent apnoea.

5. Viral gastroenteritis usually causes the combination of diarrhoea and vomiting (D&V). In the UK, rotavirus is the most common pathogen. The vomiting is not usually bile stained, and severe abdominal pain or blood and mucus in the stool suggests an invasive bacterial pathogen. The differential diagnosis includes two surgical conditions: pyloric stenosis and intussusception.

   Clinical evaluation must include an estimate of the degree of dehydration: mild, moderate, or severe. Measurements of plasma urea and electrolyte concentrations are useful in all but the mildest cases.

   The key to management is rehydration with correction of the fluid and electrolyte imbalance. In mild cases, oral rehydration with an oral rehydration solution (ORS) is appropriate. In more severe cases, intravenous rehydration is required. If there are signs of circulatory failure, immediate resuscitation is carried out with 20ml/kg of 0.9% sodium chloride or 'plasma' (human albumin, 5%).

   There is no role for antiemetics, antidiarrhoeal agents, or antibiotics in the treatment of viral gastroenteritis.

6. Nocturnal enuresis is the involuntary voiding of urine during sleep beyond the age at which dryness at night has been achieved in a majority of children. In primary nocturnal enuresis dryness has never been achieved.

   The physical examination should aim to exclude the

rare organic causes: review growth and blood pressure, palpate the abdomen to exclude an enlarged bladder, inspect the spine and examine for neurological signs in the lower limbs. Urine should be cultured and tested for proteinuria and glycosuria.

A good rapport must be established with child and parents. Parental intolerance and 'functional payoffs' should be discouraged. A diary of wetting should be kept. Further management is age-dependant. Under 5 years, reassurance, waterproof sheets, and a lifting regimen may suffice. Over 5 years, star charts are useful, and over 7 years, buzzer type alarms are worth a trial.

Desmopressin, a synthetic analogue of ADH, provides effective short-term relief, and a percentage of patients who attain dryness may remain dry when it is stopped.

7. Cerebral palsy is defined as a disorder of motor function due to a non-progressive lesion of the developing brain. In many patients the cause is unknown, but risk factors are well recognized and may be classified as :

- Antenatal, e.g. congenital infections.
- Intrapartum, e.g. birth asphyxia.
- Postnatal, e.g. hyperbilirubinaemia.

Cerebral palsy may be classified as spastic (70%), dyskinetic (10%), ataxic (10%), or mixed (10%). Spastic CP is further subdivided into hemiplegic, diplegic (lower limbs predominantly affected), and quadriplegic. It may present with delayed motor milestones, abnormal tone or posturing, feeding difficulties, or speech and language delay.

Associated problems may include sensory deficits (vision and hearing), learning impairment, and epilepsy. Management requires a multidisciplinary approach.

8. The most common cause of acute onset of a limp in a 3-year-old is transient synovitis (irritable hip). This diagnosis should be made only after excluding other important diagnoses including trauma, septic arthritis or osteomyelitis, and Perthes disease.

The history should establish the duration and existence of any prodromal illness or trauma. Important physical signs include the presence of fever, the range of movement at lower limb joints, any point tenderness or signs of inflammation over the spine or lower limbs. Useful investigations include X-rays, ultrasound of the hip joint, FBC, ESR, and blood cultures.

In Perthes disease, there is insidious onset of a limp with intermittent pain between the age of 3 and 12 years (peak 5–7 years). Hip X-rays are diagnostic, revealing flattening and fragmentation of the femoral head. Bacterial infection of bone or joint is characterized by fever, local tenderness, and a rise in acute phase reactants. In transient synovitis there is no pain at rest and limited passive abduction and rotation in an otherwise well and afebrile child.

9. Iron deficiency anaemia in infancy or childhood usually results from inadequate dietary intake rather than loss of iron through haemorrhage. Groups at risk of nutritional deficiency include preterm infants who have limited iron stores and outstrip their reserves by 8 weeks of age unless supplements are provided. Term infants will develop iron deficiency after 4 months of age if introduction of mixed feeding is delayed or unmodified cow's milk is used in excess (Both breast milk and unmodified cow's are low in iron). Children with a poor diet on account of low socio-economic status or vegetarian diets are at risk. Malabsorption syndrome may be complicated by iron deficiency.

Iron deficiency due to blood loss may occur with hookworm infestation (most common cause worldwide), menstruation, repeated venesection in babies, recurrent epistaxis, or gastrointestinal bleeding for example from a Meckel's diverticulum.

10. Acute leukaemia is a disease characterized by proliferation of immature white cells and is the most common malignancy of childhood. Acute lymphocytic leukaemia (ALL) accounts for 80% of childhood leukaemia and has a peak incidence between 3 and 6 years. ALL can be classified according to cell-surface antigens into common, non-T, non-B cell ALL (75%), T cell ALL (15%), and B cell ALL (1%). Common ALL has the best prognosis.

There is usually an insidious onset of symptoms and signs arising from infiltration of the bone marrow and other organs with leukaemic 'blast' cells. There may be bone pain (due to expansion of marrow cavity), anaemia, purpura and easy bruising due to thrombocytopenia, and infection due to neutropenia.

Diagnosis is confirmed by examination of a bone marrow aspirate which will show replacement of normal elements by leukaemic cells.

Overall, at least 65% of patients with ALL can now expect to be cured. Initial management may require blood transfusion for anaemia, broad spectrum antibiotics for infection, and allopurinol to protect the kidneys from the effects of rapid cell lysis. Typical treatment regimens are divided into three phases: induction (combination chemotherapy usually including vincristine and prednisolone), consolidation, and maintenance (further 2 years of chemotherapy). Seventy-five per cent of patients go into remission. Relapses may occur in bone marrow, CNS, or testes.

11. Insulin-dependent diabetes mellitus (IDDM) of childhood is caused by a combination of genetic and environmental factors which trigger an immune-mediated destruction of the pancreatic ß cells. A genetic aetiology is indicated by an increased incidence of IDDM in first-degree relatives (2–5% in siblings and offspring) and a concordance rate for identical twins of

30%. The HLA region constitutes a major susceptibility locus and many minor loci have been implicated. Viruses may trigger the auto immune process which is manifested by lymphocytic infiltration of the pancreas and the presence of anti-islet cell antibodies.

Insulin deficiency becomes clinically significant when 90% of the ß cell mass has been destroyed. This leads to increased lipolysis, gluconeogenesis, and hyperglycaemia. An osmotic diuresis ensues when the blood glucose concentration exceeds the renal threshold. These factors cause weight loss, polyuria, and polydipsia. As insulin deficiency worsens ketoacids accumulate and diabetic ketoacidosis supervenes, characterized by severe dehydration and metabolic acidosis.

12. The hallmarks of attention-deficit hyperactivity disorder (ADHD) are inattention, hyperactivity, and impulsiveness. Hyperkinetic syndrome is a more severe subtype in which all three features are present, persist in more than one situation, and impair function. Hyperkinetic syndrome is four times more common in boys than girls.

Inattention is manifest as frequent changes of activity, hyperactivity is an excess of movement with persisting fidgeting and restlessness, and impulsiveness leads to erratic and impetuous behaviour.

Physical examination should include a search for developmental delay, clumsiness, sensory deficits, and dysmorphic features but most children do not have an identifiable brain disorder and do not need special investigations.

About 50% of children respond to behavioural therapy including a structured environment, positive reinforcement, and measures to enhance relaxation and self-control. If this approach fails, drug therapy may be tried. Paradoxically, CNS stimulants such as dexamphetamine or methylphenidate are most effective.

13. A primary course of triple vaccine (DTP: diphtheria, tetanus and pertussis) with Hib and oral Polio vaccine is given at age 2, 3, and 4 months.

Measles, mumps, and rubella (MMR) are given between 12 and 15 months of age. Diphtheria and tetanus, together with a polio booster, and second dose of MMR are given 3 years after completing the primary course.

BCG is given to the at-risk newborn as determined by ethnicity and place of residence. Alternatively, it is given at age 10–14 years.

A further diphtheria (low dose) and tetanus with polio booster is given between 13 and 18 years.

14. Down syndrome due to trisomy 21 is the most common autosomal trisomy compatible with life with an incidence of 1 in 700 live births. The extra chromosomal material may result from non-disjunction, translocation, or mosaicism. It is often suspected at birth because of the characteristic facial appearance: round face, flat occiput, flat nasal bridge, epicanthic folds, protruding tongue, small ears and Brushfield spots on the iris. Additional features may include single palmar creases, incurved little fingers, a sandal toe gap, and generalized hypotonia. Cardiac defects are present in 50% and duodenal atresia is increased in incidence. Developmental delay occurs and there is usually severe learning impairment. Late medical complications include an increased risk of leukaemia, hypothyroidism, and atlantoaxial instability.

Down syndrome may be diagnosed antenatally by screening procedures designed to detect it in pregnancies at increased risk. Risk increases with maternal age from 1 in 900 at 30 years to 1 in 110 at 40 years. Postnatal diagnosis is confirmed by chromosomal analysis which takes several days as white cells must be examined during mitosis. Ninety-five per cent of children with Down syndrome have trisomy 21 due to non-disjunction.

15. The major problems encountered by a preterm infant are determined by the immaturity of organ systems, particularly the lungs. They include:

- Respiratory system: alveolar collapse due to surfactant deficiency (respiratory distress syndrome). Unstable respiratory drive with irregular breathing and apnoeic attacks.
- Temperature control: hypothermia may occur because heat production is low (no brown fat), and heat loss is high due to high surface area to volume ratio.
- Gastrointestinal tract: uncoordinated sucking and swallowing, gastro-oesophageal reflux and risk of necrotizing enterocolitis (NEC). 'Physiological' jaundice is more likely to be severe.
- Cardiovascular system: increased risk of ductus arteriosus remaining patent (PDA).
- Central nervous system:increased risk of intracranial haemorrhage, retinopathy of prematurity and sensorineural hearing loss.
- In addition there is an increased risk of infection, tendency to hypoglycaemia and to hyponatraemia, and a risk after several weeks of anaemia and osteopenia of prematurity.

16. The aetiology of jaundice in the newborn is best considered according to the age of onset.

Jaundice in the first 24 hours: this is always pathological. Haemolysis is the most common cause and may be due to haemolytic disease of the newborn (Rhesus or ABO incompatibility) or intrinsic red cell defects such as congenital spherocytosis or G6PD deficiency.

Jaundice between 2 days and 2 weeks: the most common cause is physiological jaundice due to the combination of liver enzyme immaturity and increased bilirubin load from red cell breakdown.

Jaundice beyond 2 weeks of age: persistent (prolonged, protracted) jaundice is usually an unconjugated hyperbilirubinaemia most commonly caused by 'breast milk' jaundice. An important cause of prolonged conjugated hyperbilirubinaemia is biliary atresia which requires early surgical treatment.

In management, the main concerns are to identify the cause and to prevent kernicterus. Treatment options include phototherapy using blue light (wavelength 450nm, not UV light), which converts bilirubin into harmless, water soluble metabolites. Exchange transfusion may be necessary if bilirubin rises to dangerous levels despite phototherapy.

17. Minor head injuries in children are extremely common. Only about 1 in 800 of those admitted develop serious complications. Causes include falls, road traffic accidents, and child abuse, especially 'shaking' injuries in infants.

The history should establish when and how the injury occurred, whether or not consciousness was lost, and the presence of subsequent symptoms such as vomiting, headache, or drowsiness. Clinical examination should focus on local signs of external injury (e.g. lacerations, haematoma), blood or CSF leak from ears or nose, level of consciousness, and focal neurological signs.

A skull X-ray is performed in all but the most minor injuries and cranial CT is indicated if there is any suspicion of raised intracranial pressure or intracranial haemorrhage. A period of observation in hospital is indicated if the injury is moderate to severe as indicated by severe headache or vomiting, declining level of consciousness, skull fracture, or suspected non-accidental injury. Severe injuries may require neurointensive care and referral to a neurosurgeon if there is evidence of an expanding haematoma.

18. A 'convulsion' is a generalized tonic–clonic seizure. The most common cause in young children is a 'febrile convulsion', but other causes at all ages include head injury, meningitis, poisoning, hypoglycaemia, and epilepsy. Hypoglycaemia is an important cause for which there is a specific treatment.

The history should include any recent trauma and whether the child is a known epileptic or diabetic. Examination should establish in particular the presence or absence of a fever, petechial rash, or meningism.

A convulsing child should be placed in the recovery position, an oral airway should be inserted and O_2 given by face mask. Blood glucose should be checked using a BM Stix and hypoglycaemia treated if present. The fit should be terminated using rectal or intravenous diazepam if it has lasted longer than 10–15 minutes as protracted convulsions may cause brain damage.

19. In general, there is no doubt that 'breast is best' but there are, in fact, a number of disadvantages in breastfeeding.

The quality of breast milk is superior in several respects to that of modified cow's milk formulae. It confers some protection against infection by virtue of containing secretory IgA, lysozyme, phagocytic cells and lactoferrin, an iron-binding agent which promotes growth of non-pathogenic flora. The nutritional content is more suited to newborn infants. The protein is easily digested, there is a low renal solute load, and a more favourable ratio of calcium to phosphate.

Potential disadvantages include uncertainty about the volume of intake and the transmission of maternal drugs such as anticoagulants and antineoplastic agents and pathogens such as HIV. Breastfed infants are at risk of two important vitamin deficiencies. Vitamin K deficiency causing haemorrhagic disease of the newborn may occur in breastfed infants unless vitamin K is given prophylactically at birth. Rickets due to vitamin D deficiency may occur, especially in dark-skinned infants, if breastfeeding is prolonged and weaning delayed.

Successful breastfeeding is an emotionally positive experience and promotes mother–infant bonding. However, failure of attempts to establish breastfeeding may cause emotional upset. Lastly, breastfeeding mothers have a lower risk of breast cancer in later life.

20. A practical definition of short stature is a height below the 0.4 centile for age, a predicted height less than the midparental target height, or an abnormal growth velocity as indicated by the height falling by more than the width of the centile band over 1–2 years.

The majority of children whose short stature has triggered concern are normal. They have either familial short stature or constitutional delay of the pubertal growth spurt.

The history should include enquiry about size at birth, parental height, and a family history of conditions such as the skeletal dysplasias. The midparental height allows calculation of a target centile range. On examination attention is paid to the height and weight, pubertal status, and the presence or absence of any dysmorphic features. Growth velocity should be calculated from at least two height measurements 6 months apart.

Potentially useful investigations include the bone age, the karyotype, and endocrine investigations such as thyroid function tests and growth hormone secretion (requires a provocation test).

Important organic causes of short stature include endocrine causes (GH deficiency, hypothyroidism), genetic disorders (Turner syndrome, Prader–Willi syndrome), and skeletal dysplasias (achondroplasia).

Management depends on the cause. Effective treatment usually involves hormone replacement using growth hormone (injected) or thyroxine if a deficiency is present.

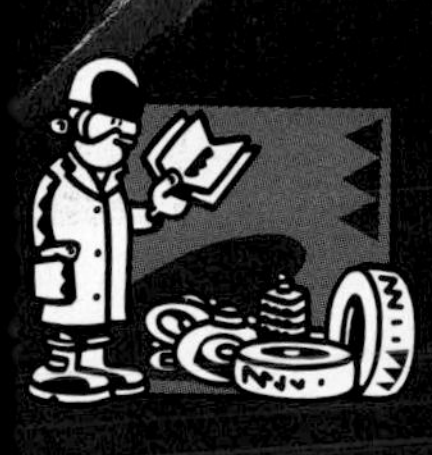

INDEX

Q

R